BSAVA
Manual of
Small Animal
Diagnostic Imaging

Second Edition

Edited by

R. Lee
BVSc, PhD, MRCVS, DVR

Published by:
British Small Animal Veterinary Association
Kingsley House, Church Lane
Shurdington, Cheltenham
Gloucestershire
United Kingdom
GL51 5TQ.

A Company Limited by Guarantee in England.
Registered Company No. 2837793.
Registered as a Charity.

Typeset and Printed by
Fusion Design, Fordingbridge, Hants.

First Edition published 1989.
Second Edition published 1995.

ISBN 0 905214 26 9

D1579726

2

Contents

4

Acknowledgements

Those reading and using this manual will realise that a considerable amount of work went into the preparation of the diagrams. In order to maintain a consistency of style this work was undertaken by a single artist, Dr. Roderick Duff, and I would like to acknowledge the considerable amount of time and effort he put into the production of all the illustrative material for this manual.

I should like to acknowledge the assistance of Brian Coles and Martin Lawton for providing the information used in compiling the chapter on the radiography of small mammals, birds and reptiles.

I should also like to thank those professional colleagues who assisted the editor by reading the manuscripts and commenting on the content and layout of the various chapter.

Finally, I should like to thank the contributors for the time and effort they have each put into the production of this manual.

R. Lee

Contributors

Dr FJ Barr,
MA, VetMB, PhD, MRCVS, DVR

Dr JV Davies,
B Vet Med, PhD, MRCVS, DVR

Mrs R Dennis
MA, Vet, MB, DVR, MRCVS

ME Herrtage
MA, BVSc, DVD, DVR, MRCVS

Prof. R Lee,
BVSc, PhD, MRCVS, DVR

DB Murdoch,
BVMS, MRCVS, DVR

Dr. M Sullivan,
BVMS, PhD, MRCVS, DVR

Dr. PM Webbon,
B Vet Med, PhD, MRCVS, DVR

Dr. SRI Duff,
BVSc, BSc, MVM, PhD, MRCVS

Foreword

No small animal practice would be considered to be offering a reasonable standard of care to patients if radiology was not available to their clients. This situation is not as it was a number of years ago. When the Manual of Radiology and radiography was published in 1989, it satisfied the demand as an up to date reference manual for the veterinary radiologist. The new edition has incorporated the expanding field of diagnostic imaging and includes ultrasonography which has now become an integral part of many small animal practices. As these fields advance, the practitioner can be assured that this manual will continue to serve as a reference book for use in a busy practice.

The new field of ultrasound has meant that those areas of the body that were difficult to visualise by X rays are now visible and it is possible to have images generated of these to assist diagnosis.

Safety for clients and staff continues to take priority in the manual. We all need to be not only aware of the regulations, but to ensure that all the necessary safeguards are taken in the working environment for the protection of those present.

The new edition also brings the next stage of imaging into the picture with information on both Magnetic Resonance Imaging (MRI) and Computed Tomography (CT) scans. It will be interesting to see how far the field of imaging moves on between this and the next manual.

The new edition with its expansion into other imaging fields will be an asset to any practice and the authors and editor are to be congratulated on their efforts.

LYNNE V HILL
President, BSAVA 1994-95

CHAPTER ONE

Introduction

Robin Lee

Radiography is a well established aid to veterinary diagnosis and is being increasingly employed by veterinary practitioners and expected by their clients.

There are already many excellent textbooks dealing with both the theory and practice of radiographic technique and the problems of radiological interpretation. However, the former tend to deal with all the available procedures for a complete radiographic study whereas in practice it is often possible to take advantage of past experience and use only those studies that are most likely to yield useful diagnostic information. Similarly, the second group of texts often deal in great detail with the niceties of radiological interpretation but may fail to provide concise guidance as to the most frequently encountered radiological signs associated with the common disease conditions.

This revised edition, now entitled the manual of Diagnostic Imaging in Small Animal Practice, apart from a number of minor corrections and additions, includes a new chapter on the use of diagnostic ultrasound and the reading list has been brought up to date. A large number of annotated line diagrams has been used to illustrate as clearly as possible the main radiological features of the conditions most likely to be encountered. In addition, check lists of signs and conditions have been used freely to aid the veterinary surgeon when reviewing radiographs of a particular region.

Some topics common to different regions may be duplicated to assist the reader in obtaining the information quickly and without frequent recourse to the index.

A manual such as this cannot deal with every combination of radiological and ultrasonographic signs likely to be encountered but it is hoped that it will provide useful assistance in the identification of conditions and that the format will make its use speedy and reliable.

The views expressed on the value or otherwise of particular techniques are those of the authors and, to a certain extent, the hints and suggestions offered will be dependent on the facilities and expertise available.

Whilst it is essential to practise good radiographic technique it is not always possible to obtain perfect film quality. The important aim must be to ensure that all films are of diagnostic quality so reducing the need for additional exposures with the attendant increase in radiation hazard. Anything less is an expensive waste of time and may lead to serious diagnostic errors.

Radiographic positioning

The variety of radiographic projections are described and the value of each projection and the indications for special views will be discussed in relation to each region.

Common pitfalls which must be avoided and practical hints of value in obtaining diagnostic films, are included where appropriate.

Equipment

In addition to satisfactory positioning, the routine production of satisfactory film quality is also dependent on:-

a) A full understanding of the available equipment and its limitations.
b) The correct choice of exposure factors.
c) Satisfactory film processing.

The X-Ray Machine

The major limiting factor in any X-ray machine is the output in terms of the maximum millamperage setting that can be obtained.

Most portable machines operate at up to 30 mA but there are now lightweight mobiles capable of up to 100mA, whereas larger mobile machines will operate at 150-500mA.

When considering the purchase of a machine it is wise to consider one with as high a milliamperage rating as cost will permit, also bearing in mind the possible requirement for portability. Care must be taken to check that the available mA is not reduced excessively as the kV is increased. A kilovoltage range of 50-70 should be adequate for the majority of small animal radiographic procedures.

Many older machines are fitted with mechanical timers which are generally satisfactory at exposure times in excess of $\frac{1}{4}$ - $\frac{1}{2}$ sec but may be inaccurate at shorter exposure times. Electronic timers are more reliable at shorter exposure times and are now routinely fitted to new equipment.

A robust stand for the head is essential in eliminating unnecessary movement artefacts and will also help to ensure standardisation of film focal distance ie. the distance from the tube head to the cassette or film.

Apart from the periodic checking of the machine for damage to plugs and cables and for obvious signs of damage, there is no maintenance or repair work that should not be entrusted to a trained engineer. If a machine fails to produce X rays or if the film density at a given setting suddenly alters without any change in processing technique, an X ray engineer should be called in to check the equipment. In addition, if for any reason personnel dosemeters indicate unexplained readings, the RPA for the practice should be informed and a check arranged through him for the possibility of radiation leakage.

It is ESSENTIAL that there is some means of collimating the X ray beam. Not only will the use of the minimum field size necessary significantly improve radiographic quality, it is of paramount importance for radiation protection.

Although many older machines are fitted with fixed or interchangeable metal cones the use of a variably adjustable light beam diaphragm is the most satisfactory arrangement. This not only allows wide variation in beam size, it also provides a visual indicator of the limits of the beam. The use of a light beam diaphragm is strongly recommended by the Ionising Radiations Regulations. If a fixed cone is used, it is essential to ensure that the maximum field size is no larger than the cassette in use. It is important to remember that the beam size produced by any cone is related to the film focal distance. (Figure 1.1).

All machines will be fitted with a mains voltage compensator to allow for variation in the mains voltage in different locations and at different times of the day. This should always be checked and adjusted prior to making an exposure, otherwise the output of the machine cannot be relied upon. If, in older equipment, it is necessary to make an exposure in order to make this adjustment, then the necessary safety precautions should be taken.

Cassettes and intensifying screens
Whilst it is not necessary to have a wide range of cassette sizes available, it is desirable on the grounds of economy to have at least two sizes. In addition, it is wise to have two cassettes of each size to permit the taking of two views without interruption.

Suggested sizes are 35 x 43 cm and 20 x 30 cm.

It should be remembered that for small regions such as bones and joints, it is more economical to take two or more views on a single film. This can be done by masking that portion of the cassette not to be exposed with a thin lead sheet or a piece of lead rubber.

Cassettes should be handled carefully and the fastening clips regularly checked to ensure that they remain light proof. To check for light leaks the cassette should be loaded with an unexposed film and then left in a normally lit room for some time (30-60 mins). The film should then be processed in the normal way, when any blackening around the edges of the film indicates that the cassette is faulty and should either be replaced or repaired.

Intensifying screens are expensive items of equipment and must be kept clean and dust, hairs etc. not permitted to accumulate in the cassette otherwise film artefacts will be seen which may obscure diagnostic information. Cassettes must never be left lying open and they should be checked regularly and cleaned according to the manufacturers instructions.

The increased intensifying factors of the rare earth screens permit a reduction in exposure factors. This effectively increases the useful range of work possible with low power equipment and is of value from the point of view of radiation safety. It is suggested that if investment is made in rare earth screens, at least one cassette fitted with Ca tungstate screens should be retained, otherwise problems of overexposure of the distal limbs of small animals may be encountered.

If different film/screen combinations are used, then it is important that the cassettes are clearly labelled as the exposure factors will vary.

Non screen films require much higher exposure factors and have very limited application but are of value for intra-oral views of the nasal cavity and mandible.

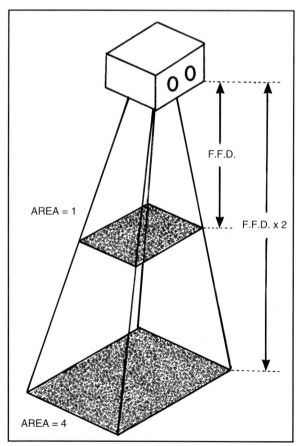

Figure 1.1: Relationship of FFD to field size.

Provided the table top is radiolucent, a film tray fitted under the table top will permit the positioning of cassettes without repeated lifting of the subject. This is particularly valuable during sequential contrast studies. Such a cassette tray does not have to be linked to a moving grid, although the use of a purpose built table fitted with a bucky grid is ideal. (Figure 1.2).

The table top or, if used, film tray, should be fitted with a piece of lead 1mm thick in order to absorb the residual primary radiation.

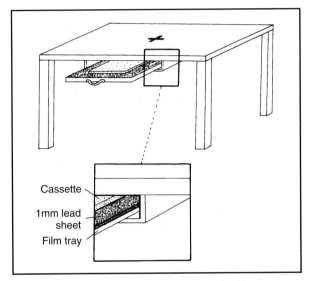

Figure 1.2: Table adapted by the addition of a film tray.

Scatter grids
A grid will help to improve film quality by the reduction of scatter radiation reaching the film so improving the radiographic contrast. A grid can be used to advantage in those situations where the region under investigation is more than 10 cm in thickness.

The grid ratio is the measure of the efficiency of the grid at removing scatter. The most suitable general purpose grid is one with a grid ratio of 8:1 and consisting of 30 lines per cm. If a focussed grid is chosen it should correspond to the FFD routinely used. A focussed grid should always be used the correct way up and all grids should be positioned perpendicular to the X ray beam.

When purchasing a grid, it is wise to choose a size to fit the largest cassette available. In order to ensure accurate centring when using smaller cassette sizes, a simple wooden or perspex tray can be used. (Figure 1.3).

The grid factor is the compensation to the mAs setting necessary to produce a film of equivalent density to one obtained without the use of the grid.

eg. Grid factor = 2
Exposure without grid = 60 kV 6 mAs
Exposure with grid = 60 kV 12 mAs

If this is not marked on the grid, it must be determined by trial and error and then used when compiling exposure charts.

If low powered equipment is being used, there may be more loss of film quality from movement resulting from the increased exposure times necessary with a grid than from the loss of contrast due to scatter. In these situations it may be more desirable to dispense with the use of a grid, even though it may otherwise be indicated.

Positioning aids
Wherever the clinical situation permits, patients should be heavily sedated or anaesthetised to reduce the risk of unnecessary radiation hazard to personnel. The choice of agents is wide and must be left to the discretion of the clinician involved.

In order to reduce the requirement for manual restraint as required under the current regulations, a variety of positioning aids are now available and should be used.

These include (Figure 1.4):-

Radiolucent positioning troughs
Foam pads and wedges
Loosely filled sandbags in a variety of sizes
Tapes, bandages etc.
Paediatric baby restrainers

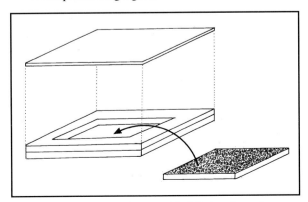

Figure 1.3: Grid holder for use with differing sizes of cassette to ensure that the cassette is always centred to the grid.

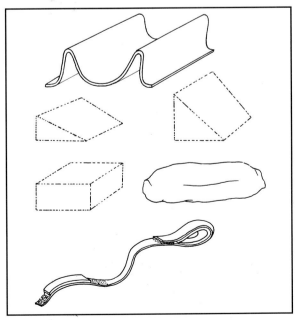

Figure 1.4: Assorted positioning aids.

Exposure Factors

In order to obtain consistent results, it is necessary to formulate an exposure chart. The limited range of kV and mA settings available on many small machines, frequently does not permit the use of fixed mAs variable kV charts so frequently advocated in American texts. The following information should provide an excellent guide to the choice of the correct factors for any given examination.

1) The region under investigation.
2) The size of the subject eg. small, medium or large; dog or cat.
3) The film focus distance.
4) The film/screen type.
5) Grid if used.
6) kV setting.
7) mA setting.
8) Exposure time.

7 and 8 may be combined as a single mAs factor.

It is not usually satisfactory to transfer an exposure chart from one machine to another, although it may provide an initial guide.

The use of an exposure chart is absolutely dependent on efficient and standardised processing technique.

Mistakes in exposure assessment will be minimised if as many variables as possible are standardised.

Variations from such an exposure chart may be necessary and, if so, the following factors will serve as a rough guide for re-calculating exposure values.

a) Divide the mAs by mA to get the exposure time. eg. 15 mAs at 10 mA = 1.5 sec.
b) If kV is raised (or lowered) by 10, the mAs should be halved (or doubled).
   E.G. 60 kV at 16 mAs = 70 kV at 8 mAs = 50 kV at 32 mAs.
c) To change FFD.
   New mAs = $\dfrac{\text{Old mAs}}{\text{Old FFD}^2} \times \text{New FFD}^2$
d) To penetrate dry POP, increase mAs x 2 wet POP, increase mAs x 4
e) To compensate for
   i) addition of a grid mAs x GF
   ii) removal of a grid mAs/GF.

GF = The Grid Factor. This is the amount by which the mAs requires to be increased in order to maintain the degree of film blackening when introducing a grid to the system. Once determined it remains a constant for that grid and is usually in the region of 2-3 X or non-grid mAs.

Film Processing

This is the one area of radiography most frequently neglected and is, consequently, the commonest cause of poor quality radiographs. It is therefore important to pay particular attention to the following points:-

1) STANDARDISE all procedures.
2) Change and replenish processing solutions at regular intervals according to the manufacturers instructions. Remember that the developer will deteriorate even when not used regularly.
3) Keep the developer tank covered to reduce oxidation.
4) Ensure that the developer is maintained at the correct operating temperature, 20°C, by the use of a thermostatically controlled heater or water jacket.
5) Develop all films for the correct time by the clock - normally 4 minutes.
6) Fix the films adequately - usually 10 minutes. Change the fixer solution regularly.
7) Practise good housekeeping in the darkroom to prevent the contamination of films and screens by chemical splashes etc. Keep the wet and dry procedures separate.
8) Wash films in running water for at least 30 minutes after fixing.
9) Dry the films in a dust free atmosphere making sure they do not touch each other.
10) Ensure that the darkroom is lightproof. Use a safelight of the correct type for the film in use. If you change to rare earth screens you may need to change the safelight - check with the manufacturer.
11) Use the correct size of bulb in the safelight - usually 25 W - and keep the safelight at the correct distance from the film.
12) Store film in light tight boxes in a dry place away from the X ray machine, excessive heat or chemicals.

If you wish to check the safety of the darkroom or safelight, place a hand or coin on an unexposed film in the darkroom, wait for 2-3 minutes then process the film. If there is an image on the film, check the light-proofing or the safelight as appropriate.

Viewing radiographs

The examination of radiographs should be done under optimum conditions. If not, then fine detail of skeletal lesions and lungfield and an appreciation of low contrast mass lesions of the abdomen, may easily be missed. The following points should be particularly noted and applied to the viewing of any radiograph.

- Ensure that the film is correctly exposed, processed and dry prior to detailed examination.
- Use a clean X-ray viewer situated away from any window and, ideally, in subdued lighting.
- Allow your eyes to accommodate for the reduced light intensity.

- Use black card masks or viewers fitted with adjustable diaphragms to reduce extraneous light from the viewer.
- Use a bright light source, eg. desk lamp with a 60W bulb, for the examination of relatively over-exposed areas of a film such as the periphery of the lungfield of the periosteal surface of the bone.
- Use a magnifying glass to examine for fine detail such as trabecular bone and periosteal reactions.
- Stand back from the film when examining large organs and mass lesions such as the liver and abdominal tumours.

If in doubt about the significance of a feature, refer to an atlas of normal radiographic anatomy or, where appropriate, a radiograph of the contralateral limb or structure of the same animal, but beware of bilateral lesions.

Advanced Imaging Techniques

In recent years the discipline of radiology has expanded to become diagnostic imaging, using a variety of other techniques to produce pictures of body tissues. These alternative techniques include ultrasonography, nuclear scintigraphy, computer tomography (CT) and magnetic resonance imaging (MRI).

Ultrasonography is being increasingly used by general practitioners in both small and large animal veterinary work, as reflected by the inclusion of a chapter on diagnostic ultrasound in this manual.

Nuclear scintigraphy involves intravenous injection of radioactively-labelled pharmaceuticals which are taken up by specific tissues depending on the chemical nature of the radioactive compounds. Subsequent imaging of the patient using a hand-held scintillation detector or a gamma camera will show "hot spots" or areas of radioactivity in sites of radioactivity accumulation. Nuclear scintigraphy is employed primarily in equine orthopaedics in which it is used to identify the site of a lesion rather than to provide accurate anatomical detail.

Computed tomography and magnetic resonance imaging are cross-sectional imaging techniques which are widely used in human medicine and which have recently become more accessible to veterinarians, especially those in referral centres. Although they are unlikely to be used routinely in first-opinion practices, an increasing number of veterinary schools and second-opinion practices worldwide have access to CT and MRI scanners either using dedicated veterinary systems or more often with out-of-hours use of medical equipment. It is therefore important for the general practitioner to be aware of the availability of such services and of the type of cases which are likely to benefit from these imaging techniques.

This section will describe in brief the principles of CT and MRI and the equipment used as well as the indications for their use in small animal patients. Both methods produce cross-sectional images or "scans" which have greatly increased tissue definition compared with conventional radiographs, allowing the internal architecture of soft tissue and bony structures to be seen. In addition, the production of multiple cross-sectional slices gives much more three-dimensional information about lesions than do radiographs, allowing more accurate planning of surgery or radiotherapy.

Computed tomography (CT)

CT scanning is a British invention, having been developed by Godfrey Hounsfield of E.M.I. in the early 1970s. It is based on conventional radiography, in which differential absorption of an X-ray beam by various body tissues produces a "shadowgraph" image on a detector placed on the opposite side of the patient. In the case of CT the X-ray tube rotates rapidly around the patient and the emergent X-ray beam is picked up by a circle of electronic detectors which also surround the patient (Figure 1.5). The electronic signal is analysed for each transient position of the X-ray tube head, with small volumes of tissue being assigned a numerical value and then a corresponding grey shade on an image depending on the degree of X-ray absorption occurring within that volume. This creates a grey-shade image of a cross-sectional slice of tissue, with bone and calcified material appearing bright and gas dark, as on conventional radiographs. The table on which the patient lies is advanced by small increments between each exposure, producing multiple images representing adjacent slices of tissue. The construction of the scanner means that true images can only be produced in a plane transverse to the way in which the patient is lying; sagittal and dorsal plane images can be produced by computer reformatting but are much poorer in detail. Contrast studies can be performed in the same way as with conventional radiography, using iodinated or barium media. Although CT scanning is rapid and non-invasive, the use of ionising radiation

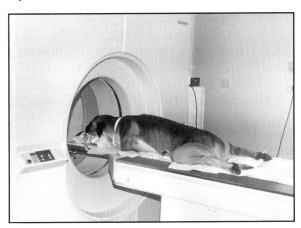

Figure 1.5: *Anaesthetised dog positioned in CT scanner for head imaging.*

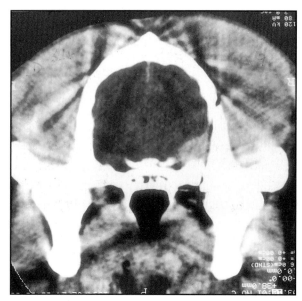

Figure 1.6: transverse CT scan of the head of a cross-bred dog which was unconscious following a road traffic accident. There is a comminuted temporal bone fracture and an adjacent area of opacity within the brain, due to haemorrhage.

means that the risk to certain types of individuals (e.g. pregnant women) must be considered.

The main use of CT in clinical veterinary work is in the diagnosis of brain lesions such as hydrocephalus, neoplasia and trauma. Within the brain, the ventricles can be seen as radiolucent cavities and haemorrhage or calcification as radiopaque areas. Tumours are visible on plain scans if they cause displacement of the ventricles or if they have central necrosis or calcification. Intravenous injection of iodinated contrast media causes opacification of lesions which have damaged the blood brain barrier, such as tumours, delineating their size and shape more clearly. The sensitivity of CT to bony tissue means that the technique is particularly useful in trauma cases in which both skull fractures and underlying brain damage can be diagnosed (Figure 1.6). Unlike MRI, CT can easily be used for such critical care patients since the short, wide gallantry allows easy access to the patient. Unfortunately, the thickness of the dog's cranium results in an artifact called "beam hardening" which degrades the image in certain areas, such as the pituitary and caudal fossae, and means that lesions here may be overlooked.

CT is eminently suited to the investigation of skeletal disease, although such applications have so far received relatively little attention in the veterinary field. Plain and myelographic spinal CT is particularly rewarding since cross-sectional images of the vertebrae and disc spaces are produced, giving information about vertebral malformation and cord compression which is not possible with radiography. CT is also likely to be of value in surgical planning of fractures because of the three-dimensional information which it produces.

In man, CT is also widely used for investigation of the extent of soft tissue masses in the head, neck, thorax, abdomen, pelvis and limbs. Areas of subtle bone involvement and metastasis to lymph nodes can be detected, and within a solid or fluid-filled organ such as the liver infiltrations with abnormal tissue can be seen. However, these applications of CT in veterinary patients are at present less common than CNS imaging.

Magnetic resonance imaging (MRI)

The phenomenon of nuclear magnetic resonance (NMR) was discovered independently by Felix Bloch and Edward Purcell, for which they jointly received the Nobel Prize in 1952. Initially, it was used to unravel the atomic structure of chemical compounds but in the 1970s the technique was modified to allow the production of two-dimensional, cross sectional images of the body. This application of NMR was renamed magnetic resonance imaging since it was felt that the word "nuclear", although referring simply to atomic nuclei, was rather to emotive for public use.

MRI is simply the production of an image by mapping out the location of protons (hydrogen nuclei) in body tissues, using a combination of magnetism and radiowaves. The body is placed in a strong magnetic field, which makes the positively-charges protons align and produce a spinning motion at a frequency determined by the strength of the magnetic field. They are then bombarded with pulses of radiowaves at a similar frequency and this has the effect of disorientating the protons. As they re-align themselves between the pulses they produce a small radiosignal themselves, the frequency emitted by each proton being determined by its position within the body. The jumble of radiosignals thus emerging is converted by a computer into a two-dimensional (or even three-dimensional) image, again displayed on a grey scale.

The MRI scanner is usually a long, cylindrical magnet into which the patient is positioned by lying on a movable table top (Figure 1.7). Scanning times are

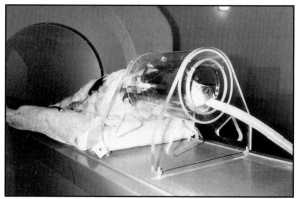

Figure 1.7: Anaesthetised dog positioned with its head in a radiofrequency coil for MRI scanning of the brain. The scanner itself can be seen in the background and the table top will be moved so that the dog lies in the centre of the scanner.

much longer than with CT and so the patient must lie absolutely still, usually necessitating general anaesthesia in veterinary patients. The magnetic field of the scanner means that no ferrous metallic objects can be brought into its vicinity and so anaesthetic and monitoring equipment must be specially designed. These factors mean that MRI is less suitable for the critically-injured patient than is CT. However, in most aspects MRI is greatly superior to CT and it is rapidly taking first place in medical imaging. The quality of the images is vastly superior, with much improved soft tissue definition, and images can be obtained in transverse, sagittal and dorsal planes with equally good definition. Different types of scan can be performed to show different tissue characteristics, and contrast studies performed using special "paramagnetic" contrast media.

In veterinary diagnosis, as with CT, most work has centred on the brain. Brain tumours have been found to be much more common in dogs than was previously thought, with a particular predilection for the boxer (Figure 1.8). Central neurological signs (such as seizures) in any middle-aged or older dog or cat warrant investigation with scanning, and since most lesions can be treated this is not simply an academic exercise. MRI can also be used to diagnose congenital disorders such as hydrocephalus and cerebellar hypoplasia, and other acquired conditions such as inflammatory brain disease.

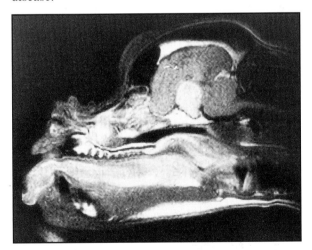

Figure 1.8: *Contrast-enhanced, sagittal, T1-weighted scan of A 7 year old boxer with a pituitary tumour. This dog responded well to radiotherapy.*

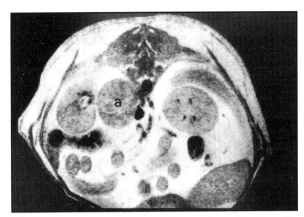

Figure 1.9: *Transverse abdominal scan of a twelve year old cross-bred bitch with a large right adrenal mass (a). The caudal vena cava is seen as a small black structure medial to the mass (dorsal=top of image, right side=left of image).*

MRI is valuable in the investigation of spinal conditions, a common application in man. Myelography is unnecessary since cerebrospinal fluid can be seen distinct from the spinal cord, and so the study is much safer and less invasive than radiography as well as producing better tissue definition and images in other planes. Other orthopaedic uses of MRI are popular in man since MRI will demonstrate articular cartilage, menisci, ligaments, tendons and other soft tissue structures not seen with radiography. Although MRI is less sensitive to calcification than CT skeletal structures are well seen, and if available MRI would certainly be of value in planning complex orthopaedic surgery. Elsewhere in the body, MRI can be used to detect masses, to assess the extent of any bone involvement before this is evident radiographically and to allow three-dimensional treatment planning (Figure 1.9).

Summary
CT and MRI are exciting, non-invasive imaging techniques which produce far better tissue definition and more three-dimensional information than radiography. For most purposes MRI produces superior images, although a choice of technique will not usually be available. The use of CT and MRI is essential for the diagnosis of brain lesions, which are surprisingly common in small animal practice. As equipment becomes cheaper and more available, these cross-sectional imaging techniques will be applied more widely to other areas of the body.

CHAPTER TWO

The Head and Neck

M. Sullivan

CONTENTS

Each area contains sections dealing with:-

- Indications
- Technique and positioning
- Evaluation of the radiograph
- Interpretation

I: THE CALVARIUM

Indications for radiography of the calvarium include:-

1) Trauma to the skull.
2) Congenital anomalies resulting in neurological abnormalities.
3) The investigation of swellings associated with either infection or neoplasia.
4) The investigation of neurological signs associated with the CNS and cranial nerves.

Technique

Both in the interests of accurate positioning and radiation protection general anaesthesia is essential. Screen films should be routinely used with use of a grid depending on the size of the animal.

There is a wide choice of views for evaluating the calvarium and associated structures. The lateral and DV views are the standard ones to use initially with other views being used to demonstrate specific regions and/or lesions. It should be remembered that the endotracheal tube will often be projected onto the area of interest and may require to be temporarily removed during the radiographic exposure. This should be borne in mind when selecting the method of anaesthesia.

Positioning

Because of the complexity of the radiographic anatomy of this region an accurate interpretation depends on well positioned films. The methods of positioning the animal and centring the beam for the major views is outlined below.

Lateral view. (Figure 2.1)

i) The animal should be placed in lateral recumbency and the nose and mandible raised with lucent pads so that the sagittal plane of the skull is parallel to the cassette.
ii) The beam should be centred mid way between the eye and the ear.

Dorso-ventral view. (Figure 2.2)

i) This is preferred to the VD view as the mandibles help to limit lateral rotation although there is some magnification of the calvarium due to the increased distance from the film.
ii) The animal is placed in sternal recumbency with the neck extended.
iii) It is often helpful to lay a sandbag over the neck to keep the hard palate parallel to the cassette especially in deep chested dogs.

Ventro-dorsal view. (Figure 2.3)

i) This is more difficult to position accurately as the sagittal crest tends to make the skull tilt laterally.
ii) The animal is placed in dorsal recumbency and the neck extended.
iii) A tape should be secured around the upper canine and fixed to the table top, or alternatively a sandbag laid over the body of the mandible, and a foam support placed under the neck ensures that the hard palate is parallel to the cassette.

Lateral oblique view. (Figure 2.4)

i) When used to demonstrate masses or lesions identified on other views the positioning - using lucent foam pads to support the head - should be such as 'skyline' the lesion under investigation.

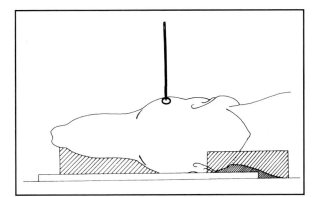

Figure 2.1: Calvarium - positioning - lateral view.

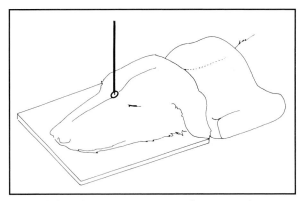

Figure 2.2: Calvarium - positioning - dorso-ventral view.

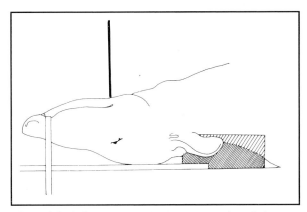

Figure 2.3: Calvarium - positioning - ventro-dorsal view.

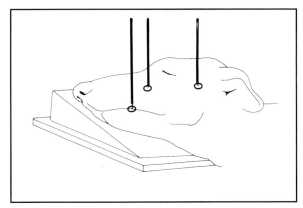

Figure 2.4: Calvarium - positioning - lateral-oblique view.

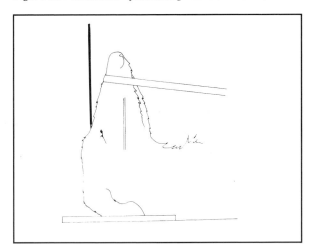

Figure 2.5: Calvarium - positioning - rostro-caudal view.

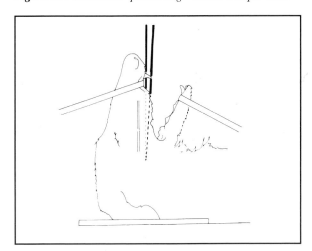

Figure 2.6: Calvarium - positioning - open mouth rostro-caudal view.

Rostro-caudal view. (Figure 2.5)

i)   This view is mainly of value in demonstrating the frontal sinuses, zygomatic arch and temporal region, and the sagittal crest. It is of less value in the cat due to the conformation of the feline skull.

ii) The animal is positioned on its back with the skull secured with a tape around the nose so that the hard palate is perpendicular to the cassette.

iii) The beam should be angled at 5-10 degrees in a rostro-caudal direction.

Open mouth Rostro-caudal view. (Figure 2.6)

i)   This is used mainly for the demonstration of the tympanic bullae and foramen magnum.

ii) Positioning is as for the rostro-caudal view but with the mouth held wide open with tapes secured to the table. The palate should be perpendicular to the cassette.

iii) The beam should be parallel to or slightly angled towards the hard palate and centred on the base of the tongue/free edge of the soft palate.

Evaluation of the Radiographs

The skull is a complicated structure composed of a large number of bones. Added to this in the dog is the wide variation in conformation found between different breeds. These can be grouped or classified into three broad categories - brachycephalic, mesaticephalic and dolichocephalic. In addition, the feline skull differs in detail from the canine skull.

It is important, if necessary with the aid of a radiographic atlas, to be able to identify the following landmarks (Figure 2.7).

1) Nuchal crest
2) Occipital condyles
3) Foramen magnum
4) Zygomatic arches
5) Temporo-mandibular joints
6) Base of skull
7) External auditory meati
8) Petrous temporal bones
9) Tympanic bullae
10) Cribriform plate and ethmoidal fossae

The skull is a symmetrical structure and on all but the lateral view, paired structures can be compared to each other and any abnormal densities or lucencies can be assessed by comparison with the opposite side of the skull.

The contents of the calvarium - the brain and meninges - are soft tissue structures and, in the absence of abnormalities of the bone of the calvarium, plain film radiographs will be of little value in identifying lesions of the CNS and cranial nerves.

Contrast studies such as cavernous sinus venography and cerebral angiography and ventriculography can provide limited assistance in the identification of intra-cranial lesions and are discussed in the appropriate section.

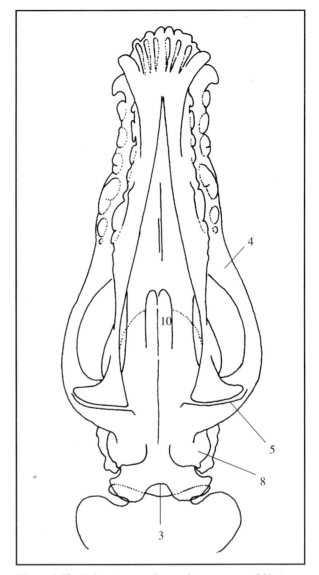

Figure 2.7b: Calvarium - radiographic anatomy - DV view.

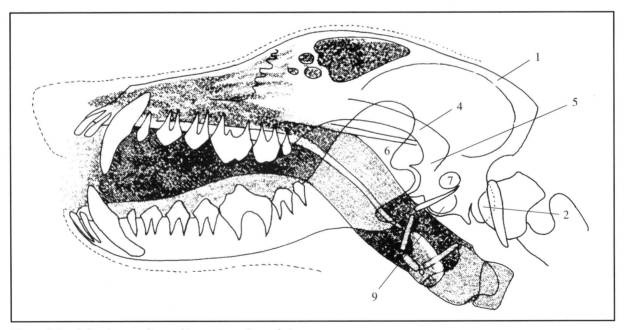

Figure 2.7a: Calvarium - radiographic anatomy - Lateral view.

INTERPRETATION

Congenital Hydrocephalus

Seen in a variety of breeds most commonly toy 'apple' headed such as Papillon, Chihuahua etc. May be asymptomatic or a variety of CNS abnormalities.

Radiological features (Figure 2.8)
- Calvarium is enlarged.
- The bones of the cranial vault are thinned with loss of the normal gyral markings.
- The fontanelle and suture lines remain open into adulthood.
- Radiological confirmation can be obtained by ventriculography or ultrasonography.

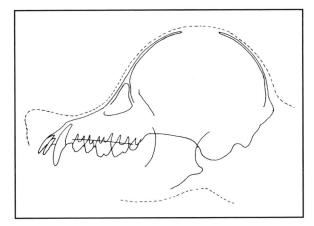

Figure 2.8: Congenital Hydrocelphalus.

Occipital Dysplasia

Seen mainly in miniature and toy breeds. May produce a variety of mid- and hind-brain CNS signs.

May be associated with congenital atlanto-axial subluxation qv.

Radiological features (Figure 2.9)
- Best demonstrated on open mouth RCd view.
- Foramen magnum 'key hole' shaped.
- C1 may be considerably shortened and ring like.
- May be associated signs of atlanto-axial subluxation qv.

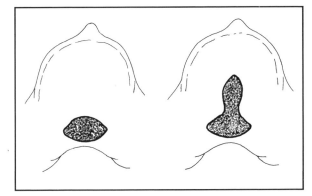

Figure 2.9a: Occipital Dysplasia.

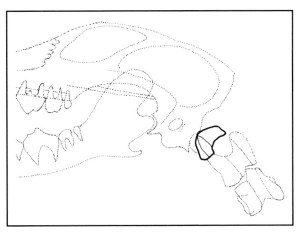

Figure 2.9b: Occipital Dysplasia.

Cranio-Mandibular Osteopathy

Most commonly seen in West Highland White terriers and related breeds. Seen in young animals 3-18 months of age. Intermittent signs of pain on handling or on opening mouth, pyrexia and malaise.

Radiological features. (Figure 2.10)
- Marked periosteal reaction around either one or both petrous temporal bones.
- May extend to involve the TMJ's.
- Often associated changes on either one or both horizontal mandibular rami.
- The dorsal aspect of the calvarium may also show evidence of thickening but rarely is there the marked periosteal reaction seen at other sites.

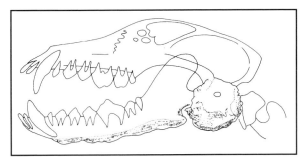

Figure 2.10: Cranio-mandibular osteopathy.

Fractures

These are relatively rare due to the strength of the canine and feline skull and the protection offered by the temporal muscles.

If of clinical significance, will be associated with CNS signs of concussion or open wounds.

Radiological features (Figure 2.11)
- Often difficult to see if undisplaced. Knowledge of and comparison with the normal radiographic anatomical detail is essential for diagnosis.
- When depressed fractures are present these are best evaluted on skyline views.

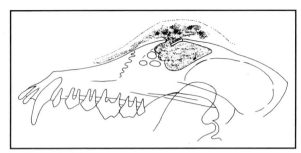

Figure 2.11: Skull fracture.

Foreign Bodies

These are generally opaque and penetrate either from the skin surface (pellets) or from the oro-pharynx (needles).

Accurate localisation usually requires at least two views and the use of radio-opaque markers may also be necessary. Occasionally, comparison of views with the mouth open and closed may be of value.

Radiological features (Figure 2.12)

• Opaque foreign bodies will be identified per se.
• Radiolucent foreign bodies may only be suspected because of associated secondary features or following the injection of contrast into a sinus tract.
• There will often be associated soft tissue swelling.
• Lucent gas tracts may be visible if there is a discharging sinus or gas forming organism present.

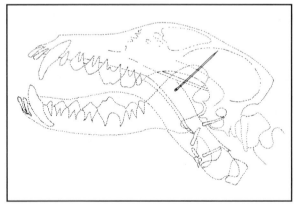

Figure 2.12a: Foreign body – lateral view.

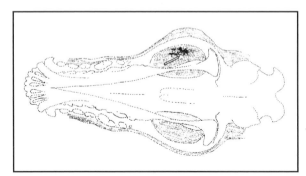

Figure 2.12b: Foreign body – DV view.

Neoplasia of the Skull

Osteosarcoma is the most common tumour. Osteomas and enchondromas are seen occasionally.

Radiological features (Figure 2.13)

• Generally marked proliferation of tumour bone with an aggressive periosteal reaction.
• Underlying bone destruction may be masked by the proliferative reaction.
• Osteomas tend to be more dense and well demarcated than osteosarcomas.

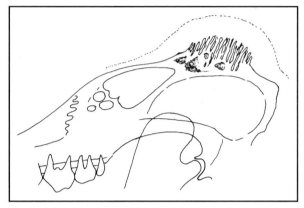

Figure 2.13: Neoplasia of the skull.

Intra-Cranial Neoplasms

These will NOT be identifiable on plain films unless there is either destruction of the calvarium or mineralisation of the tumour, which is very rare.

Contrast studies may be of assistance in a limited number of cases.

'Rubber Jaw' – Renal Secondary hyperparathyroidism

Secondary to either chronic or congenital renal disease. Clinically the teeth and jaws will feel mobile and rubbery.

Radiological features (Figure 2.14)

• Demineralisation of the skull bones.
• Initially loss of the lamina dura and radiolucent halo round all the teeth roots.
• Latterly mottled demineralisation of the mandibles, maxillae and skull.

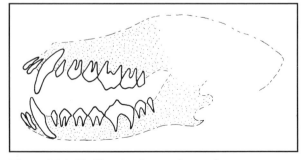

Figure 2.14: "Rubber Jaw" – renal secondary hyperparathyroidism.

II: THE EAR AND TEMPORO-MANDIBULAR JOINT

Indications for radiography of the skull to demonstrate the middle ear and/or temporomandibular joints include -

1) The investigation of swellings associated with either infection or neoplasia.
2) Abnormalities of the temporo-mandibular joints.
3) The investigation of ear disease.

Technique

Both in the interests of accurate positioning and radiation protection general anaesthesia is essential. Screen films should be routinely used with use of a grid depending on the size of the animal.

It should be remembered that the endotracheal tube will often be projected onto the area of interest and may require to be temporarily removed during the radiographic exposure. This should be borne in mind when selecting the method of anaesthesia.

Positioning

Because of the complexity of the radiographic anatomy of this region, an accurate interpretation depends on well positioned films. The methods of positioning the animal and centring the beam for the major views is outlined below.

Dorso-ventral view. (Figure 2.15)

i) This is preferred to the VD view as the mandibles help to limit lateral rotation although there is some magnification of the calvarium due to the increased distance from the film.
ii) The animal is placed in sternal recumbency with the neck extended.
iii) It is often helpful to lay a sandbag over the neck to keep the hard palate parallel to the cassette especially in deep chested dogs.

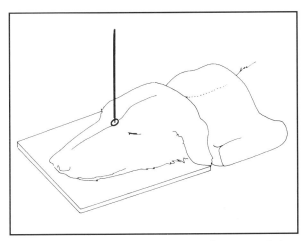

Figure 2.15: *Ear and TMJ - positioning - dorso-ventral view.*

Lateral oblique view. (Figure 2.16)

i) When used to demonstrate the temporomandibular joints or tympanic bullae the positioning - using lucent foam pads to support the head, should either tilt the head slightly about the longitudinal axis to separate the two sides or, alternatively, the nose may be tilted up by approximately 15 degrees in order to project the two sides separately.
ii) This is not an easy view to reliably reproduce from one animal to another, nor, even in the same animal, from one side to the other.

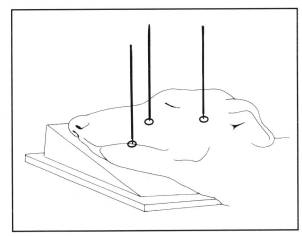

Figure 2.16: *Ear and TMJ - positioning - lateral oblique view.*

Open mouth rostro-caudal view. (Figure 2.17)

i) This is used mainly for the demonstration of the tympanic bullae and foramen magnum.
ii) Positioning is as for the rostro-caudal view but with the mouth held wide open with tapes secured to the table. The palate should be perpendicular to the cassette.
iii) The beam should be parallel to or slightly angled towards the hard palate and centred on the base of the tongue/free edge of the soft palate.

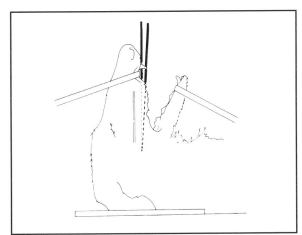

Figure 2.17: *Ear and TMJ - positioning.*

Evaluation

The tympanic bullae on the lateral and RCd open mouth views are seen as thin walled, air filled structures whereas on the DV view they appear thicker walled and denser due to superimposition on the petrous temporal bone. There is an important difference in the cat where a shelf of bone creates an inner and outer compartment to the bullae on the lateral and RCd views.

The condylar process articulates with the zygoma to form the temporo-mandibular joint. The TMJ should have an even joint space and on the lateral view the retroglenoid process can be identified as a ventral spur to the joint.

INTERPRETATION

Otitis Media

Associated with clinical evidence of external ear disease, transient head tilt, etc. Clinical signs of otitis media may be present without radiological abnormalities and vice versa.

Radiological features (Figure 2.18)
- Increased opacity of the normally air filled bulla.
- Thickening of the wall of the bulla.
- Sclerosis of the petrous temporal bone.
- Rarely increased size of the bulla.

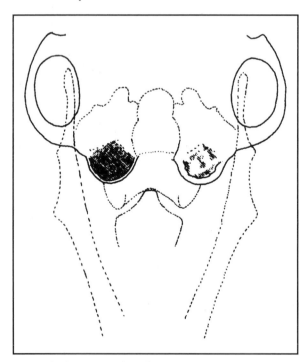

Figure 2.18: *Otitis media - dog*
a. normal tympanic bulla   b. Otitis media.

In the absence of the above signs otitis media may still be present. A strong indicator of otitis media in such a situation is the presence of ossification of the horizontal canal cartilage.

Neoplasia of the Ear

Tumours may arise either in the external ear and extend centrally or arise in the middle ear/bulla.

Radiological features (Figure 2.19)
- Lysis and distortion of the wall of the bulla.
- Soft tissue swelling of adjacent region.

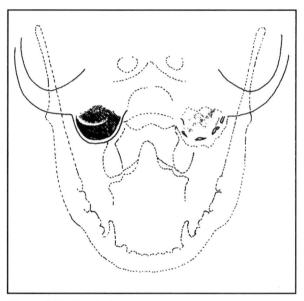

Figure 2.19: *Neoplasia of the ear - cat*
a. Normal tympanic bulla   b. Tumour of middle ear.

Dislocation of the Temporo Mandibular Joint

May be uni- or bi-lateral. More common in the cat. Sequel to some form of trauma. Malocclusion present, most obvious when uni-lateral.

Radiological features (Figure 2.20)
- May be hard to demonstrate can use either DV or lateral oblique views.
- Alternative view is lateral with nose elevated.(Figure 2.21)
- Mandibular condyle usually displaced rostro-dorsally.
- May be fracture of the mandibular condyle or glenoid rim.

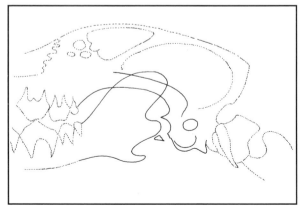

Figure 2.20a: *Fracture of retroglenoid process.*

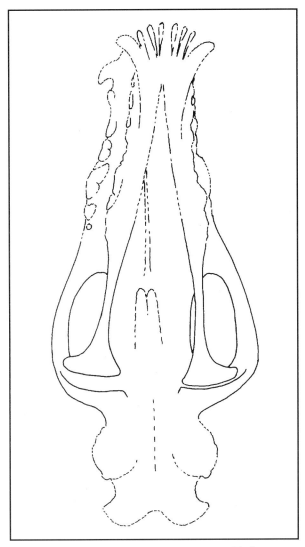

Figure 2.20b: Dislocation of the temporo-mandibular joint.

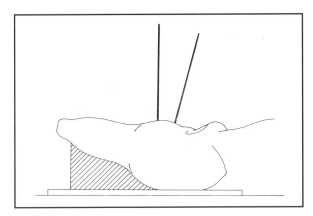

Figure 2.21: Positioning - Alternative lateral oblique view.

Tempror-Mandibular Dysplasia

Seen especially in Bassett hounds and Irish setters.

Clinical signs are open mouth jaw locking e.g. when the animal yawns.

Usually predominantly uni-lateral in which case there will be tilting of the jaw when in the 'locked' position.

Radiological features (Figure 2.22)
- If DV view taken with jaw locked then abnormal position of the coronoid process will be seen.
- If not locked then look on oblique and DV views for loss of clear joint space and abnormal conformation to the glenoid.

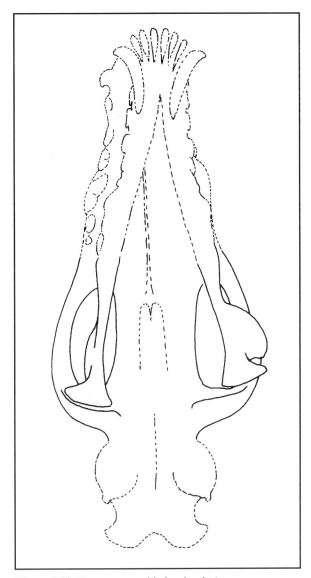

Figure 2.22: Temporo-mandibular dysplasia.

III: THE ORAL CAVITY

The indications for radiography of the oral cavity include-

1) Fractures of the mandible.
2) Congenital anomalies of the mandible or teeth.
3) The investigation of dental disease.
4) The diagnosis and pre-surgical evaluation of neoplasia.
5) The investigation of discharging sinuses associated with infection.

Technique

As mentioned under the previous section, anaesthesia is mandatory for radiographic examination of the oral cavity. Although many of the views described can be obtained using screen film, non-screen film is of value for the intra-oral views and dental films can be used for the detailed radiographic evaluation of certain dental lesions. Non-screen film also has the advantage of greatly improved image detail.

Positioning

Because of the wide variety of skull types the precise angles used for many of the views outlined below will depend on the animal under investigation but the information provided outlines the general principles to be employed.

Lateral and Dorso-Ventral views

The method for positioning for these views is described in the previous section but they are of limited value for the evaluation of the oral cavity because of the superimposition of the two sides in the lateral view and the nasal cavity in the DV view.

Lateral Oblique view (Figure 2.23)

i) The animal is placed in lateral recumbency and radiolucent foam wedges used to tilt the skull so that the dental arcade of interest is projected clear of the opposite side.

ii) For the mandible, the wedge is placed under the mandible with the side under investigation closest to the film.

iii) For the maxillary arcade the wedge is placed under the skull and nose with the side of interest closest to the film.

iv) In both instances the beam should be centred mid-way along the dental arcade and the beam closely collimated.

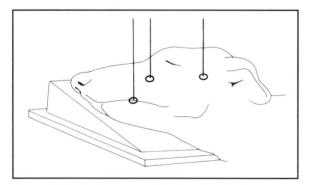

Figure 2.23: Oral cavity - positioning - lateral oblique view.

Ventral-dorsal Intra-oral view (VD/IO)
(Figure 2.24)

i) This view is used for the investigation of the body of the mandible and the mandibular incisor teeth and the rostral portions of the horizontal rami of the mandible.

ii) The animal is supported in dorsal recumbency.

iii) If only the incisor area is under investigation then cassette and screen film can be used.

iv) If the rostral portions of the horizontal rami require to be included then non-screen film is required so that the film can be positioned far enough back in the mouth.

v) The tongue should either be pushed well to one side or positioned symmetrically in midline so as not to produce any confusing variations in density.

vi) The incisor teeth require the beam to be angled about 20 degrees rostro-caudally in order to prevent undue foreshortening and permit full evaluation of the dental roots and alveoli.

vii) Care must be taken to use radiolucent gags and to position the endotracheal tube away from the area of interest.

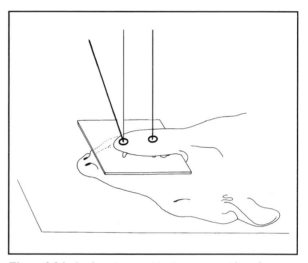

Figure 2.24: Oral cavity - positioning - ventro-dorsal intra-oral view.

Dorso-ventral Intra-oral view (DV/IO)
(Figure 2.25)

i. This view is used for the investigation of the premaxilla, the upper incisor teeth and the rostral portions of the maxilla and premolar teeth. It is essentially the same as that used for evaluation of the nasal cavity qv.

ii. The animal is supported in sternal recumbency.

iii. As with the VD/IO, screen film can be used for the incisor region but non screen film permits a fuller examination of the maxillary arcades.

iv. For examination of the incisor teeth the beam should be angled at about 20 degrees to prevent foreshortening.

v. The endotracheal tube should be tied to the lower jaw and the film placed above the tongue and tube.

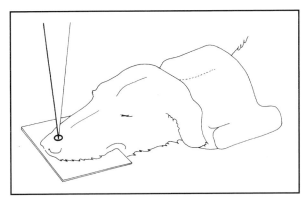

Figure 2.25: Oral cavity - positioning - dorso-ventral intra-oral view.

Evaluation of the radiograph

The dental arcades should be checked for the normal complement of teeth and for supernumerary or unerupted teeth.

The normal dental formulae are:

Dog:	Deciduous		Permanent	
	3 1 3	Total	3 1 4 2	Total
	3 1 3	28	3 1 4 3	42
Cat:	Deciduous		Permanent	
	3 1 3	Total	3 1 3 1	Total
	3 1 2	26	3 1 2 1	30

The mandible (Figure 2.28).

The following structures should initially be indentified.
  a) The body.
  b) Horizontal and vertical rami of the mandible.
  c) The coronoid process at the dorsal tip of the vertical ramus.
  d) The angular process on the ventro-caudal angle of the mandible.
  e) The condylar process which articulates with the zygoma to form the temporo-mandibular joint.
  f) The temporo-mandibular joint.
  g) The mandibular canal which forms a linear area of radiolucencies ventral to the teeth roots.
  h) The mental foraminae visible as small circular lucencies rostrally.
  i) The ventral cortex of the mandible is relatively thick and should be uninterrupted and smooth.

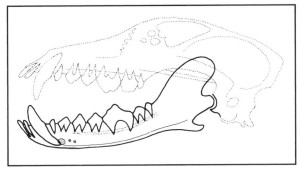

Figure 2.26: Oral cavity - radiographic anatomy.

The teeth (Figure 2.27)

Each tooth is composed of a crown lying above the gingiva and a root embedded within the supporting facial bones.

The root normally has a radiolucent centre which narrows with age.

The margin of bone forming the aveolus appears more dense than the surrounding trabecular bones and is known as the lamina dura. It should be more or less continuous round each root.

The peridontal ligament appears as a fine radiolucent line surrounding the root and lying between the root and lamina dura. This should be narrow and even in width.

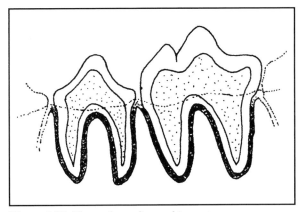

Figure 2.27: The teeth - radiographic anatomy.

INTERPRETATION

Dental anomalies

Supernumerary and missing teeth are seen occasionally in both dogs and cats.

Congenital anodontia

(Absence of all teeth) - rare.

Oligodontia (reduced numbers)

Common especially in brachycephalic breeds.

Polydontia (supernumerary teeth)

Seen occasionally.

Before removing supposedly retained deciduous teeth where no permanent tooth is identifiable clinically, it is wise to radiograph to ensure that the permanent tooth/teeth are present.

Malpositioning of teeth leading to malocclusion is best evaluated clinically.

Radiological features

  • Identification of an abnormal dental formula.
  • Presence or otherwise unerupted teeth.

Periodontal Disease

Very common in adult and elderly dogs and cats. Associated with the presence of dental calculus.

Radiological features (Figure 2.28)
- Generalised widening of the periodontal space.
- Loss of the lamina dura.
- Lysis of trabecular bone especially that lying between the roots and forming the alveolar margins and alveolar crests.
- Clubbing of the teeth roots.

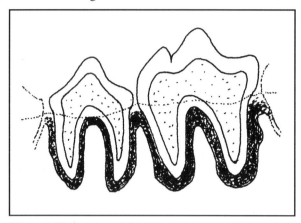

Figure 2.28: Peridontal disease.

Dental Caries

Most commonly affects the first maxillary molar. Difficulty eating. Pain on percussion of affected tooth.

Radiological features (Figure 2.29)
- Radiolucent defect in the crown of the affected tooth.
- Part of the crown may be missing - this may be best assessed clinically.
- May be associated pulpitis and peri-apical abscessation.

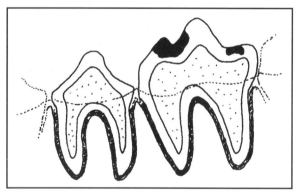

Figure 2.29: Dental caries.

Peri-Apical Abscess

May develop secondary to periodontal disease, caries or fracture of a tooth. Facial swelling and pain. Discharging sinus or fistula which may be chronic.

Radiological features (Figure 2.30)
- Prominent radiolucent halo around the root apex.
- Localised loss of the lamina dura.

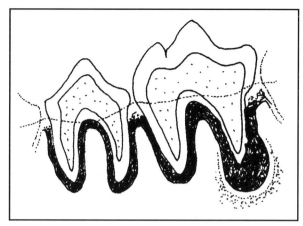

Figure 2.30: Peri-apical abscess.

- Root may appear thinner than normal and may have a ragged appearance.
- Sclerosis of the surrounding trabecular bone - this will accentuate the appearance of the lucent halo.

Oral Neoplasia

Affects a variety of breeds and ages depending on the histopathological type. Usually present with clinically identifiable masses which may become traumatised and bleed. Will eventually interfere with mastication. Precise histopathological classification requires biopsy. Range from benign to very malignant. Two main radiological types can be identified.

i) Expansile cystic types
   Usually associated with benign cysts, odontogenic tumours in young animals and dentigerous cysts.

   Radiological features (Figure 2.31)
   - Expansile lucent cavities within the affected bone.
   - Well defined margins.
   - Thinning of the overlying cortical bone.
   - Very little aggressive periosteal reaction.
   - Often one or more teeth either missing or abnormal in shape and/or position.
   - Often described as having a 'soap bubble' appearance.

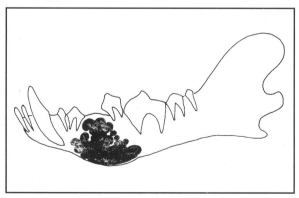

Figure 2.31a: Oral neoplasia – Expansile cystic type.

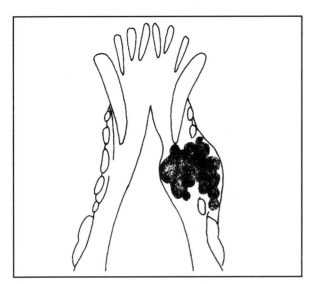

Figure 2.31b: Oral neoplasia – Expansile cystic type.

ii) Infiltrative destructive types

May arise from either soft tissue - squamous cell Ca, melanoma or bone-osteosarcoma.

Radiological features (Figure 2.32)
- Lysis of bone often irregular and mottled in appearance.
- Cortical destruction.
- Soft tissue mass usually also present.
- Displacement of otherwise normal dentition.
- Teeth may appear to be 'floating' in soft tissue due to alveolar destruction.
- Poor margination of the lesion indicative of an aggressive infiltrative lesion.
- Often marginal periosteal reaction.

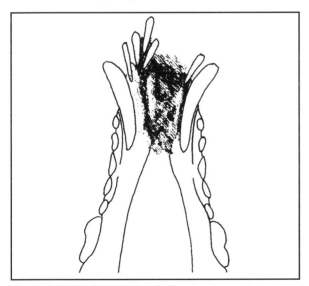

Figure 2.32: Oral neoplasia – Infiltrative destructive type.

Osteomyelitis

Mandible most frequently affected. Not very common and may be secondary to dental disease. Usually chronic low grade infection associated with swelling halitosis and possibly discharging sinus tract.

Radiological features (Figure 2.33)
- Mottled sclerosis of the affected bone.
- Moderately active periosteal reaction resulting in thickening of the cortical bone.
- May be associated signs of dental disease qv.
- Important to distinguish from neoplasia.

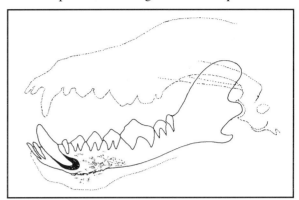

Figure 2.33: Osteomyelitis.

Fractures

Fractures of the maxillae, incisor region of the mandible (symphysis) and the horizontal rami are usually adequately evaluated by clinical examination and rarely require radiographic examination.

Fractures of the junction of the two rami and of the vertical ramus require lateral oblique and DV views to adequately assess prior to treatment because of the overlying muscle mass.

Radiological features (Figure 2.34)
- Requires well positioned radiographs and familiarity with normal anatomy. Even then may be difficult to interpret accurately.
- Indentification of radiolucent fracture lines.
- Displacement of fragments.
- Important to identify those fractures involving the TM joint.

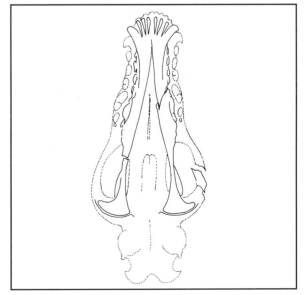

Figure 2.34: Mandibular fractures.

IV: THE NASAL CAVITY

The indications for radiography of the nasal cavity include:-

1) Trauma to the nasal structures.
2) Acute and chronic nasal discharge.
3) Persistent or recurrent epistaxis.
4) Persistent sneezing or nasal frenzy.
5) Abnormal swellings of the nose or related structures.

Technique
Both in the interests of accurate positioning and radiation protection, general anaesthesia is essential. Although screen films can be used for some of the views used to examine the nasal cavity, non-screen films are almost indispensable for the most useful view - the DV intra-oral view.

Positioning

Lateral view (Figure 2.35)

i) The value of this view for the investigation of the nasal cavity is limited due to superimposition of the two sides of the nasal cavity. It is a useful view for the identification of reactive or lytic changes affecting the dorsal bony case of the nasal cavity and for a preliminary evaluation of the frontal sinuses.

ii) Positioning is as described for the routine lateral view of the skull but the beam should be centred mid-way between the nostril and the orbit. Exposure factors will also need to be somewhat reduced due to the relative radiolucency of the nasal structures.

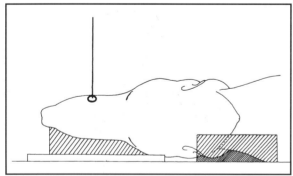

Figure 2.35: Nasal cavity - positioning - lateral view.

Dorso-ventral intra-oral view (Figure 2.36)

i) This is the most useful view for the evaluation of the nasal cavities as it allows comparison of the two sides of the nasal cavity with no superimposition of the mandibles or other structures.

ii) The animal is placed in sternal recumbency with the neck extended.

iii) It is often helpful to lay a sandbag over the neck to keep the hard palate parallel to the cassette especially in deep chested dogs.

iv) Non-screen film should be placed in the mouth with the corner projecting caudally and the film positioned as far back as possible. The use of non-screen film not only allows the maximum area of the nasal cavity to be included but also produces excellent detail. If non screen is not available, alternatives would be to wrap a piece of normal screen film in light proof black plastic in the darkroom and use this, or use a single screen/film combination without a cassette. Failing this, a VD open mouth view could be used (qv).

v) A piece of lead should be routinely placed under the skull to absorb the primary beam and prevent back scatter. Relatively high exposures are required for most types of non-screen film.

vi) The beam should be centred midway between the external nares and a line joining the eyes.

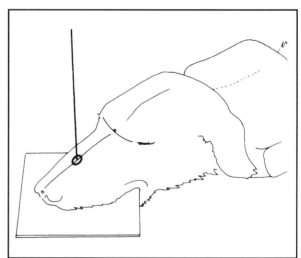

Figure 2.36: Nasal cavity positioning - dorso-ventraintra-oral view.

20 degree Ventro-Dorsal open mouth view. (Figure 2.37)

i) Used as an alternative to the Dorso-ventral intra-oral in the dog and as the preferred method for imaging the nasal cavity in the cat.

ii) The animal is placed in dorsal recumbency and the mouth held wide open with tapes attached to the table ensuring that the hard palate is parallel to the table top. The tongue and endotracheal tube should be tied to the mandible.

iii) The X-ray tube is angled 20 degrees rostro-caudally and the beam centred in the midline of the palate at the level of the third premolar teeth.

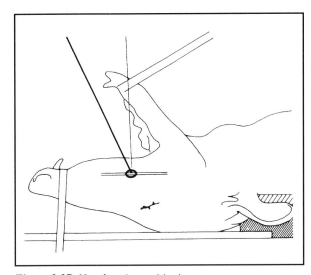

*Figure 2.37: Nasal cavity positioning -
20° ventro-dorsaopen-mouth view.*

Rostro-caudal view (Figure 2.38)
   i)   This view is mainly of value in demonstrating
        the frontal sinuses, zygomatic arch, temporal
        region and the sagittal crest. It is of less value
        in the cat due to the conformation of the
        feline skull.
   ii) The animal is positioned on its back with the
        skull secured by a tape around the nose so
        that the hard palate is perpendicular to the
        cassette.
   iii) The beam should be angled at 5 - 10 degrees
        in a rostro- caudal direction.

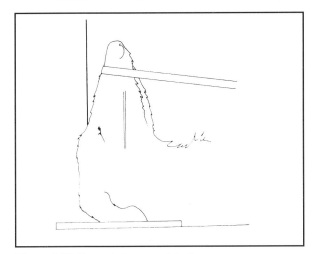

*Figure 2.38: Frontal sinus - positioning.
Rostro-caudal view.*

Evaluation of the radiographs (Figure 2.39)
The conformation of the nasal cavity can be grouped or
classified in three broad categories - brachycephalic,
mesaticephalic and dolichocephalic. The feline nasal
cavity differs considerably in detail from that of the
dog. It is important, if necessary with the aid of a
radiographic atlas,to be able to identify the following
landmarks:-

a)   The nasal septum composed of the vomer
     bone and nasal cartilage.
b)   Rostral and caudal nasal cavity - divided by
     line drawn between the cranio-medial roots of
     the carnassial teeth.
c)   The turbinates having a fine linear or reticular
     detail produced by the fine mucosal covering
     of the turbinate bones contrasted by the air
     filled interspaces of the nasal cavity.
d)   Large ventral concha and smaller dorsal
     concha in the rostral portion.
e)   Coarser scrolls of the ethmoturbinates in the
     caudal portion.
f)   The bony case of the nasal cavity composed
     of the palatine bones ventrally, the maxillae
     laterally and the nasal bones dorsally.
g)   The soft tissue density of the external nares
     with the airways outlined by gas.
h)   The naso-palatine fissure.
i)   The outline of the frontal sinuses.
j)   The frontal sinuses are also well
     demonstrated on the rostro-caudal view.
     (Figure 2.40)

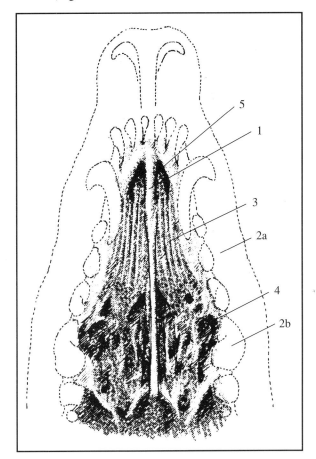

*Figure 2.39: Nasal cavity – radiographic anatomy.
1) Nasal septum
2) Rostral (a) and caudal (b) nasal cavity
3) Turbinates - ventral concha and dorsal concha
4) Turbinates - ethmoturbinates
5) Naso-palatine fissure
6) Outline of the frontal sinuses*

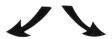

Figure 2.40: Frontal sinus - radiographic anatomy.

The nasal cavity is a symmetrical structure and, on all but the lateral views, details on each side can be compared to each other and any abnormal densities or lucencies can be assessed.

The following features should be assessed:-

a) The nasal chambers

1) Turbinate pattern
    i)   Normal
    ii)   Absent
    iii) Masked

2) Opacity of cavity
    i)   Normal
    ii)   Increased radio-opacity
    iii) Increased radio-lucency
    iv)   Mixed pattern of opacity and lucency

3) The bony case
    i)   Normal
    ii)   Bone lysis with lucent defects
    iii) Thickening
    iv)   Thinning
    v)   Periosteal reaction

4) The nasal septum
    i)   Normal
    ii)   Thinning
    iii) Deviation away from the midline
    iv)   Interrupted with defect(s)

5) Distribution of changes
    i)   Unilateral
    ii)   Bilateral

b) The frontal sinuses

1) Opacification
2) Thickening or periosteal reaction
3) Mottling of the bony wall
4) Destruction of the bony wall

Diagnostic Flowchart 1: Nasal cavity.

1.   TURBINATE BONES PRESENT

No other change

Turbinate pattern masked or coarse

Unilateral   Bilateral

Normal

Rhinarial ulceration

Cryoglobulinaemia

Idiopathic epistaxis

Coagulopathy

Foreign body

Chronic hyperplastic rhinitis

2. TURBINATE PATTERN ABSENT

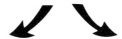

Increased lucency rostrally	Homogenous increased opacity
Increased lucency	Lysis of bony case
Mixed pattern caudally	Marginated lucencies
Punctate lucencies	Punctate lucencies
Vomer irregularity	Septal deviation and/or
	Vomer absent
	Mineralisation

DESTRUCTIVE RHINITIS   *NEOPLASIA*

Aspergillus infection
Bacterial rhinitis — cat

Diagnostic Flowchart 2: Nasal cavity.

INTERPRETATION

Nasal Neoplasia

Seen in variety of breeds but unusual in brachycephalics. Nasal discharge often associated with bleeding. Obstructed air flow down nostril. Also seen less commonly in cats - usually lymphosarcoma.

Radiological features (Figure 2.41)
- Homogenous soft tissue density.
- Turbinate destruction.
- Deviation or destruction of septum.
- Destruction of the bony case. Defects in the hard palate or nasal bones may project as sharply delineated radiolucent defect superimposed on the soft tissue density.
- May be uni- or bi-lateral involvement.
- Extra-nasal soft tissue swelling.
- Opacification of frontal sinus due to obstructed drainage.
- Feline lymphosarcoma may result in soft tissue opacification of the nasal cavity without bone destruction.

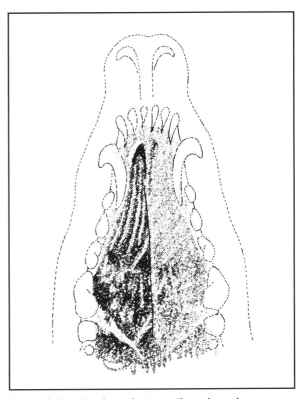

Figure 2.41a: Nasal neoplasia – unilateral neoplasm.

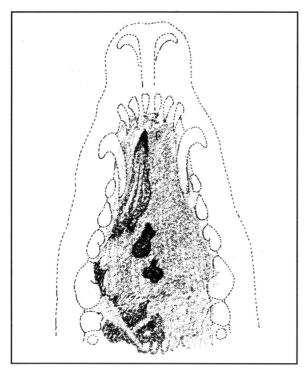

Figure 2.41b: Nasal neoplasia – extension of neoplasm through septum and palate.

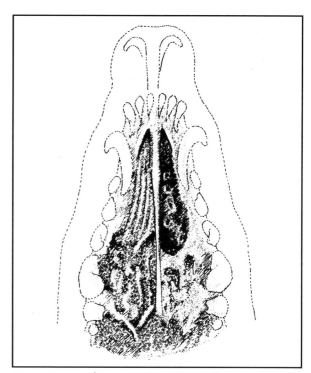

Figure 2.42b: Destructive rhinitis Aspergillus infection of the nasal cavity.

Destructive Rhinitis

Usually result of *Aspergillus* infection. More common in younger dolichocephalic and mesaticephalic breeds. Nasal discharge - initially clear then mucro-purulent occasionally haemorrhagic. May be facial pain on clinical examination.

Radiological features (Figure 2.42)

- Turbinate destruction may be uni-lateral or bi-lateral.
- Turbinate destruction usually in rostral portion but may extend caudally.
- Overall increase in radiolucency rostrally.
- Mixed pattern or increased radiolucency in caudal portion.
- Punctate lucencies may be observed.
- The vomer may appear irregular.
- May be extension into the frontal sinus(es) with opacification of the lumen.
- May be thickening and mottling of the frontal bones.

Chronic Hyperplastic Rhinitis

Similar clinical signs to destructive rhinitis but often of longer duration. An important feature distinguishing from neoplasia and destructive rhinitis is the absence of nasal bleeding.

Radiological features (Figure 2.43)

- Loss of turbinate pattern due to masking by mucosal thickening and exudate.
- Trabecular pattern of turbinate bones still visible.
- Increased radio-opacity which is often of a mottled appearance.

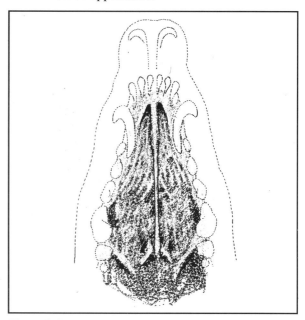

Figure 2.43: Chronic hyperplastic rhinitis.

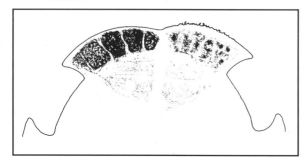

Figure 2.42a: Destructive rhinitis Aspergillus infection of the frontal sinus.

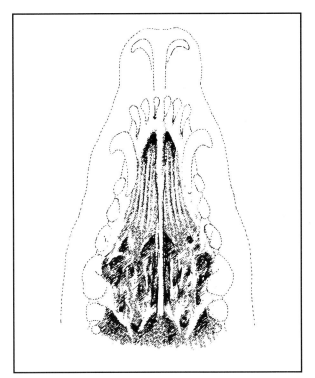

Figure 2.44

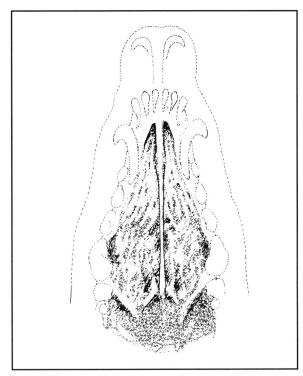

Figure 2.45

The features in both nasal foreign body and acute rhinitis may range from normal (Fig. 2.44) to uni- or bi-lateral rhinitis (Fig. 2.45).

Foreign Body

Usually but not always sudden onset of clinical signs. Sneezing may be a feature in the acute stages but may not be present when FB has been present for some time. Purulent or muco-purulent discharge in chronic cases.

Radiological features (Figure 2.44)
- May be no abnormalities seen.
- Foreign body may be identified if opaque (eg stone).
- Radiolucent FB's (pieces of wood and grass) won't be visible.
- Occasionally there is widening of the rostral end of the common meatus.
- In chronic cases may be signs of destructive or chronic hyperplastic rhinitis.

Acute Rhinitis

Acute onset of usually bilateral serous or mucoid nasal discharge.

Radiological features (Figure 2.45)
- Often normal radiological appearance.
- May be slight increase in nasal density but no loss of turbinates.
- Must differentiate from early destructive rhinitis or tumour.

Nasal Polyp

Radiological features (Figure 2.46)
- Focal increase in opacity.
- Cannot be differentiated from the early cases of nasal neoplasia.

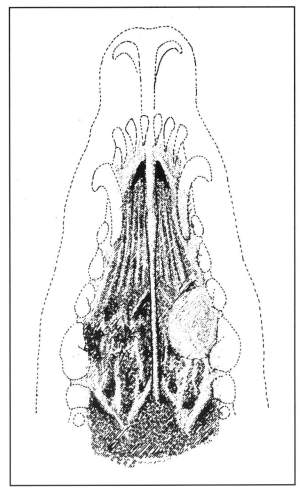

Figure 2.46: Nasal polyp.

Feline Chronic Rhinitis

Often a sequel to other respiratory infections. Can occur in any age of animal.

Radiological features (Figure 2.47)

*   Generally more difficult to evaluate radiologically than in the dog due to the more irregular turbinate pattern in this species.
*   May be turbinate destruction and disorganisation.

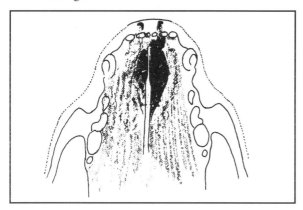

Figure 2.47: Feline chronic rhinitis.

V: THE PHARYNX AND LARYNX

The indications for radiography of the pharynx and larynx include:-

1)   Pharyngeal and laryngeal mass(es).
2)   Coughing, gagging and retching.
3)   Dysphagia and difficulty in swallowing.
4)   Swellings of the upper cervical area.

Technique

Both in the interests of accurate positioning and radiation protection, general anaesthesia is essential except in those situations where contrast examination of the pharynx is being undertaken when it will not only be hazardous to the patient but will also yield false indications of altered function. In these situations particular attention should be paid to aspects of radiation protection. Screen films should be used routinely for the examination of this region.

Positioning

Lateral view (Figure 2.48)

i)   This is the most valuable projection for evaluation of the pharynx and larynx.
ii)   Positioning is as described for the routine lateral view of the skull ensuring that the sagittal plane of the skull is parallel to the film.
iii)   The beam should be centred over the larynx.

iv)   It may be desirable to remove the endotracheal tube if present in order to obtain a true representation of the anatomical relationships. Care should be taken, especially in long eared breeds, to ensure that the ears are pulled dorsally and not superimposed on the area of interest.

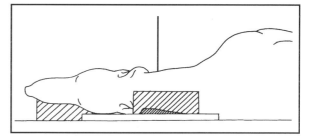

Figure 2.48: Pharynx/larynx - positioning - lateral view.

Ventro-dorsal view (Figure 2.49)

i)   This view is only occasionally of value in supplementing the lateral projections as the skull and cervical spine are superimposed on the structures of major interest.
ii)   The animal is secured in dorsal recumbency with the neck held extended and the front legs drawn caudally. Care should be taken to ensure that there is no tilting laterally and that the ears are pulled laterally
iii)   The beam should be centred on the larynx.

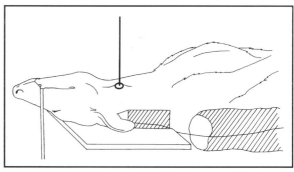

Figure 2.49: Pharynx/larynx - positioning - Ventro-dorsal view.

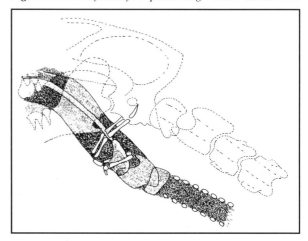

Figure 2.50: Pharynx and larynx - radiographic anatomy.

Evaluation of the radiographs

Because of the presence of air within the pharynx, larynx and trachea, the presence of the hyoid apparatus and in some animals the relative opacity of the laryngeal cartilages, it is possible to recognise a considerable amount of the normal anatomy on radiographs of this region.

It is important, if necessary with the aid of a radiographic atlas, to be able to identify the following main landmarks:-

a) The oro-pharynx naso-pharynx.
b) The soft palate separating the oro- and naso-pharynx.
c) The laryngopharynx dorsal to the larynx and bordered caudally by the crico-pharyngeal muscle at the level of the cricoid cartilage.
d) The pharyngeal isthmus starting at the top of the epiglottis and common to the respiratory and alimentary portions of the pharynx.
e) The hyoid apparatus - a group of 7 bones supporting the larynx and comprising the paired stylohoid, epihyoid and keratohyoid bones and the single basihyoid bone which is seen in end-on projection.
f) The larynx comprising the paired arytenoid, thyroid and cricoid cartilages and the unpaired epiglottis.

On good quality radiographs, not only the individual cartilages but also the laryngeal saccules will be identified.

Occasionally a small amount of gas may be identified in the proximal oesophagus.

The salivary glands and normal lymph nodes will not be identified on normal radiographs.

Contrast examinations of this region can be extremely valuable in the evaluation of pharyngeal dysfunction and also occasionally of value in the full assessment of suspected sialocoeles.

Since pharyngeal dysfunction results in a dynamic abnormality of the swallowing mechanism it requires the use of fluoroscopy for a full radiological study to be performed and this will be beyond the scope of most general practices.

The administration of barium impregnated food and the taking of an immediate 'spot' film may provide some evidence upon which to base a diagnosis of pharyngeal dysfunction but because of the need to perform these studies in the fully conscious animal which will often be distressed by the repeated attempts to swallow there are obvious radiation protection problems for the personnel involved as well as being difficult to obtain sufficiently well positioned films.

Occasionally it may not be possible to reliably diagnose a sialocoele solely on clinical grounds or to reliably determine the affected side. In these situations it is possible to cannulate the salivary ducts with a 25g. needle and outline with contrast medium the sub-mandibular and sub-lingual ducts. It is only necessary to inject about 1 ml of 60% organic iodide contrast medium (e.g. Conray 280). There are, however, a number of factors that may affect the results of such an investigation.

It is usually necessary to cannulate both the sub-mandibular and sub-lingual ducts. The former is the larger and more easily cannulated but the latter is almost invariably the one involved in the lesion. Cannulation of the sub-lingual can be difficult and time consuming. In addition the two ducts may have a common opening and thus be even more difficult than usual to cannulate individually.

If cannulation fails then an alternative procedure is to inject contrast directly into the sialocoele which is then massaged to distribute the contrast before a ventro-dorsal view of the pharynx is taken.

INTERPRETATION

Because of the ease with which the anatomical details can be seen the region should be carefully evaluated for:-
*   the presence of abnormal soft tissue densities.
*   displacement of the larynx or other identifiable landmarks.
*   loss of the normal fascial planes.
*   compression of the airways.

Fracture of the Hyoid Apparatus
A rare condition but may be seen resulting from either external trauma or choke chain injuries.

Radiological features (Figure 2.51)
*   Loss of continuity of the hyoid apparatus.
*   Caudal displacement of the larynx.

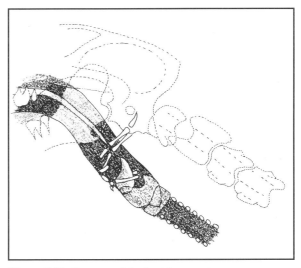

Figure 2.51: *Fracture of the hyoid apparatus.*

Pharyngeal Foreign Bodies

Associated with choking and retching if within the lumen. May be presented as a pharyngeal abscess if there is perforation of the pharyngeal wall.

Radiological features (Figure 2.52)
- Visibility depends on the nature of the foreign body. Small bones may be identified but take care not to mistake for the hyoid and vice versa.
- Pieces of wood may be visible if within the pharyngeal lumen, if embedded in peri-pharyngeal soft tissue will often not be visible.
- May be soft tissue swelling.
- Presence of radiolucent gas tract and bubbles will indicate either sinus tract or the presence of gas forming organisms.

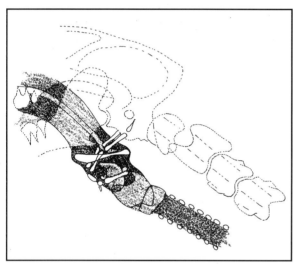

Figure 2.52: Pharyngeal foreign body.

Primary Neoplasia

Not common but may be:-

Intra-luminal e.g. naso-pharyngeal polyps in the cat.
Extra-luminal within the soft tissues e.g. thyroid adenoma and adenocarcinoma in the dog.
Involving the regional lymph nodes - multicentric lymphosarcoma.

Radiological features (Figure 2.53)
- Intra-luminal tumours - as more or less discrete soft tissue masses within either the pharynx or larynx.
- Extra-luminal tumours - usually ill defined soft tissue masses or swelling in the peri-pharyngeal and peri-laryngeal tissues.
- Obliteration of the normal fascial planes.
- Displacement of identifiable structures and possibly compression of the airways.
- Occasionally there may be mineralisation of the mass.

- Involving the regional lymph nodes - enlargement of the sub-mandibular nodes seldom identified radiographically but involvement of the retro-pharyngeal nodes will displace the pharyngeal wall ventrally and increase the size of the retropharyngeal space.

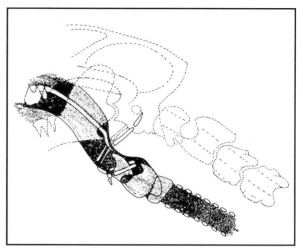

Figure 2.53a: Intra-luminal pharyngeal mass.

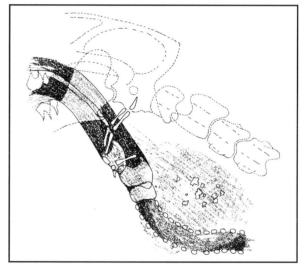

Figure 2.53b: Thyroid carcinoma.

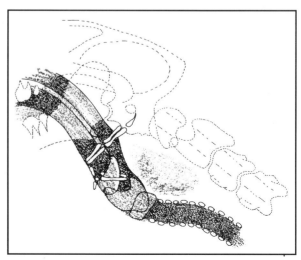

Figure 2.53c: Retropharyngeal tumour e.g. Lymphosarcoma.

Secondary Neoplasia

Most commonly affects the retro-pharyngeal lymph nodes.

Can occur secondary to a number of primary tumours affecting the oral and, less commonly, nasal cavities. Tonsillar carcinoma is a frequent cause of neoplastic enlargement of the retro-pharyngeal nodes.

Radiological features (Figure 2.54)
- Enlargement of the retro-pharyngeal nodes will displace the pharyngeal wall ventrally and increase the size of the retropharyngeal space.

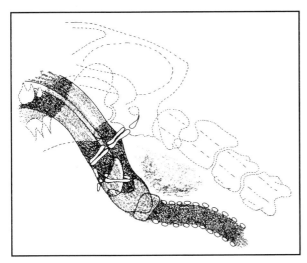

Figure 2.54: Seconday neoplasia.

Retro-Pharyngeal Abscess

Usually secondary to a penetrating wound of the pharyngeal wall.

Radiological features (Figure 2.55)
- Indentical to the retro-pharyngeal node enlargement seen in secondary neoplasia.
- Very occasionally may be gas foci present due to the presence of gas forming organisms.

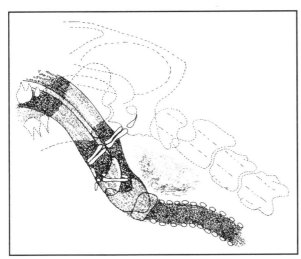

Figure 2.55: Retro-pharyngeal abscess.

Sub-Lingual Sialocoele

Presence of a soft, painless, fluctuant sub-mandibular swelling. Needle aspiration will reveal clear, straw coloured, viscid fluid.

Radiological features (Figure 2.56)
- Plain film unhelpful.
- Contrast examination following cannulation of the sub-lingual duct will result in leakage of contrast into the 'cyst' cavity.
- Normal sialogram will demonstrate acinar gland structure with no leakage of contrast.

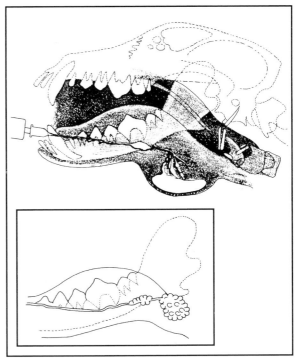

Figure 2.56: Sub-lingual sialocoele.
Inset: normal appearance of sublingual sialogram.

Pharyngeal Dysfunction and Crico-Pharyngeal Dysphagia

Either congenital problem in spaniel type breeds or acquired problem in older animals with no breed related incidence.

May be sequel to either CNS problems or neuro-muscular disease.

Radiological features (Figure 2.57)
- Plain films NAD.
- Fluoroscopic studies following barium swallow will demonstrate nasal reflux of barium.
- Retention of barium within the pharynx.
- Failure of relaxation of the crico-pharyngeal 'sphincter'.
- Aspiration of barium into the larynx and trachea.
- Incoordinated swallowing movement of the pharyngeal muscle.

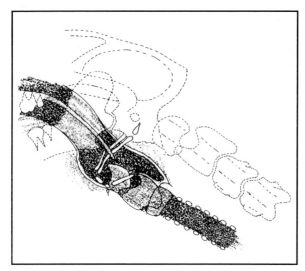

Figure 2.57: Pharyngeal dysfunction and crico-pharyngeal dysphagia.

VI: THE OESOPHAGUS

The indications for radiography of the oesophagus include:-

1)   Regurgitation of unaltered food.
2)   Dysphagia.
3)   Evaluation and diagnosis of feline dysautonomia.
4)   The investigation of myaesthenia gravis.

Technique

Whilst it is essential that wherever possible animals are sedated and restrained by mechanical means, it is frequently inappropriate to anaesthetise animals for the evaluation of oesophageal disease as it is frequently necessary to undertake some form of contrast study.

The lateral view is virtually the only view that is of value in the investigation of oesophageal disease except for selected cases of thoracic oesophageal lesions where a DV view can be of value.

Screen films should be used routinely.

Positioning

Lateral View (Figure 2.58)

i)   Lateral recumbency as for the routine lateral views of either the cervical spine or thorax.
ii)   The fore-limbs may be drawn caudally for examination of the cervical oesophagus or cranially for the thoracic oesophagus.
iii)   For evaluation of the cervical oesophagus the beam should be centred over the mid cervical area and collimated to include the pharynx and thoracic inlet.
iv)   For evaluation of the thoracic oesophagus the beam should be centred over the fifth intercostal space and collimated to include both the thoracic inlet and diaphragm.

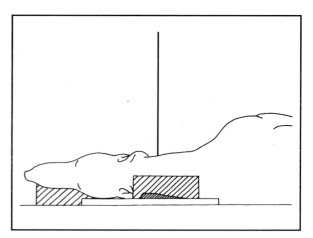

Figure 2.58: Oesophagus - positioning - lateral view.

Whereas a number of oesophageal conditions will have plain film radiological features, it is frequently necessary to undertake contrast examinations.

Plain film studies are a pre-requisite to any contrast study.

Following the administration of contrast, radiographs should be taken immediately.

Initial examination with a liquid barium swallow may be adequate but oesophageal strictures and dilations are often more adequately demonstrated by the administration of barium mixed with food. Barium paste can be used for the evaluation of mucosal defects, but its value is limited in the dog and the cat. If perforation of the oesophagus is suspected, then an aqueous organic iodide such as gastrograffin should be used rather than Barium sulphate suspension to prevent any unnecessary foreign body tissue reaction.

Full evaluation of oesophageal motility and certain strictures require the use of dynamic studies provided by Image Intensified fluoroscopy which will not be routinely available in practice.

Evaluation of the radiographs

Because the oesophagus is a soft tissue structure with no normal luminal contents and surrounded by tissue of similar density, it is not normally identified on plain films. Occasionally very small accumulations of gas may be seen in the proximal oesophagus or cranial to the aorta. In anaesthetised animals it is also not unusual to see larger accumulations of gas within the oesophagus which must not be mistaken for abnormalities.

INTERPRETATION

Congenital and Acquired Mega-Oesophagus

Congenital megaoesophagus is seen in Irish Setters, German Shepherd Dogs and Great Danes. Clinical signs are regurgitation of unaltered food without retching or discomfort. Usually signs first noticed after weaning. May occasionally be symptom free. Acquired megaoesophagus is seen in adult animals and may result in regurgitation or may be symptom free.

The aetiology may be undetermined or the oesophageal dysfunction related to myasthenia gravis, neuro muscular disease or feline dysautonomia. Both forms of megaoesophagus may have the clinical signs and radiological features of aspiration pneumonia.

Radiological features (Figure 2.59)
- Dilated air or ingesta filled oesophagus.
- Oesophageal wall may be highlighted by the intra-luminal gas.
- Heart base and trachea displaced ventrally.
- If associated with myasthenia gravis, dysautonomia and neuromuscular disease the dilation may not be apparent without contrast studies.

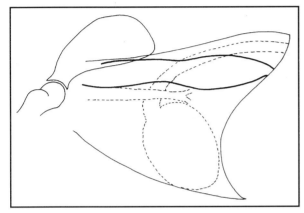

Figure 2.59: Congenital and acquired mega-oesophagus.

Vascular Ring Anomalies

Similar clinical signs to congenital megaoesophagus.
Commonest lesion is a dextraposed aorta but other vascular anomalies may be present.

Radiological features (Figure 2.60)
- Dilation of cervical and cranial thoracic oesophagus.
- Lumen distended with either gas or ingesta.
- Abrupt narrowing of lumen at heart base although a lateral pouch may project caudally mimicking congenital megaoesophagus - DV view useful to distinguish.
- If due to anomalous origin of the subclavian artery then the oesophageal narrowing is cranial to the aortic arch.

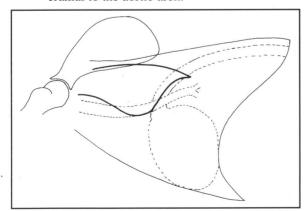

Figure 2.60: Vascular ring anomalies.

Oesophageal Foreign Body

Commonest cause of oesophageal obstruction in the dog. Frequently due to the impaction of chop bone. Any breed but more common in terrier breeds.

Radiological features (Figure 2.61)
- Presence of more or less mineralised foreign body.
- Most commonly lodge midway between the heart base and diaphragm.
- Occasionally lodge at thoracic inlet or over the heart base.
- The oesophagus proximal to the obstruction may contain gas or small quantities of fluid or ingesta.
- If there has been oesophageal perforation there will be mediastinitis with increased mediastinal density loss of clear delineation of the caudal thorax and possibly free pleural fluid.
- Radiolucent or poorly mineralised FB may require contrast examination in which case aqueous organic iodides preferred because of the possibility of perforation.

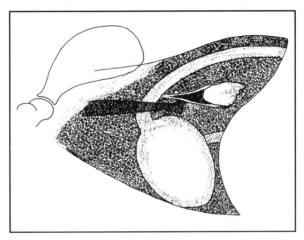

Figure 2.61: Oesophageal foreign body.

Oesophageal Perforation

Sequel to foreign body obstruction in thoracic oesophagus. Sequel to penetrating wound from lumen e.g. stick.

Radiological features (Figure 2.62)
- Cervical oesophagus -
- Soft tissue swelling.
- Loss of normal fascial planes.
- Interstitial emphysema which may extend to thoracic inlet and result in pneumomediastinum.
- Subcutaneous emphysema.
- Thoracic oesophagus -
- Mediastinitis with increased opacity loss of thoracic definition increased mediastinal width reverse fissuring etc.
- Free pleural fluid.

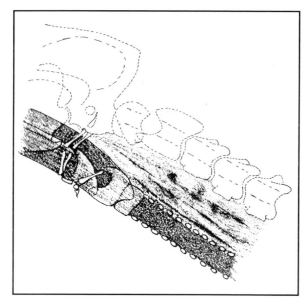

Figure 2.62: Oesophageal perforation.

Oesophageal Neoplasia

Extremely rare in the dog in the UK - may be associated with parasitic infections in tropics. Very occasionally encountered in the cat.

Radiological features (Figure 2.63)
- Occasionally soft tissue mass identified.
- Narrowing and luminal irregularity on contrast examination.

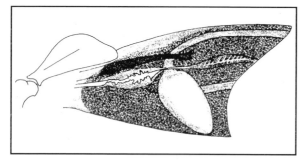

Figure 2.63: Oesophageal neoplasia - cat.

VII: THE TRACHEA.

The indications for radiography of the trachea include:-

1) Dyspnoea.
2) Coughing.
3) Collapse on exercise associated with cyanosis.
4) Inspiratory and expiratory noise.

Tecnique

Whilst it is essential that wherever possible animals are sedated and restrained by mechanical means, it is frequently inappropriate to anaesthetise animals for the evaluation of tracheal disease.

The lateral view is virtually the only view that is of value in the investigation of tracheal problems although where facilities for fluoroscopy are available this can be valuable in cases where tracheal collapse is suspected.

Screen films should be used routinely.

Positioning

Lateral view (Figure 2.64)
i. Lateral recumbency as for the routine lateral views of either the cervical spine or thorax.
ii. The fore-limbs may be drawn caudally for examination of the cervical trachea or cranially for the thoracic trachea.
iii. For evaluation of the cervical trachea the beam should be centred over the mid cervical area and collimated to include the pharynx and thoracic inlet.
iv. For evaluation of the thoracic trachea the beam should be centered over the fifth intercostal space and collimated to include both the thoracic inlet and diaphragm.
v. An extended lateral, positioned as above but with the head and neck extended, may be of value in the assessment of tracheal collapse.

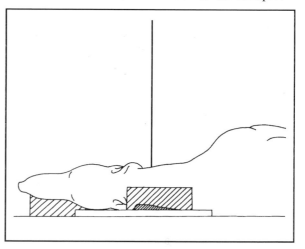

Figure 2.64: Trachea - positioning - Lateral view.

Tangential rostro-caudal view of the thoracic inlet. (Figure 2.65)

i) This view has been described to outline the lumen of the trachea at the thoracic inlet.
ii) The animal is placed in sternal recumbency with the head and neck extended.
iii) The beam is directed rostro-caudally toward the base of the neck.
iv) This view has the obvious disadvantage of difficulty in positioning without producing of exacerbation of the respiratory obstruction.

Although contrast studies can be used to evaluate the mucosal surface of the tracheal lumen their use is very limited.

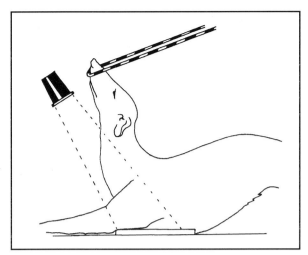

Figure 2.65: Trachea - positioning - Tangenital rostro-caudal view of the thoracic inlet.

Evaluation of the Radiographs

As the trachea is an air filled structure, its lumen is easily seen on the plain film. However, as it is surrounded by soft tissue densities, it is not normally possible to identify the outer surface of the trachea although the trachea rings will be more or less identifiable depending on their degree of mineralisation which increases with age.

Obese animals may appear to have narrowed tracheas due to surrounding fat, particularly at the thoracic inlet.

Marked extension of the neck will result in the tracheal lumen being displaced laterally and superimposed on the ventral cervical muscles at the thoracic inlet giving a false appearance of tracheal narrowing.

Flexion of the neck will result in dorsal displacement of the distal portion of the trachea.

Features which should be looked for as indications of tracheal disease include:-

a) The tracheal lumen should be an even diameter throughout its length.
b) The lumen should be free of abnormal opacities.
c) The mucosal surface should appear smooth.
d) Tracheal rings should correspond to the diameter of the lumen.
e) There should be no abnormal ballooning of the lumen.
f) The lumen should normally be at least as wide as the proximal end of the third rib.
g) The outer wall of the trachea should not normally be visible.

INTERPRETATION

Tracheal Collapse

Very common condition of small brachycephalic breeds, the Yorkshire terrier and miniature and toy poodle.

Although probably congenital in origin, the clinical signs of dyspnoea on exercise or excitement may not develop until adulthood.

Radiological features. (Figure 2.66)
*   Changes usually seen at the thoracic inlet and the distal cervical trachea, but may extend distally as far as the tracheal bifurcation.
*   Lumen appears to gradually narrow.
*   Features of luminal narrowing depend on the phase of respiration.
*   Comparison of films taken at inspiration and expiration will show narrowing during inspiration and ballooning during expiration - this may require fluoroscopy.
*   The above features may be exacerbated by pinching the nostrils.
*   Rostro-caudal tangenital view will demonstrate an oval or 'C' shaped tracheal lumen.

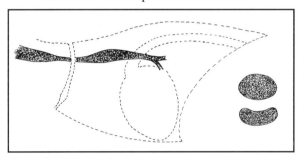

Figure 2.66: Tracheal collapse.

Filaroides Osleri

Clinical signs are of persistent chronic cough.

Radiological features. (Figure 2.67)
*   May be possible to see nodules confluent with the tracheal mucosa in the distal thoracic trachea but these are often not apparent on plain films.
*   Contrast studies can be used to outline the nodules but endoscopy is probably the preferred technique of demonstrating them.

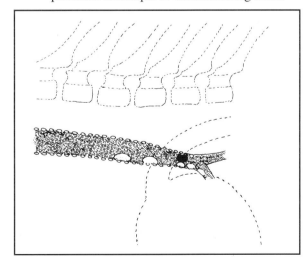

Figure 2.67: Filaroides osleri.

Tracheal Foreign Body

Relatively rare. Usually vary in position so can produce intermittent signs severe of respiratory obstruction and dyspnoea.

Radiological features. (Figure 2.68)
- Small lucent foreign bodies frequently not identified on plain radiographs.
- Larger soft tissue, dense FBs and radio-opaque FBs will be identified as masses within the tracheal lumen.

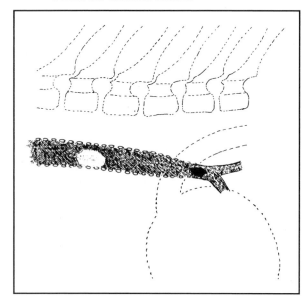

Figure 2.68: Tracheal foreign body.

Tracheal Hypoplasia

Seen as congenital problem in young dogs.

Radiological features. (Figure 2.69)
- The tracheal lumen is evenly narrowed throughout the whole of its length, measuring less than the width of the proximal end of the third rib.

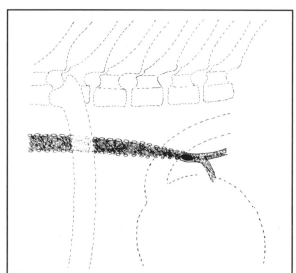

Figure 2.69: Tracheal hypoplasia.

Peri-Tracheal Disease

Radiological features (Figure 2.70)
- Masses adjacent to the trachea will result in displacement or deviation of the trachea due to its relatively rigid nature.
- The presence of gas within the surrounding tissues will highlight the external surface of the trachea, e.g. pneumo-mediastinum, interstitial emphysema.

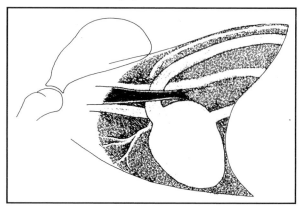

Figure 2.70a: Peri-tracheal disease - pneumo-mediastinum.

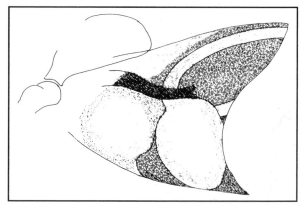

Figure 2.70b: Peri-tracheal disease - mediostinal mass.

Submucosal Thickening/Infiltration

Occasionally in association with coagulopathies and diffuse neoplasia, e.g. lymphosarcoma.

Radiological features (Figure 2.71)
- The tracheal lumen will appear narrowed but the tracheal rings will maintain their normal diameter.

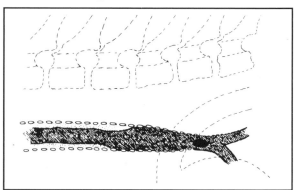

Figure 2.71: Submucosal thickening/infiltration.

CHAPTER THREE

The Thorax

M. E. Herrtage and R. Dennis

CONTENTS

I: INDICATIONS AND RADIOGRAPHIC TECHNIQUE FOR THORACIC RADIOGRAPHY

Indications

Radiography of the canine and feline thorax is an invaluable aid to the diagnosis of many thoracic diseases and lesions as it allows assessment of the lower airways, lung parenchyma, heart, mediastinum, pleural cavity, thoracic wall and diaphragm. Radiography of the thorax does, however, pose particular problems, especially relating to positioning and prevention of movement blur, and these are discussed below.

The indications for thoracic radiography include the following clinical presentations -

1) Coughing
2) Dyspnoea
3) Cardiovascular disease
4) Thoracic trauma
5) Assessment of primary and secondary neoplasia
6) Lesions of the chest wall.
7) Regurgitation of food
8) Investigation of other abnormalities detected by palpation, auscultation or percussion
9) Miscellaneous

A check list of the conditions which may be associated with these various clinical presentations is presented in Table 3.1 and the common radiological features of each condition are described and illustrated.

Restraint for Thoracic Radiography

The Ionising Radiations Regulations (1985) require that animals may only be manually restrained for radiography when clinical consideration precludes the use of sedation or anaesthesia. The spectrum of diseases affecting the thorax includes many that would make anaesthesia hazardous and indeed a full evaluation of the heart and lungs may be clinically desirable prior to anaesthesia. This would include severely dyspnoeic animals and those with cardiovascular disease. If manual restraint is required then all measures to protect personnel detailed in Chapter 9 must be taken.

With gentle and sympathetic handling, most patients can be restrained using moderate sedation and positioning aids such as troughs, sandbags, foam wedges and ties. General anaesthesia may be safer than frantic struggling and may prevent unnecessary repeat radiography due to inadequate films.

Radiographic Technique

Movement blur due to respiration or panting is a particular problem in thoracic radiography and is of especial importance when the lung fields are under investigation. Sedation or general anaesthesia will reduce the respiratory rate and if the animal has been intubated will even allow for the temporary cessation of respiratory movement during the exposure. The use of fast film/screen combinations and in particular of rare earth screens will permit the exposure times to be kept to a minimum and in addition will increase the capabilities of low powered equipment. This is because rare earth screens are more sensitive to primary radiation than are calcium tungstate screens.

A grid should be used to reduce the effect of scattered radiation if the chest is more than 15-20 cm thick; however this will require an increase in exposure time of approximately 2-3 fold. Rare earth screens are less sensitive to scatter than conventional screens and will often permit a grid to be dispensed with without detracting from image contrast. If the use of a grid requires exposure times to be increased to such a degree that movement blur is inevitable, it is probably more satisfactory to accept some loss in image contrast but with minimal movement unsharpness.

Large cassettes - up to 43 x 35 cm - are preferable for large dogs so that the whole thorax can be included in a single film. It is harder to interpret two or three smaller films and there is an unnecessary increase in

Table 3.1

COUGHING

Acute or chronic bronchitis

Bronchopneumonia

Allergic lung disease (feline asthma, allergic bronchitis, pulmonary infiltrate with eosinophilia)

Bronchiectasis

Left-sided heart failure (pulmonary congestion and oedema)

Filaroides osleri infection

Aleurostrongylus abstrusus infection (cat)

Inhaled tracheal/bronchial foreign body

Pressure on the airway (e.g enlarged left atrium, pulmonary neoplasia)

Primary and secondary pulmonary neoplasia

Pulmonary abscess/granuloma

DYSPNOEA

i) **Pleural disorders:**

   Pleural effusions

   Pneumothorax

   Diaphragmatic rupture

   Mediastinal masses (+/- pleural fluid)

ii) **Pulmonary disorders:**

   Pulmonary oedema (acute or chronic left sided heart failure)

   Pulmonary haemorrhage (coagulopathies or trauma)

   Bronchopneumonia

   Feline asthma

   Widespread pulmonary neoplasia (miliary metastases)

   Pulmonary thromboembolism

   Paraquat poisoning

   Pulmonary emphysema

   Heart worm disease (imported dogs)

iii) **Airway obstruction:**

   Tracheal foreign body

   Filaroides osleri infection

   Intraluminal tracheal/bronchial tumour

CARDIOVASCULAR DISEASE

Murmurs in young dogs

Murmurs in adults with associated circulatory impairment

Congestive heart failure

Unexplained alteration in cardiac rate or rhythm

THORACIC TRAUMA

Pneumothorax or pneumomediastinum

Pulmonary haemorrhage or contusion

Haemothorax

Diaphragmatic rupture

Rib fractures

NEOPLASIA

Evaluation of primary thoracic and multicentric tumours

Evaluation of pulmonary metastases

THORACIC WALL LESIONS

Rib tumours

Discharging sinuses

Subcutaneous emphysema

Thoracic deformity

REGURGITATION

Megaoesophagus

Oesophageal foreign bodies

Vascular ring anomalies

Oesophageal stricture

Oesophageal diverticuli

Oesophageal and perioesophageal neoplasia

Oesophagitis

Hiatal hernia

MISCELLANEOUS

Pyrexia of unknown origin

Assessment of lung changes in Cushing's syndrome

radiation hazard due to the greater number of exposures. Close collimation of the beam will reduce scattered radiation and improve detail but the margins of the lung field should not be coned out as they may contain useful diagnostic information.

The exposure factors should be chosen so as to keep the exposure time to the minimum. This is best achieved by using a high kV low mAs technique. This results in a radiograph with a wide latitude of contrast most suitable for an area where there is a wide range of tissue densities.

Exposure factors will need to be increased if pleural fluid or diffuse lung pathology are present and reduced if a pneumothorax is present.

The exposure should be made on full inspiration so that the lung fields are fully expanded and aerated. This may be difficult in animals that are panting or if breathing is shallow; however temporary occlusion of the nostrils may cause the animal to inhale deeply on removal of the occlusion at which time the exposure should be made. Alternatively blowing on the nostrils may cause momentary breath holding to the same effect. In the anaesthetised animal the lungs may be held inflated by use of the rebreathing bag taking care to avoid overdistension. Films taken at expiration should be recognised as such as the relatively poor aeration results in increased opacity which may mimic diffuse pathological changes.

Positioning

Standard radiographic views
Although in some instances a single lateral view will provide a diagnosis, it is advisable in many cases to obtain dorsoventral (DV) or ventrodorsal (VD) views in order to permit full evaluation of the nature and distribution of lesions. Small pulmonary changes such as metastases or focal pneumonia may be missed on a single lateral projection due to superimposition of the lung fields and pleural effusion and pneumothorax are easier to assess on the DV view.

Lateral view (Figure 3.1 a, b and c)
Right lateral recumbency is preferred since:-

i) The heart lies in a more consistent position.
ii) There is more air-filled lung between the heart and the lower chest wall giving better cardiac detail.
iii) The diaphragm obscures less of the caudal lung field.

As the dependent lung field is less well aerated small soft tissue density changes may be masked and only demonstrated if a second film in left lateral recumbency is taken. The non-dependent lung will contain more air which will provide better contrast with any pathological process. The two views may be surprisingly different with lesions evident on one film and not on the other.

Occasionally animals in respiratory distress may not tolerate lateral recumbency and this may indeed be hazardous for the animal. In these situations the lateral view should be dispensed with and a DV - NOT VD -

Figure 3.1: Thorax - positioning - lateral view.

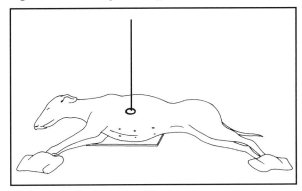

Figure 3.1a: Note position of legs.

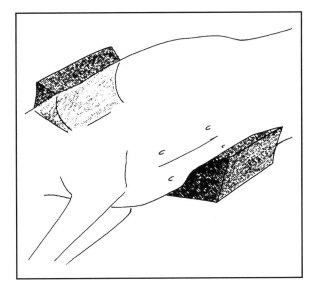

Figure 3.1b: Use of foam supports.

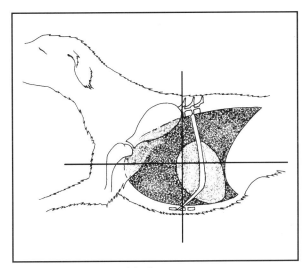

Figure 3.1c: Centring of the beam.

film obtained. A horizontal beam standing lateral view may be of value in rare instances - see below.

i) The subject should be positioned in lateral recumbency with the forelegs drawn forwards and held by sandbags or ties so as to avoid superimposition of the triceps muscle mass over the cranial lung field.

ii) The head and neck should be gently extended - not flexed or overextended.

iii) Many animals require the use of a radiolucent foam wedge placed under the sternum to prevent rotation of the chest about the longitudinal axis of the body. Barrel chested breeds may require support in the other direction with a foam wedge placed under the spine.

iv) The beam should be centred over the 5th rib or level with the caudal border of the scapula and midway between the sternum and the thoracic spine bearing in mind that the spine may be some distance ventral to the dorsal body wall. A useful guide is midway between the caudal border of the scapula and the sternum.

v) The beam should be collimated so as to include the thoracic inlet, thoracic spine, sternum and the full extent of the diaphragm including the cranial abdomen. If, in large subjects, this cannot be achieved on a single film, two will be necessary for a full study.

Dorsoventral/Ventrodorsal views

The DV projection is essential if the heart is under investigation as it will then be lying in an anatomically correct position whereas in the VD view it will frequently rotate to one side and its size and shape will be distorted. In addition this view is mandatory for animals in respiratory distress as they may not tolerate lateral recumbency and dorsal recumbency would be extremely hazardous.

For the investigation of the lung field either position may be used although positioning for the DV may

be difficult for animals with orthopaedic problems in the hindlegs. For both views it is important to ensure symmetrical positioning with the spine and sternum superimposed.

DV view (Figure 3.2)

i) For the DV view the subject is placed in sternal recumbency with elbows symmetrically abducted and drawn forwards. The head and neck are held down with sandbags - taking care not to compromise a dyspnoeic patient.

ii) Radiolucent foam wedges or a radiolucent trough may be used under the sternum to assist in positioning but sandbags are not suitable as they are radiodense.

iii) The hindlegs are flexed into the normal crouching position and if necessary supported by sandbags to ensure there is no rotation.

iv) The beam should be centred in the midline at the level of the caudal prominences of the scapulae.

v) The beam should be collimated so as to include the thoracic inlet and the diaphragm including the cranial abdomen. A right or left marker should be included on the film.

VD view (Figure 3.3)

i) For the VD view the subject is positioned on its back either supported by foam wedges or a radiolucent trough.

ii) The forelegs should be drawn well forwards and secured either by tapes or by sandbags placed behind the elbows. The hindlegs may be either extended or allowed to remain in the flexed position provided they are supported and the pelvis not allowed to rotate to either side.

iii) The beam should be centred midway along the sternum.

iv) The beam should be collimated so as to include the thoracic inlet and the diaphragm/cranial abdomen as for the lateral view.
A right or left marker should be included on the film.

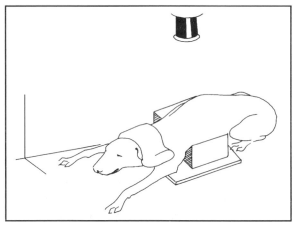

Figure 3.2: Thorax - positioning - dorso-ventral view.

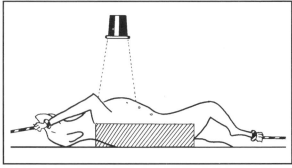

Figure 3.3a: Thorax - positioning - ventro-dorsal view. Note position of the legs.

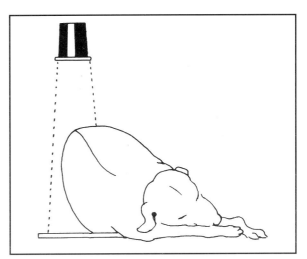

Figure 3.4: Thorax - positioning - oblique dorso-ventral view (a similar technique can be used VD).

Horizontal beam standing lateral view (Figure 3.5)

i)   This view may be required occasionally in animals with such severe respiratory compromise that they cannot be restrained safely in any other way.

ii) The subject stands or sits on the X-ray table with a cassette supported vertically against the thoracic wall. Small dogs and cats may be restrained in narrow cardboard boxes or perspex cages.

iii) It is difficult to ensure that the front legs are adequately drawn forwards and great care must be taken with regard to protection of personnel as this is potentially a hazardous procedure.

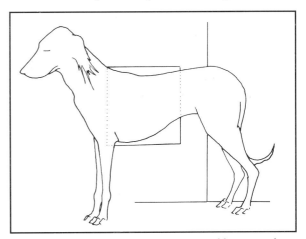

Figure 3.5: Thorax - positioning - horizontal beam standing lateral view.

Decubitus lateral view (Figure 3.6)

i)   This view is rarely required but can be of value in assessing small pleural effusions, pneumothorax or pleural lesions.

ii) With the animal in lateral recumbency a VD view or DV view is taken using a horizontal beam. Again, particular attention should be paid to aspects of radiation protection.

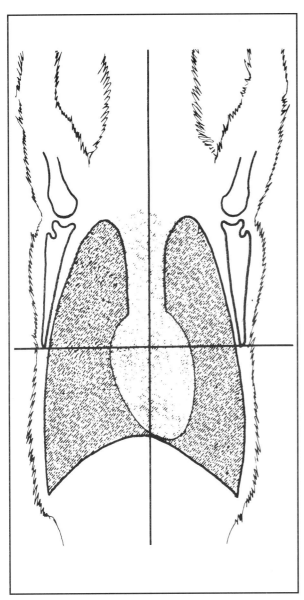

Figure 3.3b: Thorax - positioning - ventro-dorsal view. Centering of the beam.

Additional views

The following additional views of the thorax may occasionally be of value:

Oblique DV view (Figure 3.4)

i)   This is of value for the assessment of lesions of the thoracic wall e.g. rib tumours.

ii) The subject is positioned in ventral recumbency and then rotated either to the left or right as appropriate so that the X-ray beam projects the most prominent aspect of the lesion tangentially.

iii) The degree of obliquity must obviously be dependent on the precise location of the lesion.

iv) The exposure factors usually need to be reduced significantly.

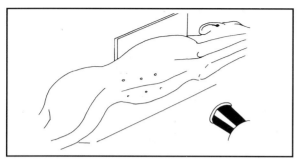

Figure 3.6: Thorax - positioning - decubitus lateral view.

Erect VD view (Figure 3.7)

i)   Rarely indicated. May be of value in assessing cranial mediastinal lesions.

ii) The subject is positioned vertically on its hindlimbs and a horizontal VD view obtained. Again this is potentially very hazardous.

All the above projections utilising horizontal beams should only be used when absolutely essential and the protocol for such studies should have been previously discussed with the practice's RPA.

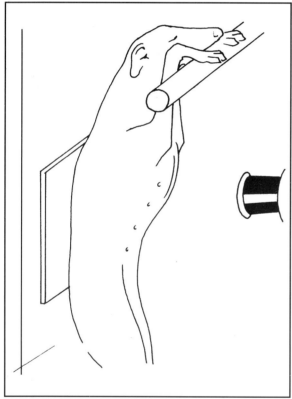

Figure 3.7: Thorax - positioning - erect VD view.

Contrast Techniques for Thoracic Radiography

The indications for the use of contrast studies of the thorax and the techniques used are discussed in the appropriate section.

II: THE EVALUATION OF THORACIC RADIOGRAPHS

A systematic and thorough evaluation of the thoracic and extrathoracic structures is essential to avoid overlooking important radiographic changes. Although the precise technique employed will vary from individual to individual a complete interpretation must include:-

1)   Consistent placing of the radiographs on the viewing box as this enhances familiarity with the normal anatomy and makes it easier to compare similar areas on different radiographs. Lateral radiographs are viewed with the head to the left and DV or VD radiographs are positioned with the patient's right side to the viewer's left.

2)   Evaluation of the radiograph for technical quality, particularly symmetrical positioning and proper exposure factors.

3)   Determination of whether or not the radiograph was made at inspiration or expiration by observing the positioning of the diaphragm.

4)   Evaluation of the extrathoracic structures including the spine, sternum, diaphragm, ribs, thoracic wall and liver.

5)   Evaluation of the position and diameter of the trachea and carina.

6)   Evaluation of the cranial and caudal mediastinum for evidence of widening, abnormal density or the presence of a mass.

7)   Evaluation of the aorta, aortic arch and caudal vena cava.

8)   Evaluation of the cardiac borders (cranial, caudal, left and right) and the position of the apex of the heart.

9)   Evaluation of the main pulmonary artery and the size and shape of the pulmonary arteries and veins.

10) Evaluation of the lung fields, which for descriptive purposes can be divided into three areas - central, middle and peripheral.

For more detailed descriptions of the precise features to be looked for refer to the relevant sections below.

Normal Thoracic Anatomy

The main features of the radiographic anatomy of the normal thorax should be noted.

Lateral view (Figure 3.8)
Trachea: normally diverges from the thoracic spine except in the case of some shallow-chested breeds in which it may run parallel to the spine. Apparent tracheal narrowing mimicking tracheal collapse may be

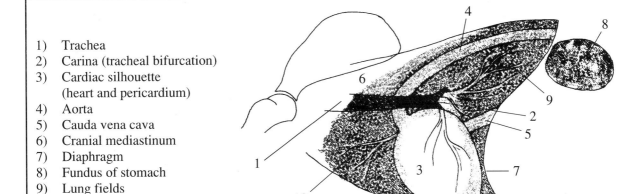

1) Trachea
2) Carina (tracheal bifurcation)
3) Cardiac silhouette
   (heart and pericardium)
4) Aorta
5) Cauda vena cava
6) Cranial mediastinum
7) Diaphragm
8) Fundus of stomach
9) Lung fields
10) Pulmonary vessels

Figure 3.8: *Thorax - radiographic anatomy - lateral view.*

seen at the thoracic inlet due to overlying soft tissue densities from the ventral neck muscles or oesophagus.

Carina (tracheal bifurcation): should be level with the 5th intercostal space. It is closely associated with the heart base. A dark circular area may be seen just cranial to the carina representing the end on projection of the common origin of the left cranial/middle lobe bronchus.

Cardiac silhouette (heart and pericardium): is egg-shaped with the base dorsally and the apex ventrally. May be raised from the sternum by fat in obese animals. Occupies relatively more of the thorax in barrel-chested dogs. For assessment of heart size see section on cardiovascular system.

Aorta: aortic arch usually visible. Descending aorta may be obscured by pulmonary markings. Normal diameter is similar to the height of the thoracic vertebral bodies.

Caudal vena cava: emerges through right crus of diaphragm and normally slopes slightly cranioventrally before merging with the caudal outline of the heart. Normally parallel-sided and similar in size to the aorta. May get wider towards the heart.

Cranial mediastinum: soft tissue density cranial to heart and dorsal to the cranial lung lobes. Consists of cranial vena cava, left subclavian artery, brachiocephalic trunk, lymph nodes, oesophagus and trachea. The trachea is the only structure to be identified. In the anaesthetised animal the oesophagus may contain some air.

Diaphragm: consists of two crura, right and left and the ventral dome or cupola. In lateral recumbency the dependent crus moves cranially resulting in a variation in the appearance of the diaphragm in left and right recumbency.

The diaphragmatic line is straighter and more caudal in a film taken during inspiration. (Figure 3.9).

Figure 3.9: *Variations in shape of the diaphragm.*

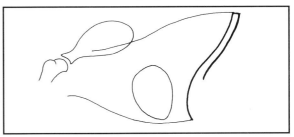

Figure 3.9a: *Right lateral inspiratory film.*

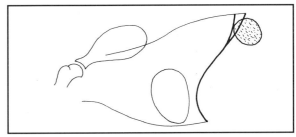

Figure 3.9b: *Left lateral inspiratory film.*

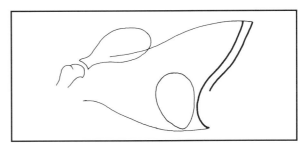

Figure 3.9c: *Right lateral expiratory film.*

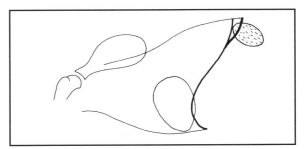

Figure 3.9d: *Left lateral expiratory film.*

Fundus of stomach: usually gas-filled and can be seen caudal to the left crus of the diaphragm, which overlies the caudal lung field in left lateral recumbency.

Lung fields: normally lucent with pulmonary blood vessels seen as either linear or focal densities. Bronchial markings usually only apparent in older animals or as a result of pathological change. Interlobar divisions are not normally seen except in the cranial extremity of the thorax or over the apex of the heart. In cats, the dorsal outline of the caudal lobes deviates away from the spine. (Figure 3.10)

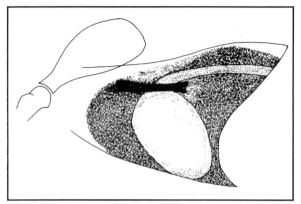

Figure 3.10: Dorsal margin of lung in the cat.

Pulmonary vessels: the arteries and veins are paired and branch towards the periphery of each of the seven lobes of the lung. The arteries and veins are normally of similar size and run on either side of the bronchi. The arteries are situated dorsally and the veins ventrally. The vessels are normally smaller than the diameter of the proximal third of the fourth rib. Superimposition of the larger vessels over ribs may result in composite shadows mimicking nodular pulmonary densities. Vessels seen in end-on projection are seen as small circular radiodensities.

Dorsoventral view (Figure 3.11)

Trachea: is not always seen. It often lies slightly to the right of the midline at the thoracic inlet, especially in chondrodystrophic breeds but may be superimposed on the dorsal spine and sternum.

Carina: again not always well seen; superimposed on heart base at level of 5th thoracic vertebra.

Cardiac silhouette: lop-sided egg shape with apex to the left of midline. The aortic arch is usually seen as a slight bulge on the cardiac outline at 1 o'clock; caudal to this it is superimposed on the dorsal spine and sternum.

Cranial mediastinum: usually parallel-sided and of homogenous soft tissue density except for the tracheal lumen.

Caudal mediastinum: runs from apex of the heart to the diaphragm slightly to the left of midline. Often incorrectly referred to as the cardiophrenic ligament.

Diaphragm: the shape of the diaphragm varies markedly with positioning, variation in centring of the beam, phase of respiration and conformation of the patient. The right side is often more cranially positioned with a greater degree of contact with the cardiac silhouette on expiration. On the DV view the diaphragm is seen as a single dome shape whilst on the VD the two crura and cupola are often seen as separate convexities. (Figure 3.12)

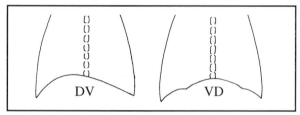

Figure 3.12: Variations in shape of the diaphragm.

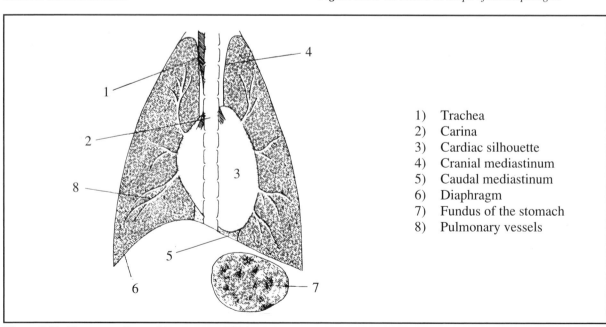

1) Trachea
2) Carina
3) Cardiac silhouette
4) Cranial mediastinum
5) Caudal mediastinum
6) Diaphragm
7) Fundus of the stomach
8) Pulmonary vessels

Figure 3.11: Thorax - radiographic anatomy - DV view.

Fundus of stomach: often contains gas in the DV view but may not in the VD view.

Thymus: not normally seen in the adult. In young dogs a thin, triangular, soft tissue density representing the thymus is sometimes seen projecting from the cranial mediastinum to the left of the midline and just cranial to the cardiac silhouette. This is called the 'thymic sail' (Figure 3.13).

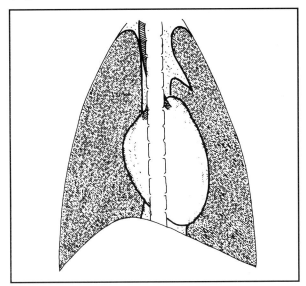

Figure 3.13: Thymic 'sail' in young animal.

Pulmonary vessels: best seen running caudally over the liver shadow. The arteries lie lateral to the veins.

In deep chested breeds, skin folds extending caudally from the axillae onto the lateral thoracic walls are frequently projected as dense linear opacities across the lateral portions of the left and right lung fields. This appearance may mimic the presence of a pneumothorax and must be recognised as a normal feature. The folds extend beyond the thoracic wall and on examination of the peripheral lungfield with a bright light pulmonary vascular markings will be observed extending to the thoracic wall. (Figure 3.14)

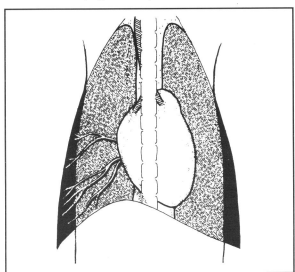

Figure 3.14: Pseudo-pneumothorax due to skin folds.

III: THE CARDIOVASCULAR SYSTEM

Normal Heart Size

a) The dog
Heart size and shape varies greatly between different breeds of dog e.g. in deep-chested breeds such as setters the heart is tall, narrow and upright whereas in barrel-chested breeds such as bull terriers it is almost globular.

Lateral view (Figure 3.15)
The **width of the heart** is usually 2.5 - 3.5 times the width of the intercostal space. However, it must be stressed that the heart may be pathologically enlarged in a given animal and yet still measure within these limits.

The **height of the heart** from base to apex is usually two-thirds the height of the thoracic cavity measured at the same level. In barrel-chested breeds, it may appear relatively taller.

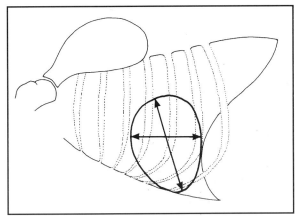

Figure 3.15: Normal heart size – lateral view – dog.

DV view (Figure 3.16)
The width of the heart is normally approximately two-thirds of the width of the thoracic cavity at the level of the fifth intercostal space. The craniocaudal length of the heart varies greatly with the breed and the shape of the chest.

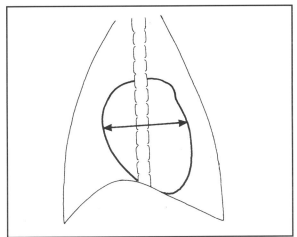

Figure 3.15: Normal heart size – lateral view – dog.

b) The cat

Heart size and shape is much less variable in the normal cat than in the dog.

Lateral view (Figure 3.17)

The heart is positioned at a more sloping angle within the thoracic cavity than in many dogs and so the **craniocaudal diameter** is measured at right angles to the longitudinal axis and then compared to the horizontal width of the intercostal spaces.

The normal measurement is two intercostal spaces (from rib 3 - 5).

The height of the heart is two thirds of the height of the thoracic cavity as for the dog.

DV view

The width of the heart on the DV view is also two thirds of the width of the thoracic cavity, at the level of the fifth intercostal space.

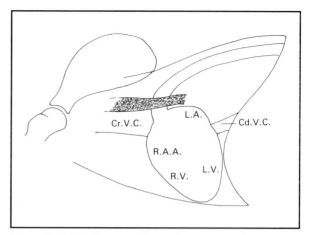

Figure 3.18: The heart - radiographic anatomy - lateral view.

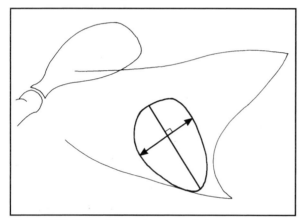

Figure 3.17: Normal heart size - lateral view - cat.

The relative position of the heart chambers

On the lateral view the cranial border of the heart consists of the right auricular appendage and the right ventricle. The cranial vena cava within the cranial mediastinum may be seen to merge with the right auricular appendage forming an angle of about 90 degrees - the so-called 'cranial cardiac waist'.

The caudal heart border consists of the left atrium and left ventricle. A small notch may be visible at the junction of these two chambers and is referred to as the 'caudal cardiac waist'. (Figure 3.18)

On the DV view the cardiac silhouette may be likened to a clock face with the various component chambers and vessels positioned as follows (Figure 3.19):-

11 to 1 o'clock - the aortic arch

1 to 2 o'clock - the pulmonary artery

2 to 3 o'clock - the left auricular appendage

2 to 5 o'clock - the left ventricle

5 to 9 o'clock - the right ventricle

9 to 11 o'clock - the right atrium.

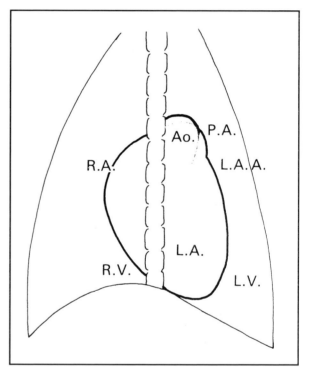

Figure 3.19: The heart - radiographic anatomy - dorso-ventral view.

Increased Heart Size (Cardiomegaly)

Radiography is the single most useful technique for the evaluation of heart disease in the dog and cat but it must be supplemented by a thorough clinical examination and where available ECG findings. More sophisticated techniques such as echocardiography, angiography and blood gas and pressure measurements, where available, can also provide useful information and in some cases may be necessary before a definitive diagnosis can be made.

With a sound knowledge of cardiac anatomy and breed variations, many diagnoses may be derived from first principles. It is important to decide which heart chambers are enlarged and to look for secondary evidence of either right- or left-sided cardiac failure.

Left-Sided Cardiomegaly

This develops secondary to:-

i)   Mitral incompetence resulting from either chronic valvular disease in older dogs or mitral dysplasia in young dogs.

ii) Congenital aortic stenosis, although in many cases the cardiac silhouette appears normal.

iii) Cardiomyopathy which is seen primarily in giant breeds, doberman pinschers, boxers and cocker spaniels. This is primarily a left-sided problem but there may also be right-sided involvement.

Radiological features (Figure 3.20)

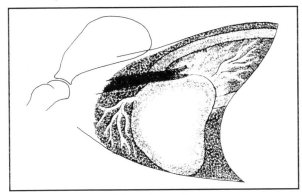

Figure 3.20a: Left-sided cardiomegaly.

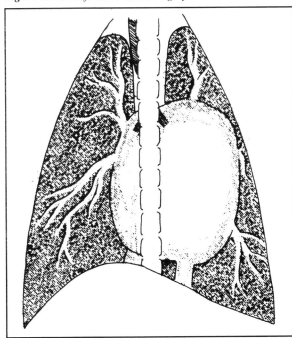

Figure 3.20b: Left-sided cardiomegaly.

Lateral view
- The heart is taller than normal resulting in tracheal elevation.
- The caudal cardiac border is straighter and more erect than usual.
- The left atrium bulges caudodorsally.
- There is loss of the caudal cardiac waist and elevation of the caudal vena cava.

DV view
- There may be increased width of the cardiac silhouette.
- The left cardiac border is rounded.
- An enlarged left auricular appendage may be identified at 2 - 3 o'clock.
- The heart apex may be displaced to the right.
- The dilated left atrium is superimposed on the cardiac silhouette and represented by a relative increase in opacity.
- In cases of aortic stenosis a prominent post stenotic dilation may be identified as a bulge in the 12 - 1 o'clock position.

Secondary features of left sided failure include:-
- Engorgement and tortuosity of the pulmonary veins compared to the arteries (see page 78).
- Patchy increase in lung density particularly in the perihilar region and sometimes with visible air bronchograms representing pulmonary oedema.

Right-Sided Cardiomegaly

This develops secondary to:-

i)   Tricuspid incompetence resulting from either chronic valvular disease in older dogs or tricuspid dysplasia in young animals.

ii) Congenital pulmonic stenosis.

iii) Chronic pulmonary disease; the cardiomegaly is then referred to as cor pulmonale.

iv) Parasitic cardiovascular disease. Angiostrongylus vasorum usually in dogs imported from Ireland. Dirofilaria immitis which is seen in dogs from North and South America, Southern Europe, Asia and Australia.

Radiological features (Figure 3.21)

Lateral view
- The heart is enlarged craniocaudally.
- Rounding of the cranial border.
- Increased sternal contact (however, it must be stressed that there is considerable breed variation in the degree of sternal contact in normal animals).
- As a result there is a more acute angle than normal between the cranial vena cava and the cranial border of the heart.
- There may be elevation of the cranial lobe bronchi and vessels or of the trachea just cranial to the carina.

DV view
- Increased width of the heart.
- Rounding of the right cardiac border producing a reversed 'D' shape to the cardiac outline.
- The apex may be displaced further to the left than normal.

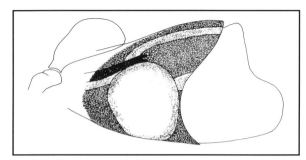

Figure 3.21a: Right-sided cardiomegaly.

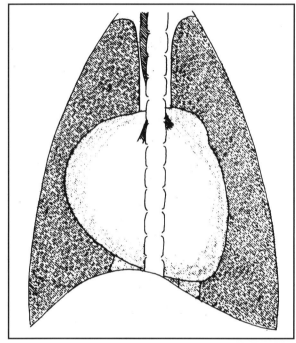

Figure 3.21b: Right-sided cardiomegaly.

Secondary features of right-sided failure include:-

- Engorgement and enlargement of the caudal vena cava.
- Hepatic enlargement.
- Ascites resulting in a 'ground glass' increase in abdominal density with loss of visceral detail.

Generalised Cardiac Enlargement

By the time cardiac disease is recognised clinically the heart is often showing radiographic evidence of both right- and left-sided enlargement irrespective of the underlying cause.

Common causes of bilateral cardiac enlargement include:-

i) Concurrent left- and right-sided A/V valve disease.
ii) Congenital cardiac defects resulting in shunts e.g. patent ductus arteriosus and ventricular septal defects.
iii) Cardiomyopathy.
iv) Chronic anaemia.

Radiological features (Figure 3.22)

- The radiological signs of both left- and right-sided enlargement will be present with the heart enlarged in all directions.
- In the presence of left-to-right shunts there may be evidence of severe pulmonary overperfusion with enlarged and tortuous vessels.
- Pulmonary oedema may also be present.

It is important to differentiate from an enlarged cardiac silhouette associated with pericardial effusion or peritineo-pericardio-diaphragmatic hernia.

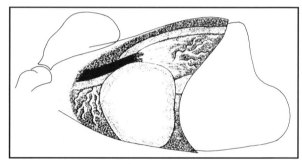

Figure 3.22: Generalised cardiac enlargement.

Pericardial Effusion

This term is used to cover the accumulation of fluid of whatever type within the pericardial sac.

Causes:

i) Pericardial haemorrhage may be idiopathic in certain large breeds (St. Bernard, Golden Retriever, Great Dane).
ii) Pericardial haemorrhage may also occur secondary to haemangiosarcoma of the atrium or heart base tumours.
iii) Pericardial effusions may be associated with right sided heart failure in the dog and cardiomyopathy in the cat.
iv) Septic pericarditis may be either haematogenous or secondary to penetrating foreign bodies.
v) Exudates may occur in conditions such as F.I.P.

It is not possible to identify the nature of the fluid from the radiological findings.

Radiological features (Figure 3.23)

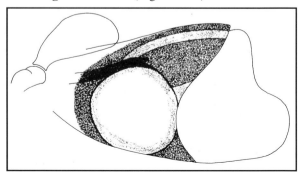

Figure 3.23a: Pericardial effusion.

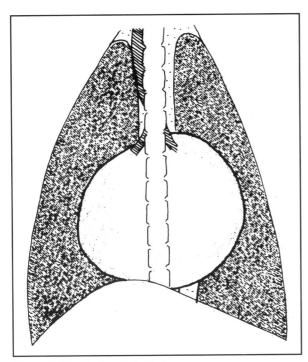

Figure 3.23b: Pericardial effusion.

- The whole cardiac silhouette is usually grossly enlarged.
- The silhouette appears globular in shape in both views.
- The outline of the cardiac shadow is very distinct as there is no movement unsharpness due to the heart beat.
- Secondary features of right-sided failure will occur before left-sided failure due to cardiac tamponade.
- If pleural or mediastinal fluid is also present diagnosis may be difficult due to masking of the cardiac shadow.
- Where available echocardiography provides a very sensitive modality for the accurate identification of pericardial fluid and possibly neoplastic masses. Pneumo-pericardiography may also be used for the identification of masses within the pericardial sac.

Decreased Cardiac Size (Microcardia)

This is much less frequently identified than cardiac enlargement.

Causes:
i) Hypovolaemic shock secondary to haemorrhage or severe dehydration.
ii) Hypoadrenocorticism (Addison's disease) resulting in dehydration and electrolyte changes.

Radiological features (Figure 3.24)
- The heart size is reduced in all directions.
- The heart apex may be raised from the sternum.

- The cardiac shape appears more triangular than normal.
- There is hyperlucency of the lung field due to pulmonary undercirculation.
- The caudal vena cava may be reduced in size.

Feline Cardiomyopathy

Two types of cardiomyopathy are commonly recognised in the cat which produce different radiological appearances; hypertrophic and congestive.

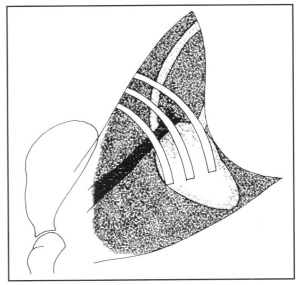

Figure 3.24: Decreased cardiac size - microcardia.

Radiological features (Figure 3.25)

Hypertrophic cardiomyopathy
- The plain films may show no abnormality if all the hypertrophic changes are concentric.
- The DV view may have a characteristic 'valentine heart' shape due to enlargement of the right and left atria.
- Failure is usually left-sided with associated pulmonary oedema (often interstitial).

Congestive (dilated) cardiomyopathy
- There is generalised cardiomegaly.
- Failure is usually right-sided with pleural effusion, hepatomegaly and ascites.

Angiocardiography

Under general anaesthesia an iodine-containing contrast medium may be injected as a bolus either directly into one of the chambers of the heart or into one of the great vessels. Serial films are then taken over a short period of time in order to follow the passage of the contrast medium through the heart chambers and pulmonary circulation.

This technique allows features which cannot normally be seen on plain films to be assessed, such as the precise size and position of the heart chambers, the thickness of the myocardium, the integrity of valves and abnormal shunting of blood.

As it is necessary to change the films rapidly over a period of a few seconds it requires the use of either a sophisticated angiography table or a simple, improvised cassette tunnel.

Non-selective angiocardiography: This is the technique most applicable to use in general practice. Contrast is injected into a peripheral vein (e.g. jugular vein) as rapidly as possible to produce a bolus of undiluted contrast. This passes directly to the right heart, through the pulmonary circulation and thence to the left heart and aortic outflow.

This technique is simple to perform but is not suitable for all studies due to dilution of the contrast medium and superimposition of the right and left chambers. It is ideal for the demonstration of pulmonic stenosis but will not adequately assess left-to-right shunts such as VSD and PDA.

Selective angiocardiography: This depends on the surgical positioning of an intravascular catheter directly into either the right heart - via the jugular vein, or the left heart - via the carotid or femoral artery. Blood samples for blood gas analysis and intra-cardiac pressure readings can also be taken. Highly sophisticated equipment is, however, necessary both for the accurate placement of the catheters and for the recording of the results.

IV: THE LUNGS

Normal Lung Pattern
The normal lungs are composed primarily of air. The remaining portion of the lungs contains the pulmonary vasculature, bronchi, bronchioles, alveolar ducts, alveoli, interstitial tissue, lymphatics and pleurae. The major pulmonary vessels and bronchi are usually vis-

ible in the central zone near the hilus, but only the pulmonary vessels are seen in the middle zone. The other structures provide general background density. The pulmonary vessels and bronchi that are observed should be parallel-sided, branch and taper gradually towards the periphery.

The normal lung pattern can be shown diagrammatically (Figure 3.26).

Note that if the bronchial walls are not visible, the space between the paired pulmonary artery and vein does not necessarily represent the bronchial lumen.

It is difficult to describe what the normal lung opacity should be since the appearance of the lung can be readily altered by a number of factors other than the presence of a disease process. These include:-

Incorrect exposure:
Underexposure may create artifactual lung opacities. Overexposure may mask increases in lung density. The correct exposure technique cannot be assessed by evaluation of the lung parenchyma. It must be determined by the relative opacities between bone and soft tissue. In general, thoracic radiographs should be sufficiently penetrated to see the form of the thoracic vertebral bodies but not their internal trabecular pattern.

Phase of respiration:
Radiographs should be taken, whenever possible, at full inspiration. Expiratory films show a marked increase in the background density. Conversely, over-inflation of the lungs of an anaesthetised patient causes hyperlucency, which may obliterate lung pathology. It may be difficult to obtain full inspiration in obese patients or in patients that are breathing rapidly. Brachycephalic dogs (especially bulldogs) also have increased pulmonary density associated with poor inspiration.

Figure 3.26: *Lungs - radiographic anatomy.*

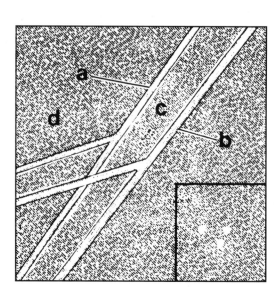

a) pulmonary artery
b) pulmonary vein
c) bronchial lumen
d) pulmonary parenchyma

Inset shows end on view
of pulmonary vessels

Prolonged lateral recumbency:
This may lead to partial collapse of the dependent lung either as a result of general anaesthesia or inability of the patient to maintain sternal recumbency. As a result there will be increased lung opacity that could either mimic or obliterate primary lung pathology. Further radiographs taken after a period of sternal recumbency or assisted ventilation will confirm that the affected lung has returned to normal.

Age of the animal:
Older animals show an increased interstitial density associated with pulmonary fibrosis.

Experience in viewing radiographs facilitates the differentiation of pulmonary pathology from artifacts due to technical errors and other factors.

Abnormal Lung Patterns

The identification of abnormal lung patterns on radiographs is essential to the diagnosis of the underlying cause. Examine the radiographs for the presence of lung patterns that differ from the normal appearance. These will initially be identified as linear, nodular, ill-defined or homogenous in appearance depending on the underlying pathological changes.

By characterising the pulmonary patterns into bronchial, vascular, alveolar, interstitial and mixed, and by identifying the distribution of these changes it is possible to make a list of differential diagnoses that could possibly explain the changes seen. With additional information from the history, physical examination, laboratory findings and other data, it is usually possible to make a specific diagnosis.

As the radiographic appearances of different types of lung disease are often very similar it is not helpful to list and describe each condition individually. Therefore the following section describes the various types of radiographic pattern which may be seen, indicates the pathological changes and clinical conditions associated with each pattern and points out features which may result in misinterpretation.

Bronchial pattern

With a bronchial pattern, the bronchial density becomes more prominent and extends further into the middle lung zone. The increase in density may result from bronchial wall thickening, peribronchial infiltration and/or mucosal thickening. The pulmonary vessels may be lost in the peribronchial infiltrate. The appearance of the affected bronchi is shown diagrammatically and has been likened to 'doughnuts' when viewed end-on and to 'tram lines' when projected laterally(Figure 3.27).

A bronchial pattern is usually associated with bronchitis, either chronic or less frequently acute, irrespective of whether the cause is infectious, inflammatory, allergic or irritant. The severity of the clinical signs

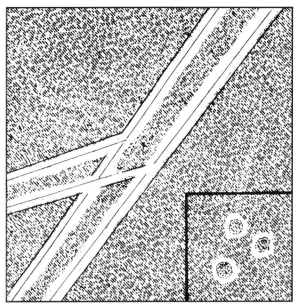
Figure 3.27: *Bronchial pattern. Inset shows end-on view of the bronchi*

does not always correlate with the radiographic findings and some cases of clinical bronchitis show no radiographic abnormality.

Bronchial calcification is a normal finding in old dogs. It is also seen frequently in hyperadrenocorticism (Cushing's disease). It results in well-defined, fine, linear shadows, which are obviously different from the ill-defined linear shadows found with bronchitis (Figure 3.28).

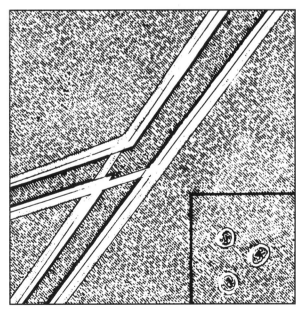
Figure 3.28: *Bronchial calcification. Inset shows end-on view of the bronchi.*

Other important details of an abnormal bronchial pattern include changes in diameter with saccular or cylindrical dilation, irregularity of the bronchial lumen and loss of the normal gradual tapering towards the

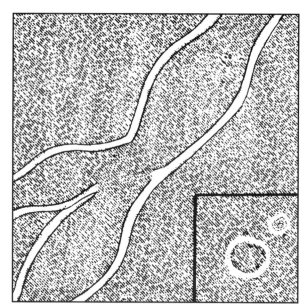

Figure 3.29: Bronchiectasis. Inset shows end-on view of the bronchi.

periphery of the lung field. These changes are seen with bronchiectasis although frequently it is necessary to perform bronchography (see Chapter 7) to confirm the diagnosis (Figure 3.29).

Vascular pattern
The normal pulmonary vessels should be clearly visible in the central and middle zones of the lung field, tapering uniformly towards the periphery. Only in larger dogs are the vessels clearly seen in the peripheral zone.

On a lateral radiograph, the pulmonary artery is dorsal to the bronchus and to the pulmonary vein. The arteries are usually more clearly delineated than the veins. The right cranial lobar artery, bronchus and vein are seen most frequently, particularly in left lateral recumbency, when aeration of the non-dependent lobe produces better contrast. The left cranial lobar vessels are usually superimposed over the cranial mediastinum and are thus less easy to interpret.

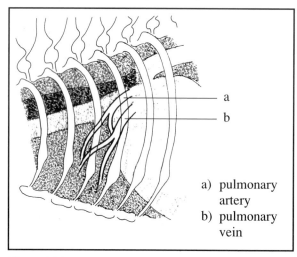

a) pulmonary artery
b) pulmonary vein

Figure 3.30: Normal size of right lobar artery and vein - lateral view.

The right cranial lobar artery and vein should be approximately equal in size and their diameter at the fourth intercostal space should not exceed the smallest diameter of the proximal part of the fourth rib (Figure 3.30).

In the other plane, the pulmonary vessels are best seen on the dorsoventral rather than the ventrodorsal projection. The right and left caudal lobar arteries and veins can be identified. The arteries are lateral to the veins, should be approximately equal in size and should not exceed the diameter of the ninth rib where they cross (Figure 3.31).

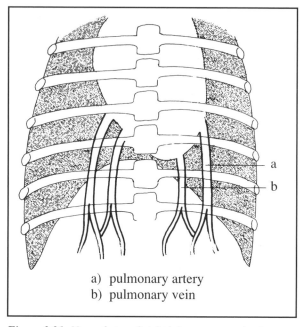

a) pulmonary artery
b) pulmonary vein

Figure 3.31: Normal size of right lobar artery and vein - dorso ventral view.

The pulmonary vessels should also be assessed for:-
i)   Tortuosity - seen in heartworm disease, congestive cardiac failure, feline cardiomyopathy and pulmonary hypertension (Figure 3.32).

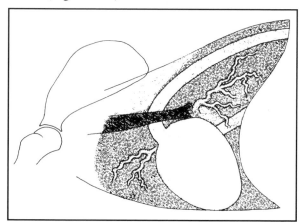

Figure 3.32: Increased tortuosity of pulmonary vessels.

ii) Pruning - seen in heartworm disease, cor pulmonale, pulmonary artery hypoplasia and pulmonary thromboembolism (Figure 3.33).

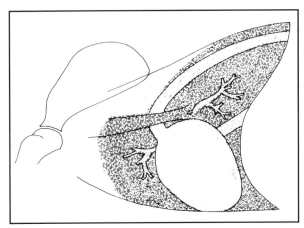

Figure 3.33: 'Pruning' of pulmonary vessels.

iii) Loss of margination - seen in early alveolar
or interstitial oedema (Figure 3.34).

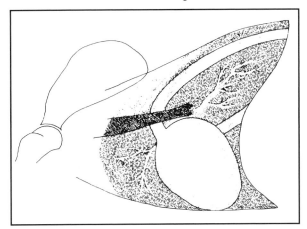

Figure 3.34: Loss of margination of pulmonary vessels.

Many cardiopulmonary disorders result in radiographic
changes involving either the pulmonary arteries, veins
or both. An increased vascular pattern - hypervascularity
or overcirculation - is associated with increased opacity of the lung field, whereas when the vascular pattern
is reduced - hypovascularity or undercirculation - the
lung fields appear more radiolucent.

Conditions which may **increase the size** of the
pulmonary arteries and veins include:-

i) Left-to-right shunts causing overcirculation
of the lungs e.g. patent ductus arteriosus,
ventricular septal defect.
ii) Congestive heart failure - in this case the
veins will be larger than the arteries.
iii) Heartworm disease (Dirofilaria immitis and
Angiostrongylus vasorum) - in this case the
arteries will be larger than the veins.
iv) Iatrogenic fluid overload.

Conditions which may **reduce the size** of the pulmonary arteries and veins include:-

i) Right-to-left shunts resulting in
undercirculation of the lungs e.g. Tetralogy of
Fallot.

ii) Severe pulmonic stenosis.
iii) Hypovolaemia resulting from shock,
dehydration or hypoadrenocorticism
(Addison's disease). In this case the heart is
also frequently reduced in size.
iv) Lung lobes affected by pulmonary
thromboembolism.

Alveolar pattern

An alveolar pattern is seen when the alveoli become
filled with fluid (oedema, blood or exudate), cellular
debris or neoplastic infiltration and when they are
collapsed due to lack of normal aeration.

The radiological features may include:-

i) Fluffy, ill-defined patchy densities
(Figure 3.35).

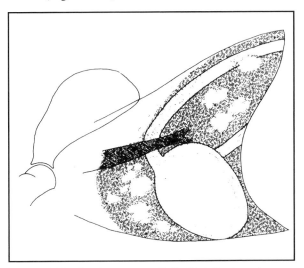

*Figure 3.35: Alveolar pattern - fluffy, ill-defined patchy
densities.*

ii) Areas of increased opacity that tend to
coalesce (Figure 3.36).

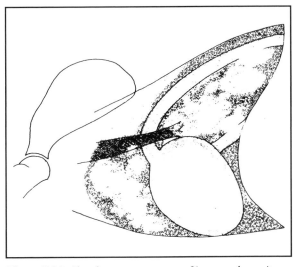

*Figure 3.36: Alveolar pattern - areas of increased opacity
that tend to coalesce.*

iii) Areas of increased opacity that frequently
      affect the entire lobe or portion of the lobe.
      As a result the borders of the lobe, which are
      not normally seen, become visible where they
      contrast with adjacent normal lung (Figure 3.37).

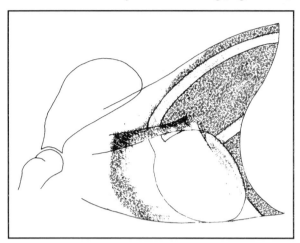

Figure 3.37a: Alveolar pattern - lateral view. Right middle
lobe consolidation.

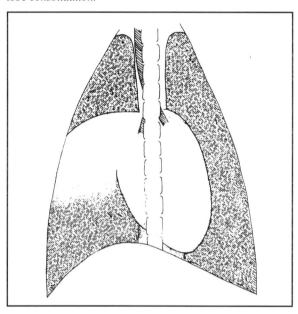

Figure 3.37a: Alveolar pattern - dorsal view. Right middle
lobe consolidation.

iv) The presence of air bronchograms where the
     air-filled lumen of the bronchus is contrasted
     against the dense, consolidated lung tissue
     (Figure 3.38). The vascular structures and
     bronchial walls are not visible in the affected
     areas. If the bronchus also becomes filled
     with fluid or exudate the affected lobe will be
     totally consolidated with a homogenous soft
     tissue density.

v)   The presence of air alveolograms where
     groups of normally aerated alveoli are
     interspersed amongst affected alveoli. This
     gives the infiltrate a mottled and sometimes
     granular appearance (Figure 3.39).

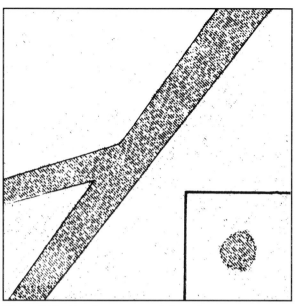

Figure 3.38: Alveolar pattern - air bronchograms.
Inset shows end on views of bronchi.

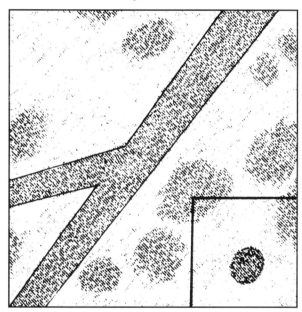

Figure 3.39: Alveolar view - air alveolograms.
Inset shows end on views of bronchi.

Conditions which may be associated with an alveolar
pattern include:

i) Pulmonary oedema: usually cardiogenic. When
acute this has a widespread, patchy distribution. When
chronic it tends to affect mainly the perihilar and
dependent portions of the lung lobes.

ii) Pulmonary haemorrhage: seen following thoracic
trauma and in association with coagulopathies (Warfa-
rin poisoning, von Willebrand's disease etc.)

iii) Pneumonia of various types:
•   Bronchopneumonia, where the changes tend
     to be mainly peribronchial in distribution and
     usually affect all lobes. The tracheobronchial
     lymph nodes may be enlarged.

- Lobar pneumonia, where the changes are usually restricted to one or two lobes with outlining of the lobe borders. Lobar pneumonia is commonly seen in association with inhaled foreign bodies.
- Aspiration pneumonia, where the cranioventral lobes are the most frequently affected.

iv) Less frequently pulmonary thromboembolism: primary or secondary neoplasia and atelectasis (failure of lobar inflation).

Interstitial pattern

Having checked for the presence of bronchial, vascular and alveolar patterns, any remaining changes must be interstitial. Apart from a discrete nodular pattern, interstitial patterns tend to be more difficult to recognise than the preceding patterns.

An interstitial pattern is seen when the supporting tissue of the lung is infiltrated with fluid, fibrous tissue or neoplastic deposits. The pattern may be generalised or localised and linear/curvilinear or nodular.

a) Linear/curvilinear patterns

These non-bronchovascular markings produce an increase in lung opacity with general loss of contrast. The heart, pulmonary vessels and aorta can usually still be seen but may appear less well defined. There are no air bronchograms or air alveolograms and occasionally the appearance may take on a reticulated or honeycomb appearance (Figure 3.40).

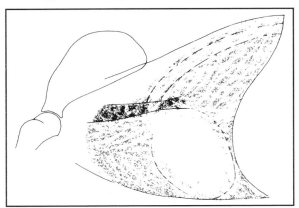

Figure 3.40: *Interstitial pattern - linear/curvilinear pattern.*

Conditions which may be associated with a linear/curvilinear interstitial pattern include:
  i)   Interstitial pulmonary oedema - especially in cats with heart failure.
  ii) Interstitial pneumonia - usually viral e.g distemper.
  iii) Interstitial haemorrhage - seen following thoracic trauma or associated with coagulopathies.
  iv) Pulmonary fibrosis - this is a normal ageing change but also occurs in the healing phase of many disseminated pulmonary diseases.
  v)   The later stages of paraquat poisoning.

It is important to differentiate this pattern of change from the appearance resulting from underexposure, expiratory or underinflated lungs, increased opacity due to obesity.

b) Nodular interstitial patterns

Nodular densities are usually circular and can vary widely in size, number, density and distribution within the lung. Small numbers of nodular densities, usually greater in diameter than 5mm may be individually identified. These must be distinguished from end-on views of blood vessels, superimposed nipples and enlarged lymph nodes (Figure 3.41).

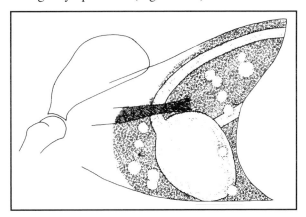

Figure 3.41: *Interstitial pattern - nodular pattern.*

Large numbers of nodular densities smaller than 5mm may become superimposed and create either an overall granular pattern or the appearance of larger irregular/ill-defined nodular densities (Figure 3.42).

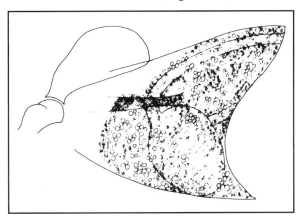

Figure 3.42: *Interstitial pattern - multiple miliary nodular pattern.*

Conditions which may be associated with the presence of discrete nodules >5mm in diameter:-
  i)   Metastatic neoplasia - this is by far the commonest cause.
  ii) Primary lung neoplasia - usually only solitary masses which may range in size from 5mm to several cms. They may be so extensive as to take on the shape of an entire lung lobe.
  iii) Pulmonary abscesses or granulomas - relatively rare.

Conditions which may be associated with the presence of multiple miliary nodules usually less than 5mm in diameter:

i)   Metastatic neoplasia - this is the commonest cause.
ii) Pulmonary lymphosarcoma.
iii) Aleurostrongylus abstrusus infection in cats.
iv) Granulomatous fungal diseases e.g. blastomycosis - these are not usually seen in the U.K.
v)   Primary lung neoplasia - usually alveolar cell carcinomas.

Care must be taken not to mistake normal end-on vascular shadows and calcified pleural plaques, frequently seen in adult and aged dogs, for significant pathological lesions.

Occasionally well-circumscribed, encapsulated radiolucent areas may be identified within the lung field. These may be intrapulmonary or sub-pleural bullae or blebs. They may also be associated with cavitating lesions e.g. neoplasia or tuberculosis (Figure 3.43).

In pulmonary emphysema, one or more lobes will appear more radiolucent than normal with a loss of the normal lung pattern. The pulmonary vessels in the affected lobes are pruned and truncated and the normal bronchial pattern cannot be identified.

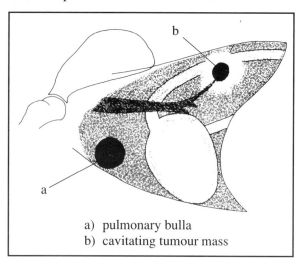

a)   pulmonary bulla
b)   cavitating tumour mass

Figure 3.43: Encapsulated radiolucent shadows in the lungfield.

Mixed pattern
In many cases more than one pattern may be identified. This is not surprising because of the inter-relationship between the various structures within the lung. For example, in congestive heart failure there may be vascular, interstitial and alveolar patterns present on the same radiograph. By using the differential lists as well as clinical, laboratory and other data it should be possible to reach a diagnosis.

It is important not to over-read radiographs of the lung fields and thus attach pathological significance to normal variations in appearance or to appearances resulting from technical artifacts. A common error is to misinterpret the lucent space of the bronchial lumen as an air bronchogram since it is bordered by a dense pair of pulmonary vessels.

Serial radiographs can be of particular value in reaching a diagnosis on thoracic radiographs and in monitoring treatment as lung patterns, particularly the alveolar pattern, can change dramatically over a short period of time.

V: THE PLEURAL CAVITY

Pneumothorax

Causes:
i)   Traumatic rupture of lung parenchyma or more rarely a bronchus.
ii) A sequel to perforating wounds of the thoracic wall and iatrogenically following thoracocentesis.
iii) Less commonly may result from rupture of lung bulla, lung abscess or cavitating neoplasm.

Radiological features (Figure 3.44)
*   Retraction of lung lobes from chest wall, increased opacity of collapsed lung lobes - may mask pathological change.
*   Collapsed lobes surrounded by radiolucent (dark) area containing no lung markings.
*   Cardiac silhouette may be 'elevated' from sternum on recumbent lateral view with radiolucent gas density between heart and sternum.
*   Usually bilateral as the mediastinum is fenestrated or easily perforated in normal animals.
*   If pneumothorax is unilateral there may be evidence of pleural thickening due to fibrosis.

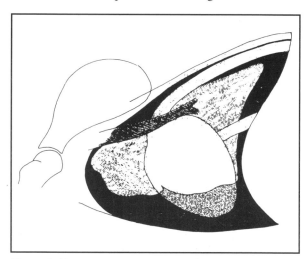

Figure 3.44: Pneumothorax - lateral view.

Tension Pneumothorax

Causes:
This occurs when damage to the lung results in a valve-like action permitting air to be pumped into the pleural cavity raising intra-pleural pressure above atmospheric.

Radiological features (Figure 3.45)
- Appearance similar to that described above but lung lobes severely compressed.
- The thorax is overdistended with the ribs and costal cartilages perpendicular to the spine.
- The diaphragmatic line is markedly flattened.
- Tension pneumothorax requires immediate thoracocentesis to relieve the intra-pleural pressure.

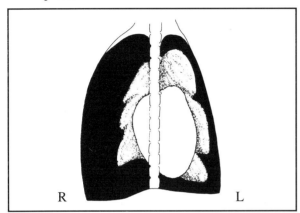

Figure 3.45: Pneumothorax - view with appearance of tension pneumothorax on the right side.

Pleural Effusion/Hydrothorax

Causes:
Many causes and a variety of fluid types may be present but these cannot usually be differentiated solely on the radiological signs unless some other causative lesion such as a mediastinal mass, ruptured diaphragm or fractured ribs can be identified. Most effusions are bilateral as the mediastinum is usually incomplete. Unilateral effusion may indicate an inflammatory response resulting in pleurisy and mediastinal thickening e.g. pyothorax or chylothorax.

i)   Transudates and modified transudates may result from congestive cardiac failure, neoplasia, diaphragmatic rupture and incarceration of liver, hypoproteinemia, lung lobe torsion and pulmonar thromboembolism.
ii) Haemothorax may be seen following trauma or in coagulopathies.
iii) Chylothorax may occur spontaneously or as a sequel to trauma.
iv) Pyothorax may result from penetrating foreign bodies or from haematogenous spread e.g. Nocardiosis. Non-septic exudates may occur in FIP in cats.

Radiological features (Figure 3.46)
- Retraction of lung lobes away from the chest wall with a surrounding soft tissue (fluid) density. The DV view is the most helpful if the amount of fluid is small.
- Interlobar fissures of soft tissue density visible on both views (these must be differentiated from the normal costal cartilages).
- Rounding of the retracted lung lobes producing a 'scalloped' appearance and rounding of the costo-phrenic angle on the DV view.
- Cardiac and diaphragmatic outlines obscured.

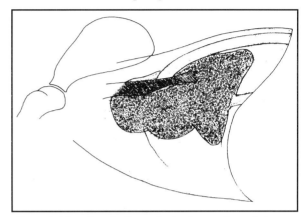

Figure 3.46a: Pleural effusion/hydrothorax - lateral view.

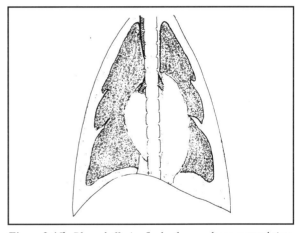

Figure 3.46b: Pleural effusion/hydrothorax - dorso-ventral view.

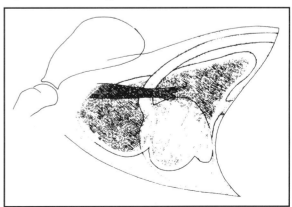

Figure 3.46c: Pleural effusion/hydrothorax - cortication of the lung lobes.

NB Animals with suspected pleural effusions should NOT be placed in dorsal recumbency as this may result in severe respiratory compromise.

Once a moderate or severe pleural effusion has been identified further radiographic examination following thoracocentesis is indicated.

This will facilitate the identification of any underlying causative lesions. When there is an inflammatory response resulting in pleurisy the lung lobes may fail to expand fully following drainage of the pleural cavity and the lobes will retain a rounded outline with a radiodense margin - this is referred to as 'cortication'.

Diaphragmatic Rupture

Causes:
i) Usually the result of trauma such as an RTA.
ii) Rarely congenital herniation.

When a diaphragmatic defect is suspected, it is advisable to position the animal for a lateral recumbent view with the normal hemithorax upwards to minimise respiratory embarrassment. It is therefore wise to obtain a DV view initially so that the affected side can be determined.

Radiological features (Figure 3.47)
* Loss of all or part of the diaphragmatic outline. NB this will also occur due to the presence of pleural fluid or severe pulmonary disease resulting in loss of normal contrast.
* Loss of visibility of the normal intrathoracic anatomy with a reduction of the amount of aerated lung and displacement of the heart.
* The presence of abdominal viscera within the thorax. Stomach and intestines are recognised by the presence of ingesta and gas, liver and spleen as homogenous soft tissue masses.
* Absence or displacement of viscera within the abdomen.
* Possibly the presence of free pleural fluid especially if liver or spleen in incarcerated in the defect. NB. Small defects with only solitary liver lobes displaced may produce large amounts of fluid and can be very hard to diagnose radiographically.
* Fractured ribs may be seen as a coincidental finding.
* If there is a congenital hernia the viscera may be contained in a peritoneal sac so resulting in the presence of a discrete thoracic mass in continuity with the diaphragm.
* If the plain films are equivocal then the administration, with due care, of a small amount of barium 30-60 minutes prior to radiography may confirm the presence of herniated viscera or displacement of abdominal viscera.

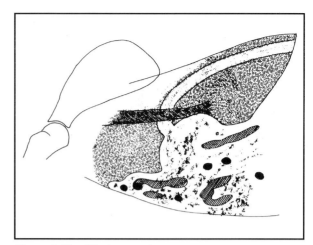

Figure 3.47a: Diaphragmatic rupture.

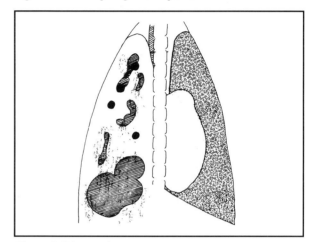

Figure 3.47b: Diaphragmatic rupture.

VI: THE MEDIASTINUM

The mediastinum is the potential space in the midline between the right and left pleural sacs. It contains the heart, trachea, major blood vessels, oesophagus, lymph nodes, vagus and phrenic nerves, the thoracic duct and, in young animals, the thymus.

It is continuous cranially with the cervical fascial planes and caudally with the retroperitoneal space via the aortic hiatus. In most dogs and cats the mediastinum is fenestrated allowing free communication between the two pleural sacs. Normally only the heart, aorta, caudal vena cava and trachea are visible on a radiograph as identifiable features. The remaining structures are not seen due to either their small size of the fact that they are surrounded by tissues of similar radiographic density.

Pneumomediastinum

Causes:
i) May result from tracheal rupture or alveolar damage with air then tracking alongside the major bronchi into the mediastinum.

ii) Oesophageal rupture or the caudal extension of cervical subcutaneous and interstitial emphysema will also result in pneumomediastinum.

iii) Rarely gas may extend forward from the retroperitoneal space or develop due to gas-forming organisms in an infected mediastinum.

Radiological features (Figure 3.48)
- The presence of mediastinal air results in increased contrast and so highlights structures not normally identified such as the oesophagus, azygos vein and cranial blood vessels etc.
- Both the luminal and extraluminal outline of the trachea can be identified.
- The heart may be displaced from the sternum in a recumbent lateral view as in pneumothorax but the lung margins will be seen to extend to the periphery of the thorax.

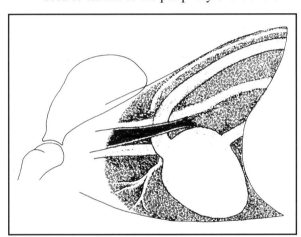

Figure 3.48: Pneumomediastinum.

Mediastinal Fluid

Causes:
i) Accumulations of fluid within the mediastinum may be seen as a result of mediastinal infections e.g. due to oesophageal rupture.
ii) Associated with congestive cardiac failure.
iii) Feline infectious peritonitis.
iv) Mediastinal masses.
v) Coagulopathies.
vi) Trauma.

Radiological features (Figure 3.49)
- Increased width of mediastinal shadow on the DV view.
- 'Reverse fissures' - i.e. interlobar fissures of fluid density but extending outward from the midline.

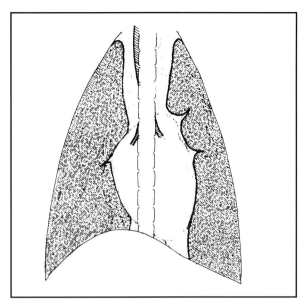

Figure 3.49: Mediastinal fluid.

Cranial Mediastinal Masses

Causes:
i) Tumours such as thymic lymphosarcoma, ectopic thyroid tumours, heart base tumours.
ii) Lymphadenopathy of the cranial mediastinal nodes due to either infection or tumour metastases.

Radiological features (Figure 3.50)
- Increased width of the cranial mediastinal soft tissue density located in midline on the DV view.
- Caudal displacement of the heart, elevation and deviation of the trachea cranial to the heart and loss of the cranial cardiac outline.
- Caudal and lateral displacement of the cranial lung lobes which may also be collapsed. This may result in the cranial soft tissue density appearing 'diamond' shaped on the DV view.
- Possibly the presence of associated pleural or mediastinal fluid.

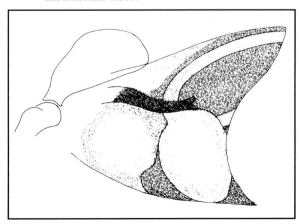

Figure 3.50a: Cranial mediastinal mass.

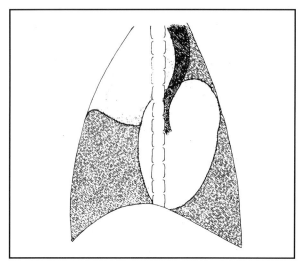

Figure 3.50b: Cranial mediastinal mass.

Peritoneo-Pericardial Diaphragmatic Hernia

Causes:

i)   Usually a congenital defect resulting in communication between the peritoneal and pericardial sacs.

ii) May be associated with umbilical hernias and/or sternal abnormalities.

iii) Abdominal viscera, usually small intestine, are displaced into the percardial sac resulting in respiratory, cardiovascular or alimentary problems.

Radiological features (Figure 3.51)

• An enlarged cardiac silhouette which merges caudally with the diaphragmatic outline.

• Differential densities within the cardiac silhouette.

• Gas-filled intestinal loops may be identified superimposed on the cardiac shadow, and this may be confirmed by the administration of barium.

• There is an absence of the radiographic signs of heart failure in cases of peritineo-pericardio-diaphragmatic hernia.

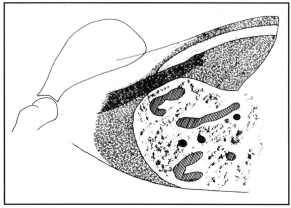

Figure 3.51: Peritoneo-pericardial diaphragmatic hernia.

VII: THE THORACIC WALL

The thoracic wall consists of skin, subcutaneous fat, muscle, ribs, sternum and parietal pleura. Stippled mineralisation of the costal cartilages is frequently observed in both young and older animals and is generally of no clinical significance. The chest wall should be evaluated on both the routine views of the thorax; lateral and DV.

Oblique views of the thoracic wall may be necessary for the full radiographic examination of those lesions suspected but inadequately demonstrated on the routine views, or lesions apparent on clinical examination. The precise positioning must depend on the location of the area of interest but should ideally 'skyline' the region by means of a 'lesion-orientated oblique view'.

Conditions which may be diagnosed radiographically include:

Fracure of Ribs

Rib fractures are usually transverse and tend to involve multiple adjacent ribs.

If a series of ribs are fractured this may result in a 'flail' chest with paradoxical chest wall movement during respiration.

Lateral, DV and occasionally oblique views are necessary to evaluate rib fractures completely.

Check that there is no underlying bone pathology e.g. osteoporosis, multiple myeloma.

Radiological features (Figure 3.52)

• Lucent defect to rib continuity with or without displacement.

• If not recent there may be evidence of periosteal reaction.

• Subcutaneous emphysema may be identified as linear lucent (dark) shadows in the subcutaneous and fascial planes.

• Pneumothorax or pulmonary contusion/haemorrhage may be present (qv).

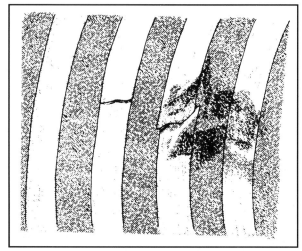

Figure 3.52: Fractures of the ribs.

Fracture of the Sternum

Sternal fractures are often seen as incidental findings and seldom cause clinical problems.

Radiological features (Figure 3.53)
- Displacement of adjacent sternebrae possibly with associated rib fractures.

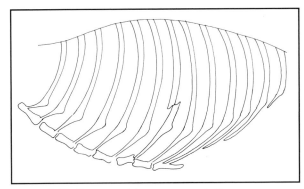

Figure 3.53: Fracture of the sternum and rib.

Tumours of the Chest Wall

Primary tumours affecting the ribs (osteosarcoma or chondrosarcoma) are seen most commonly.

Occasionally soft tissue tumours may arise in or infiltrate the chest wall.

Radiological features (Figure 3.54)
- An expansile lesion of the rib usually close to the costo-chondral junction.
- Associated bone destruction and periosteal reaction - this is best evaluated on the DV projection but oblique views may be of value.
- Soft tissue swelling causing displacement of adjacent ribs and extension into the thorax as an extra pleural mass.
- Adjacent ribs may exhibit periosteal reaction.
- Occasionally there may be pleural effusion present.
- Soft tissue tumours may show only swelling, displacement of ribs and associated sub-pleural mass and/or fluid.

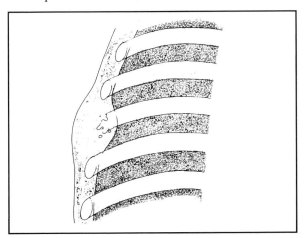

Figure 3.54: Tumour of the chest wall showing soft tissue swelling and destruction of the rib.

Pectus Excavatum

A congenital deformity of the sternum affecting cats and dogs.

It is not usually associated with clinical signs but has been seen in association with peritoneo-pericardial hernia (qv).

Radiological features (Figure 3.55)
- The sternum is displaced dorsally into the thoracic cavity.
- The caudal portion of the sternum is usually most severely affected.
- There is associated abnormal curvature of the ribs and costal cartilages.
- The heart and mediastinum will be displaced dorsally and usually to one side.

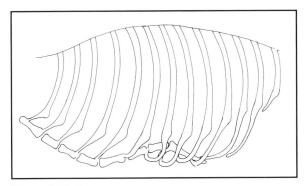

Figure 3.55: Pectus excavatum.

Osteomyelitis of the Sternum

Uncommon but may be a sequel to penetrating wounds or bites. An intermittently discharging sinus may be present.

Radiological features (Figure 3.56)
- Periosteal reaction around affected sternebra.
- May be either lysis or sclerosis of the sternebra.
- Soft tissue swelling ventral to sternum - lucent gas tracts may be seen if there is a discharging sinus.

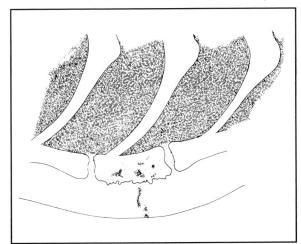

Figure 3.56: Osteomyelitis of the sternum.

CHAPTER FOUR

The Abdomen

D. B. Murdoch

CONTENTS

I: THE INDICATIONS FOR ABDOMINAL RADIOGRAPHY

The indications for radiography of the abdomen include the following clinical presentations -

1) Persistent vomiting.
2) Abdominal pain.
3) Haematuria/dysuria.
4) Evaluation of an abdominal mass.
5) Evaluation of abdominal distension.
6) Tenesmus.
7) Jaundice.
8) Persistent diarrhoea.
9) Incontinence.
10) Evaluation of an external swelling.
11) Owner and Veterinary Surgeon's peace of mind!

1) Investigation of Persistent Vomiting

Value: Almost always helpful in persistent vomiting

Initial views: Depends upon the history. It should be possible to establish the pattern of vomiting, i.e. retching, regurgitation or true vomiting.

For retching, a lateral view of the pharynx would be indicated - see appropriate section.

For regurgitation, lateral views of the neck and thorax to check for oesophageal abnormalities would be indicated - see appropriate section.

For true vomiting, initially a lateral view of the abdomen is indicated. Either a right or left lateral view is acceptable, but it is advisable to get into the habit of taking the same view each time, in order that one becomes familiar with that view. Always check the corner of thorax for the presence of megaoesophagus.

Further views: A ventro-dorsal view may be useful if an equivocal lesion is noted on the lateral. This view will also help accurate location of an abnormality noted on the initial view. A barium swallow may be helpful if a specific problem is suspected.

2) Investigation of Abdominal Pain

Value: Very important, especially after abdominal trauma. Many cases of abdominal pain require prompt surgical correction.

Initial views: Lateral abdomen.

Further views: A barium swallow, especially where cranial abdominal pain is present, to differentiate between pancreatitis, acute intestinal obstruction, diaphragmatic rupture etc.

Urinary catheterisation, plus contrast studies to check for ruptured bladder.

Occasionally may need to use a horizontal beam to identify free abdominal air. This is most easily detected with the animal in left lateral recumbency, so that the free air rises to a position between the costal arch and the right liver lobes.

N.B. This view is inconvenient and increases the radiation hazard.

3) Investigation of Haematuria/Dysuria

Value: Useful.

Initial view: Lateral abdomen.

Further views: Lateral abdomen with hind legs drawn forward to touch the ventral abdominal wall. This view allows clearer visualisation of the region of the ischial and penile urethra.

Contrast studies on the bladder (usually a pneumocystogram is sufficient) to determine the relationship between the prostate and the bladder, the thickness and appearance of the bladder wall, the presence of blood clots and calculi etc.

Occasionally, contrast studies (positive contrast) are necessary to show up radiolucent calculi.

Intravenous infusion urography may be necessary to visualise the kidneys in more detail.

4) Evaluation of a Palpable Mass

Value:
a) To determine which organ is affected.
b) To establish whether the mass is normal, e.g. foetuses, kidneys and faecoliths can all be mistaken for pathological masses.
c) To decide whether surgery is feasible.

Initial view: Lateral abdomen.

Further views:
a) Ventro-dorsal - important to determine the location and size.
b) Barium swallow useful to evaluate liver size.
c) Pneumocystogram to identify bladder and prostate.
d) Rarely, may perform infusion urography to identify kidneys.

5) Evaluation of Abdominal Distension

Value:
a) Rarely of value when the abdomen is distended by fluid (parencentesis is much more useful).
b) Radiography very useful in determining the presence of a small quantity of fluid.
c) Will differentiate between fat, fluid and foetuses (from around the 45th day of gestation foetuses are sufficiently radiodense to be identified. Prior to this time, an enlarged uterus will be obvious.
d) Can identify abdominal distension as a result of changes in abdominal musculature, e.g. hyper-adrenocorticism.

Initial view: Lateral abdomen.

Further views: Barium swallow may be useful to determine the size of the liver.

6) Investigation of Tenesmus

Value:
a) To differentiate the cause of constipation.
b) To determine whether the clinical signs are originating from the urinary or alimentary tracts.
c) To determine the contents of a swelling associated with tenesmus, e.g. perineal hernia.

Initial view: Lateral abdomen.

Further views:
a) Ventro dorsal view to look for pelvic injuries, masses etc.
b) Contrast studies to determine the position of the bladder and its relationship with the prostate.

7) Investigation of Jaundice

Value:
a) To differentiate the causes of hepatomegaly.
b) To determine the presence of an extra-hepatic mass, e.g. pancreatic carcinoma.
c) To detect small quantities of fluid especially in association with traumatic damage to the biliary tree.

Initial view: Lateral abdomen.

Further view: Barium swallow to determine the position of the stomach in relation to the liver.

8) Investigation of Persistent Diarrhoea

Value: of limited value in diarrhoea cases with the following exceptions:-
a) The diagnosis of intussusception.
b) To investigate intestinal tumours.
c) Occasionally helpful in the diagnosis of chronic generalised intestinal disease, e.g. lymphosarcoma.

Initial view: Lateral abdomen.

Further views:
a) Barium enema may be useful in the diagnosis of lower intestinal diarrhoea, e.g. intussusception, colitis.
b) Barium swallow helpful with some intestinal lesions.

9) Investigation of Incontinence

Value: Plain radiographs of limited value. Contrast studies are essential for the diagnosis of most causes of incontinence.

Initial view: Lateral abdomen to eliminate gross lesion, e.g. cystic calculus.

Further views:
a) Infusion urography to identify kidneys, bladder, ureter.
b) Often helpful to combine infusion urography with a pneumocystogram.
c) Retrograde vagino-urethrography is a valuable technique for the evaluation of the urethra, bladder neck and will often demonstrate ureteral ectopia.
d) Double contrast studies, using water soluble contrast media and air, are often useful especially with bladder tumours.

10) Evaluation of an External Swelling

Value:

a) To determine whether an external swelling contains viscera.

b) With traumatic hernias, to find out where the wall is damaged.

c) To differentiate ruptures/swellings from other abdominal masses, e.g. neoplasia, haematomas etc.

Initial view: Lateral abdomen.

Further views:

a) Ventro dorsal view.

b) Barium study to identify the gastro-intestinal tract.

c) Pneumocystogram to locate the bladder.

11) Owner and Veterinary Surgeons Peace of Mind!

Although often used as an indication for abdominal radiography, it is questionable if this is justifiable.

Positioning

Lateral recumbent views (Figure 4.1)

i) This may be either left lateral or right lateral. The appearance will vary slightly between the two and you should be aware of these differences.

ii) Position animal in lateral recumbency on the chosen side.

iii) Ensure that the hind limbs are drawn caudally and secured with ties, and the fore limbs drawn cranially and similarly secured.

iv. Depending on the shape of the abdomen, it may be necessary to use foam wedges to prevent rotation about the longitudinal axis.

v) Centre the beam appropriately.

a) For small dogs and cats, the whole abdomen can satisfactorily be examined on a single film and the beam should be centred over mid abdomen - mid-way between the umbilicus and the level of the lumbar spine. NB this is about $1/3$ of the way between the ventral and dorsal skin surfaces, particularly in obese animals.

b) For larger animals, two films may be required. For the cranial abdomen - liver, stomach etc, centre over the costal arch. For examination of the caudal abdomen - bladder, prostate, uterus, colon - centre midway between the last rib and pelvic inlet.

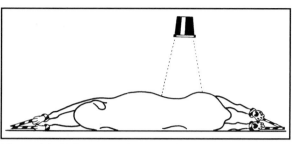

Figure 4.1: Abdomen - positioning - lateral view of abdomen.

Ventro-dorsal view (Figure 4.2)

i) This view is preferable to the DV view for the examination of the abdomen, with the exception of the contrast studies of the stomach.

ii) The animal should be positioned in dorsal recumbency - preferably supported in a radiolucent trough or supported by sandbags, ties etc.

iii) The forelimbs should be drawn cranially and secured with ties and the hind limbs extended.

iv) Care should be taken to ensure that there is no rotation to either side.

v) Centre the beam appropriately.

a) For small dogs and cats, the whole abdomen can satisfactorily be examined on a single film and the beam should be centred over mid abdomen - the level of the umbilicus.

b) For larger animals, two films may be required. For the cranial abdomen - liver, stomach etc, centre over the mid line level with the last rib. For examination of the caudal abdomen - bladder, prostate, uterus, colon - centre midway between the last rib and pelvic inlet.

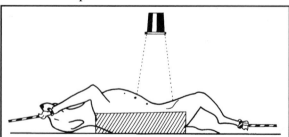

Figure 4.2: Abdomen - positioning - ventro-dorsal view.

Decubitus lateral view (Figure 4.3)

i) Rarely indicated and requires special attention with regard to radiation protection. May be useful for the detection of free abdominal gas.

ii) The animal is placed in left lateral recumbency and the X-ray beam aligned horizontally and centred on mid ventral abdomen.

iii. The film is positioned vertically adjacent to the back and held with either a suitably designed cassette holder or sandbags - it must NOT be hand held.

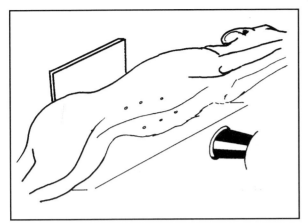

Figure 4.3: Abdomen - positioning - decubitus lateral view.

Oblique views of the caudal abdomen and pelvis

i)   These are occasionally of value in the demonstration of the distal ureters following intravenous urography.

ii) Positioning is as for the standard VD view but two films are taken with the caudal abdomen slightly rotated to left and then right side.

Lateral view of caudal abdomen with legs drawn cranially (Figure 4.4)

i)   This view is particularly used for the demonstration of the ischial portion of the urethra.

ii) The animal is placed in lateral recumbency and the legs drawn forwards and held with ties or sandbags.

iii) The beam is centred over the ischial arch.

iv) It will be necessary to adjust the exposure values to prevent over exposure of the region of interest.

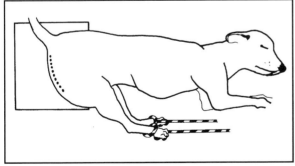

Figure 4.4: Abdomen - positioning - lateral view of caudal abdomen with legs drawn cranially.

II: THE EVALUATION OF ABDOMINAL RADIOGRAPHS

The radiological diagnosis of abdominal disorders, as in the thorax, depends on an analysis of the radiological features which must then be considered in relation both to each other and to the history and relevant clinical findings.

The following section will deal with both the radiological principles underlying these signs, together with the anatomical and pathological reason for these appearances.

In addition, as in the other chapters of this manual, the radiological features of specific conditions will be outlined and illustrated. However, it must be pointed out that quite frequently in abdominal radiology it is not possible to reach a definitive diagnosis on radiological evidence alone. Often the radiologist is presented with one or more possible differentials to explain the observed features. Hence the importance of an analytical approach and an understanding of the basic principles of image formation.

Obtaining a Clear Image

The radiographic image is a collection of shadows. As regards soft tissue radiography, all these shadows have similar densities so the viewer is attempting to sort out subtle gradations of shades of grey rather than a clear differential between black and white.

The following should be considered when attempting to achieve a clear image on a radiograph.

1)   Reduce Scatter

Reduce the kV (if variable):

•   this will reduce the amount of scatter but may result in an unacceptable exposure time. (see later).

•   when the kV rises above 70, the amount of scatter increases markedly.

Use a grid:

•   a grid (either a stationary or a Potter-Bucky) will help if the area to be radiographed is greater than 15 cm - it is not usually necessary to use a grid for cats or small dogs.

•   a grid may increase the exposure time to such an extent that movement blur becomes a significant problem. This is a more serious complication than scatter, so if using the grid is going to result in unacceptably long exposure, dispense with the grid.

Use collimation by means of a light beam diaphragm (or a cone if LBD not fitted).

•   The beam should always be confined to the area under investigation, not only to reduce scatter, but to reduce the risk to the radiographer. It is bad practice to attempt 'whole animal' radiographs on one plate; much better to cone down and take several views.

Use rare earth intensifying screens whenever possible.

•   this results in a reduction in mA, kV and exposure time.

2) Minimise Movement Blur

This is achieved by using as short an exposure time as possible.

Use a general anaesthetic.

- obvious exceptions to this rule are where a G.A. is clinically contra-indicated, or if alimentary contrast studies are planned. In these situations it has been found that acetyl promazine can be used without interfering with the rate of passage of alimentary contrast.
- under G.A., respiration can be suspended in inspiration by squeezing the rebreathing bag (this refers to thoracic radiographs).
- take abdominal radiographs in expiration. Abdominal musculature is stationary for three times as long in expiration as inspiration.

Increase the kV.

- this will reduce the exposure time but remember that this may increase the scatter.

Use as high an mA as possible.

Use rare earth intensifying screens.

Dispense with the grid if the exposure time is unacceptably long.

- most grids require an increase in mAs (i.e. mA multiplied by the exposure time) by a factor of at least four. The loss of clarity due to movement blur is usually more serious than that resulting from scatter.

3) Patient preparation

Starvation.

- if performing a planned, elective, radiographic examination of the abdomen, withhold food and water for at least 12 hours prior to radiography.

Make sure the coat is clean.

- water and dirt in the coat will produce confusing radiodensities on the films.

Perform an enema.

- a water enema prior to radiography will improve visualisation of the viscera by removing the confusing shadows of colonic contents. This is especially important when investigating the bladder, performing infusion urography or proceeding to a barium enema.

Interpreting the Image

It is important to remember that the radiographic appearance of a tissue depends upon its atomic number and specific gravity. (Figure 4.5).

When looking at soft tissue structures, the appearance will depend upon the shape of the structure, its

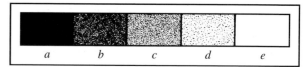

Figure 4.5: Relative densities of body tissues. a: gas. b: fat. c: soft tissue. d: bone. e: mineral.

Tissue	Atomic No.	Specific Gravity
Air	7.6	0.001
Fat	5.9	0.9
Soft tissue	7.4	1.0
Bone	14.00	1.8
Lead	82.00	11.3

relation to the direction of the x-ray beam and the tissues surrounding that structure, as well as its radiographic density.

1) Tubular structures containing fluid, e.g. loops of fluid filled bowel may appear as parallel sided linear or curved densities or circular densities depending upon their relation to the x-ray beam. (Figure 4.6).

    If however, a tubular structure contains material less dense than the walls, e.g. a loop of bowel containing gas, it will appear as parallel densities separated by a lucent space in one projection but as an annular opacity in the other.

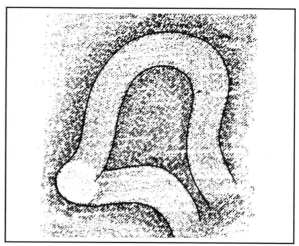

Figure 4.6: Radiographic appearance of tubular structures containing fluid.

2) The presence of differing material surrounding an object or filling the lumen of a hollow structure will greatly influence the radiographic appearance. (Figure 4.7).

    a) In a lean or immature animal there will be little or no omental, falciform or retro-peritoneal fat to provide inherent radiographic contrast. As a result, very little visceral detail will be appreciated on the radiograph.

Figures 4.7a and 4.7b: Radiographic appearance of gas filled bowel surrounded by: a. - normal omental fat, or b.- peritoneal fluid.

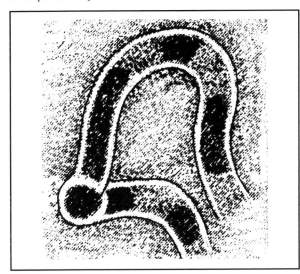

Figure 4.7a.

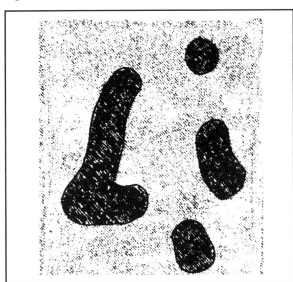

Figure 4.7b.

b) Gas densities within the intestinal lumen will be visible and if there is adequate visceral definition the serosal surface of the bowel wall will also be identifiable. However, if the inherent contrast is lost due to the presence of peritoneal fluid, then only the luminal gas will be identified.

c) The outline of the parenchymal organs, kidneys, liver and spleen and fluid filled viscera such as the bladder, will be identified in an abdomen with normal visceral contrast, but will not be identified if there is diminished contrast due to emaciation or free peritoneal fluid.

3) If two structures overlap, the appearance of the composite shadow will much more dense, e.g. kidneys. (Figure 4.8)

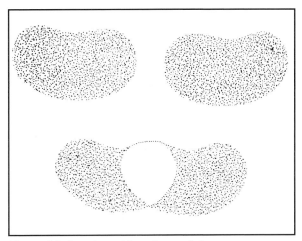

Figure 4.8: Superimposition of two soft tissue structures.

4) A flattened piece of material, whether soft tissue or mineralised, will show up poorly if the beam is perpendicular to the line of the object or structure but will be projected as a very dense linear opacity if the beam projects it edge-on. (Figure 4.9)

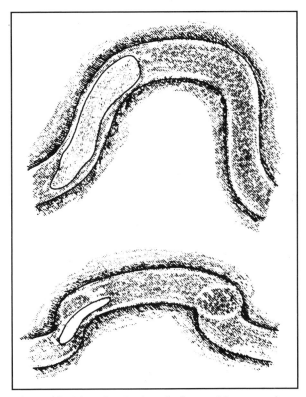

Figure 4.9: Edge of projection of a flattened fragment of bone within the bowel.

5) The significance of the silhouette sign should not be overlooked. If two soft tissue densities are confluent e.g. mass projecting from the capsule of the kidney then the outline of the composite shadow will be continuous. If they are are not confluent even if closely adjacent or touching, two distinct outlines will be seen. (Figure 4.10)

Figure 4.10a and b: The silhouette sign.

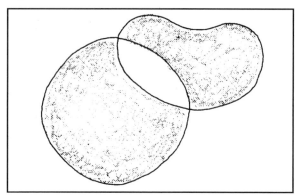

Figure 4.10a: Mass superimposed on the kidney.

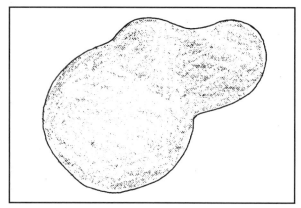

Figure 4.10b: Mass confluent with the kidney.

Normal Radiographic Anatomy

The radiograph should be systematically evaluated to identify all the viscera visible. The normal anatomy of the abdomen is illustrated in the annotated line diagrams. It must be realised that for the reasons indicated some or all these features may not be identified on a particular radiograph. (Figure 4.11-13)

It is important to identify each organ and evaluate it for -

Size:
- Enlarged or reduced in size?
- Is the organ abnormally obvious?

Shape/contour:
- Is there more or less tissue present?
- Does it contain abnormal tissue?
- Are there changes due to adjacent pathological lesions?

Changes in density:
- Is the density increased or decreased?
- Are these changes generalised or localised?
- Are they homogeneous or mottled?
- Are they clear or ill defined?

Changes in postition:
- Is it displaced by adjacent structure(s)?
- Is it displaced through abnormal openings?
- Has damage to the organ allowed movement?

Figure 4.11: Radiographic anatomy - left lateral recumbent view of the abdomen.

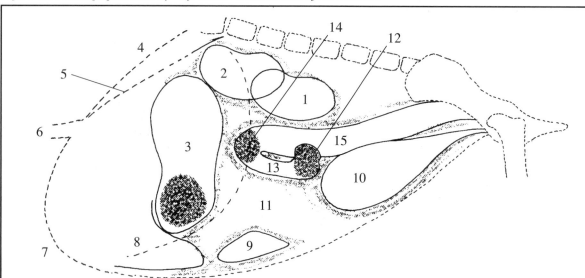

1) Left kidney - dorsal to the right.
   Right kidney - cranial to the left.
2) Kidneys closer together than on right lateral.
3) Body of stomach fills with ingesta (and barium). Usually two gas bubbles.
4) Right crus of diaphragm - lies behind and crosses left.
5) Inter-crural line usually visible.
6) Caudal vena cava - located halfway between sternum and spine.
7) Single, distinct diaphragmatic cupola visible.

8) Liver in a more anatomically normal position than in right lateral.
9) If the spleen visible, the tail may appear as a triangular opacity.
10) Bladder.
11) Small intestines - may obscure the spleen.
12) Caecum.
13) Ascending colon.
14) Transverse colon.
15) Descending colon.

Figure 4.12: Radiographic anatomy - right lateral recumbent view of abdomen.

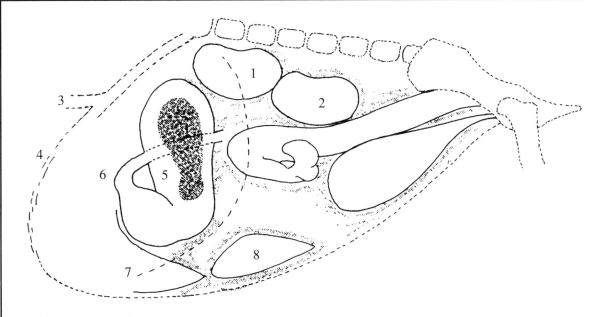

1) Right kidney - cranial and dorsal to the left.
2) Right crus of diaphragm - cranial and parallel to the left crus.
3) Caudal vena cava - located at a point between the sternum and spine.
4) Indistinct diaphragmatic cupola (may appear double).
5) Both pyloric antrum and fundus may fill with ingesta (and barium). Usually only a single gas bubble.
6) Proximal loop of descending duodenum - usually cranial to the pylorus.
7) Left lateral lobe of liver - may displace ventrally to give a false impression of hepatomegaly.
8) Splenic shadow - usually visible as a flattened triangular opacity on abdominal floor.

Figure 4.13: Radiographic anatomy - ventro-dorsal view of abdomen.

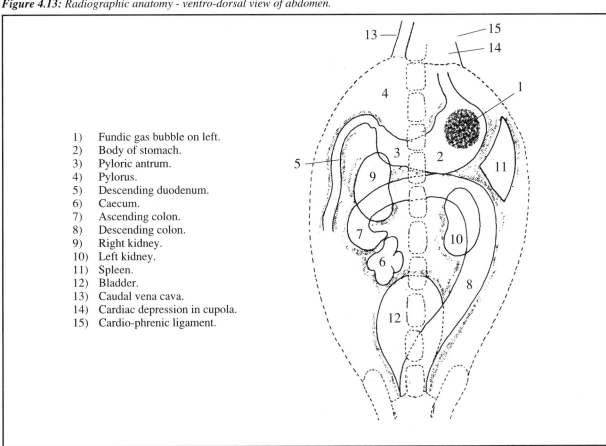

1)   Fundic gas bubble on left.
2)   Body of stomach.
3)   Pyloric antrum.
4)   Pylorus.
5)   Descending duodenum.
6)   Caecum.
7)   Ascending colon.
8)   Descending colon.
9)   Right kidney.
10) Left kidney.
11) Spleen.
12) Bladder.
13) Caudal vena cava.
14) Cardiac depression in cupola.
15) Cardio-phrenic ligament.

III: THE ALIMENTARY TRACT

Stomach

Radiographic anatomy. (Figure 4.14)

Radiographic pitfalls.
*   Gastric F.B.'s are very common and following identification on a radiograph, check that there are no other causes of vomiting before deciding upon surgery.
*   Beware of diagnosing peristaltic waves as filling defects.
*   The pylorus is circular and is filled with fluid or gas depending which side of the animal is adjacent to the plate. This annular structure may be erroneously diagnosed as a foreign body.
*   The rugal pattern in the dog is very prominent and it is diffficult to diagnose gastritis radiologically. As a rough guide the width of a rugal fold should not be greater than the distance between the adjacent rugae.
*   Contrast media should not be administered to an animal which has not been starved, as food in the stomach results in delayed gastric emptying of the contrast medium and numerous filling defects.

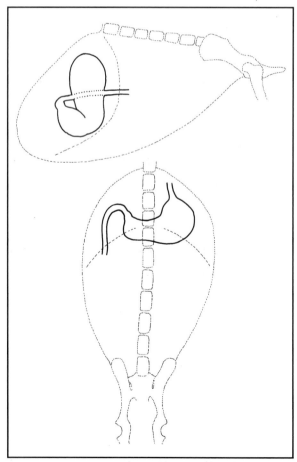

Figure 4.14: Stomach - Radiographic anatomy.

Gastric Enlargement

Causes:
   i)   Gastric dilation (gas).
   ii)   Gastric torsion (gas).
   iii) Post prandial (food and liquids).
   iv)   Respiratory distress with aerophagia (gas).
   v)   Outflow obstruction (food and/or liquids).

Radiological features (Figure 4.15)
*   Enlargement of the gastric shadow.
*   Contents may be entirely gas, food or fluid or a mixture.
*   In all cases except torsion the fundus, antrum and pylorus will be in a normal position.
*   In gastric torsion the anatomical relationships may be altered depending on the degree of rotation - 180, 270 or 360 degrees.
*   A linear soft tissue density formed by the gastric wall may be identified in torsion.
*   In outflow obstruction there may be an accumulation of opaque ingesta in the antral area.

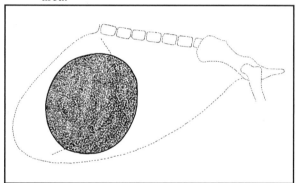

Figure 4.15a: Gastric enlargement. Gaseous distention of the stomach.

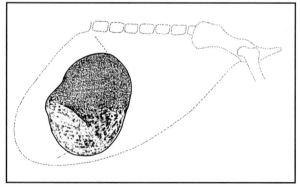

Figure 4.15b: Gastric enlargement. Distension with gas, food and fluid.

Caudal Displacement

Causes:
   i)   Hepatomegaly due to CCF, hepatitis etc.
   ii)   Hepatic neoplasia - primary or secondary.
   iii) Hepatic cysts.

Radiological features (Figure 4.16)
*   Caudal displacement of the gastric shadow - may need contrast to confirm. Alteration in angle of the gastric axis with the antrum more caudal than the fundus.

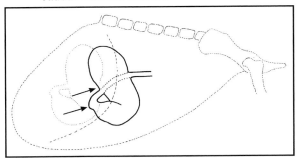

Figure 4.16: Stomach - Caudal displacement.

Cranial Displacement

Causes:
i)   Reduced hepatic size due to cirrhosis/fibrosis.
ii) Porto-systemic shunts with reduced liver size.
iii) Herniation of viscera through a diaphragmatic defect.
iv) Mid abdominal mass.

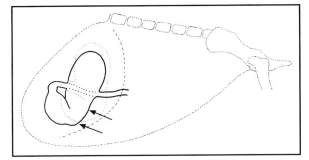

Figure 4.17: Stomach - Cranial depression.

Radiological features (Figure 4.17)
*   Cranial displacement of the gastric shadow.
*   Alteration in the gastric axis with the antrum more cranial than the fundus.

Delayed Gastric Emptying

In the dog, barium should start to enter the duodenum by 30 minutes post administration and the stomach should empty by 90. These times are much shorter in the cat.

Causes:
i)   Intestinal obstruction - see later
ii) Gastric outflow obstruction
         - pyloric foreign body
         - pyloric stenosis
         - pylorospasm
         - gastric neoplasia.
         - gastric ulceration with secondary fibrosis.
         - chronic hypertrophic gastritis.
iii) Acute alimentary inflammation - e.g. canine parvo virus.
iv) Inflammation adjacent to pyloric canal - hepatitis, pancreatitis etc.

Thickened Stomach Wall/Gastric Carcinoma

May result from ulceration plus fibrosis or neoplasia. The commonest site for gastric neoplasia in the dog is the pyloric antrum and lesser curvature of the stomach.

Radiological features (Figure 4.18)
*   Contrast will be necessary in almost all cases.
*   Image intensified fluoroscopy is an invaluable aid.
*   Without fluoroscopy great care must be taken when interpreting radiographs of gastric barium studies.
*   Significant lesions must be demonstrable on at least two sequential radiographs.
*   The pyloric antrum may not dilate fully.
*   The mucosal surface will be irregular.
*   There may be intra-luminal filling defects - more commonly seen in tumours other than carcinomas e.g. polyps, lymphosarcoma.
*   It can be very difficult to differentiate between gastric neoplasia and ulceration radiographically.
*   Uncomplicated gastric ulceration is best seen following double contrast gastrography.
*   There is persistent staining of the ulcerated area with barium and a surrounding 'lucent' ring with no adherent barium.

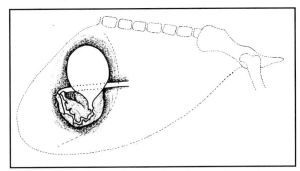

Figure 4.18a: Thickened stomach wall - gastric carcinoma.

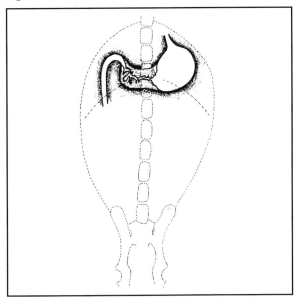

Figure 4.18b: Thickened stomach wall - gastric carcinoma.

Duodenum

Radiographic anatomy (Figure 4.19)

1) Normal gastric peristaltic waves.
2) Normal narrowing at the pylorus.
3) Descending duodenum runs parallel to the right body wall.

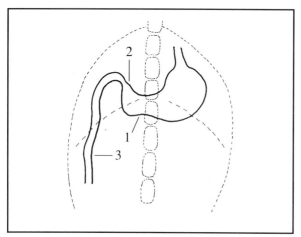

Figure 4.19: Duodenum - Radiographic anatomy.

Radiographic pitfalls
- Pseudoulcers are very common in the duodenum. These should not (Figure 4.20) be diagnosed as duodenal ulcers.
- Duodenal segmentation is very common especially in the cat. (Figure 4.21)

Intra Luminal Duodenal Lesions

Causes:
i) Neoplasia.
ii) Foreign bodies.
iii) Duodenal ulceration.

Radiological features (Figure 4.22)
- Contrast examination mandatory unless radiopaque foreign body.
- Intra-luminal filling defect.
- Irregular outline and attached to mucosal surface if neoplastic (see SI).
- Outlined by contrast if intraluminal foreign body.
- Duodenal ulcers very difficult to identify and distinguish from either early neoplasm or normal pseudoulcer.

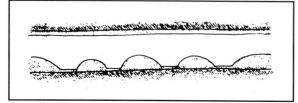

Figure 4.20: Pseudoulcers in the duodenum.

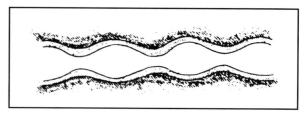

Figure 4.21: Duodenal segmentation.

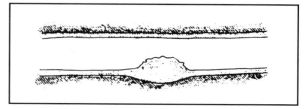

Figure 4.22a: intra-luminal mass.

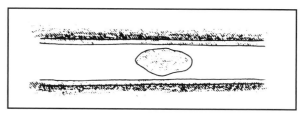

Figure 4.22b: intra-luminal foreign body.

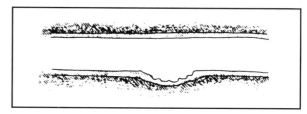

Figure 4.22c: mural ulceration.

Displacement of the Duodenum by Abdominal masses

Causes:
i) Cranial abdominal masses - pancreatic and splenic tumours.
ii) Dorsal masses - renal and adrenal.
iii) Mid abdominal masses - mesenteric node tumours.

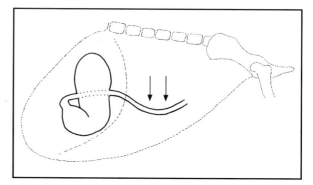

Figure 4.23: Displacement of the duodenum.

Radiological features (Figure 4.23)
• Cranial intra-abdominal masses e.g. pancreatic or splenic tumours will cause lateral displacement on the VD view.
• Dorsal masses e.g. renal tumours etc, will result in ventral and lateral displacement.
• Cranial abdominal masses are often poorly delineated.

Duodenal Appearance in Pancreatitis

Radiological features (Figure 4.24)
• The duodenal lumen is often dilated, C-shaped and displaced close to the right abdominal wall.
• Fluoroscopically will appear fixed and immotile. There is delayed passage of contrast.
• There is localised peritonitis with mottled increase in density in the right cranial quadrant of the abdomen.

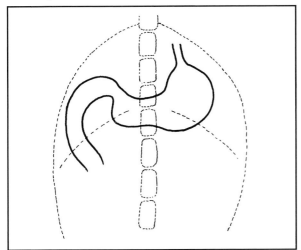

Figure 4.24: Duodenal appearance in pancreatitis.

Jejunum/Ileum

Radiographic anatomy.
No loop of ileum should be more than twice the diameter of an adjacent loop, another rough guide is that no loop should be wider that two rib widths. It is common for the area where the column of barium is in contact with the intestinal mucosa to appear 'fuzzy'.

The mass of small intestine should be located in mid abdomen on both lateral and VD views.

Radiographic pitfalls.
• Normal peristalsis can resemble the classic apple core appearance associated with intestinal neoplasia. (Figure 4.25)
• Peristalsis may result in normal narrowing along a length of intestine.
• It is not uncommon for a considerable length of the intestine to appear narrowed like a piece of string.

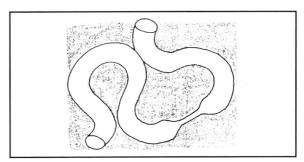

Figure 4.25a: Normal peristalsis patterns.

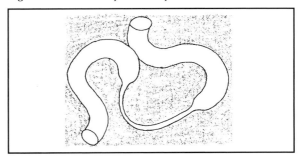

Figure 4.25b: Normal peristalsis patterns.

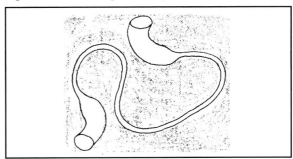

Figure 4.25c: Normal peristalsis patterns.

Intestinal Obstruction

Causes:

Localised ileus.
  a) Intestinal obstruction - foreign body.
     Intussuception.
     Intestinal neoplasia.
     Hernial incarceration.
  b) Intestinal infarction - post traumatic.

Generalised ileus.
  a) Acute enteritis.
  b) Chronic low intestinal obstruction.
  c) Paralytic ileus due to intestinal volvulus, peritonitis or any abdominal catastrophe.

Radiological features (Figure 4.26)
• Small intestinal loops are dilated (see above) with fluid and/or gas - ileus pattern - may be localised or generalised.
• The descending colon may appear empty i.e. no faecoliths present -
• Gravel sign. There are tiny pieces of material in most diets which appear radiodense. These are normally cleared by intestinal peristalsis

but when intestinal obstruction is present, this material builds up and resembles gravel. This sign suggests a chronic, partial obstruction.
- Contrast material in the gut may appear pale and grey (rather than dense white) as it diffuses into the fluid sequestrated in the gut.
- There is a delay in the passage of contrast medium down the gut. The following times may be taken as a guide to the normal rate of passage.
  - Stomach starts to empty within 30 mins.
  - Barium enters the ileum within 60 mins.
  - Barium will reach the ileo-caecal junction after 2 hours.
  - Little barium should be left in the stomach by 1$\frac{1}{2}$ hours.
    N.B. ALL THESE TIMES ARE SHORTER IN THE CAT.

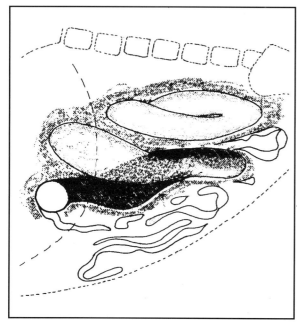

Figure 4.26: Intestinal obstruction.

Caudal Displacement of Small Intestine

Causes:
i) Anterior abdominal mass
   - usually hepatic, splenic or gastric.

Radiological features (Figure 4.27)
   All the small intestine shadows restricted to the caudal abdomen.

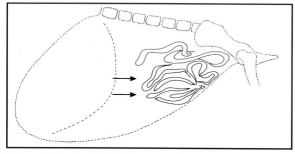

Figure 4.27: Caudal displacement of SI mass.

Cranial Displacement of Small Intestine

Causes:
i) Caudal abdominal mass.
ii) Uterine enlargement.
iii) Bladder distension.
iv) Enlarged prostate.
v) Prostatic cyst.

Radiological features (Figure 4.28)
- All the small intestine shadows restricted to the cranial abdomen.
- Presence of distended viscus or mass in caudal abdomen.

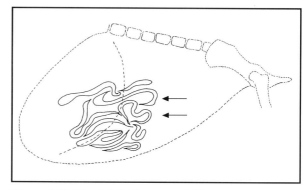

Figure 4.28: Cranial displacement of SI mass.

Deviation of Small Intestines Laterally to Left or Right Abdomen

Causes:
i) Unilateral abdominal masses -
ii) Splenic enlargement/neoplasia.
iii) Renal enlargement - cyst, neoplasia, abscess.
iv) Adrenal tumour.
v) Ovarian tumour.
vi) Retained tumified testicle.

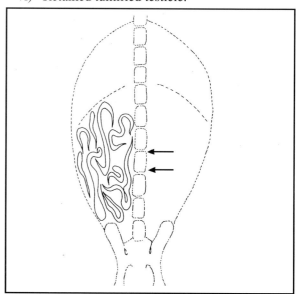

Figure 4.29: Deviation of SI mass laterally to left or right abdomen.

Radiological features (Figure 4.29)
- Small intetines displaced to one side of midline on VD view.
- Splenic tumours tend to lie to left side and displace the small intestines to the right.
- Other masses may be situated on either side of the abdomen and displace the SI accordingly.

Deviation of Small Intestines Ventrally

Causes:
- i)   Dorsal/retroperitoneal mass -
- ii) Renal enlargement - cyst, neoplasia, abscess.
- iii) Adrenal tumour.
- iv) Ovarian tumour.

Radiological features (Figure 4.30)
- Small intestines restricted to the ventral abdomen on a lateral view.
- Dorsal abdominal mass more or less well defined.

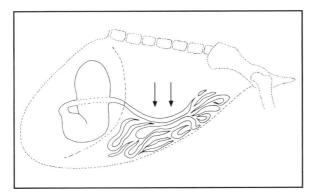

Figure 4.30: Deviation of the SI mass ventrally.

Small Intestines Appear 'Bunched Up' or Plicated in Central Abdomen

Causes:
- i)   Linear foreign bodies e.g. string, fabric etc.
- ii) Chronic enteritis.
- iii) Chronic peritonitis e.g. as a sequel to biliary tract damage.

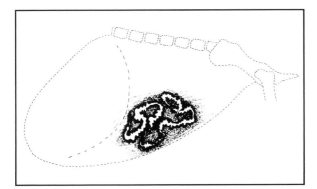

Figure 4.31a: SI mass appears 'bunched up' or plicated in central abdomen.

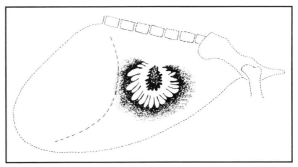

Figure 4.31b: SI mass appears 'bunched up' or plicated in central abdomen.

Radiological features (Figure 4.31)
- Small intestines appear restricted to the central abdomen.
- After contrast examination appears plicated or 'flounced'.
- May be 'stacking' of linear gas shadows.
- Often signs of peritonitis with mottled increase opacity and loss of visceral detail.

Intra-Luminal Filling Defects

Causes:
- i) Localised intestinal neoplasia.
- ii) Radiolucent foreign bodies.

Radiological features (Figure 4.32)
- Contrast examination necessary.
- Filling defect within the lumen usually with distension of the bowel proximally.
- If defect confluent with intestinal mucosa then likely to be neoplastic.
- Surface may be irregular and either to one side or annular.
- If defect surrounded by contrast and not confluent with wall then FB.

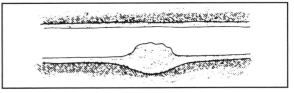

Figure 4.32a: Intra-luminal filling defects - intra-luminal mass.

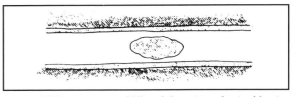

Figure 4.32b: Intra-luminal filling defects - intra-luminal foreign body.

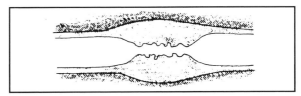

Figure 4.32c: Intra-luminal filling defects - mural ulceration.

Intramural Thickening

Causes:
  i)   If localised - intestinal neoplasia.
  ii) If generalised - chronic inflammatory
       intestinal disease, lymphosarcoma.

Radiological features (Figure 4.33)
  •   If localised - unilateral or annular.
  •   If generalised infiltrative lesion then intestinal
      lumen will be variable in diameter with
      mucosal roughening.
  •   Barium will often flocculate.

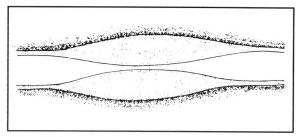

Figure 4.33a: *Intramural thickening. Localised with smooth mucosa.*

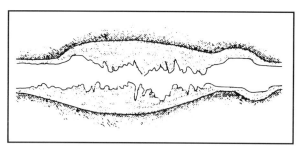

Figure 4.33b: *Intramural thickening. With mucosal roughening.*

Intussusception

Radiological features (Figure 4.34)

Plain film:
  •   MAY see elongated soft tissue mass.
  •   May be signs of intestinal obstruction - see
      above.

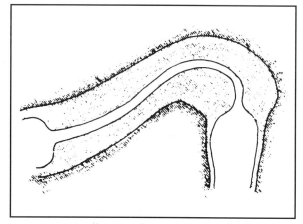

Figure 4.34a: *Intussusception - narrowing of the central lumen.*

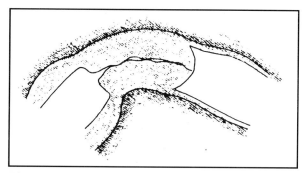

Figure 4.34a: *Intussusception - contrast outlining the proximal and distab. ends of the intussusception.*

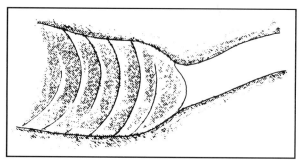

Figure 4.34a: *Intussusception - 'coiled spring' appearance following Ba enema.*

Following contrast examination:
  •   Persistently narrowed segment of intestinal lumen.
  •   Contrast may outline the proximal intra-
      luminal bulges of the intussusception.
  •   Contrast may pass through the narrowed
      bowel and then track back between the
      intussusceptum and intussuscipiens to
      produce the appearance of a 'coiled spring'.
      This appearance is more frequently seen
      following a barium enema.

Large Intestine

Radiographic anatomy (Figure 4.35)
  •   The transverse colon should almost contact
      the caudal aspect of the stomach.
  •   In the dog the caecum is commonly seen as a
      gas filled 'comma' shaped structure ventral to
      the third lumbar vertebra in the lateral view
      and to the right side of the abdomen in the
      VD view. It is rarely seen in the cat.
      The descending colon runs distally in the
      dorsal abdomen on the lateral view and to the
      left of midline on the VD view.

Radiographic pitfalls.
  •   Following contrast examination by barium
      enema filling defects are common if the
      patient has not been adequately prepared by
      starving and enemata.
  •   As with the small intestine, peristaltic waves
      may produce an appearance similar to those
      caused by neoplastic lesions.

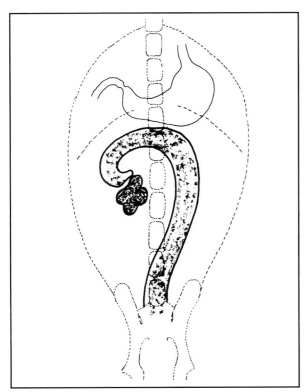

Figure 4.35a: Large intestine - radiographic anatomy.

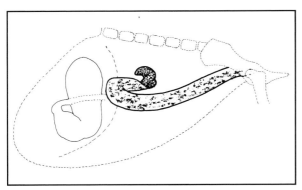

Figure 4.35b: Large intestine - radiographic anatomy.

Displacement of the Colon

Causes:

Any abdominal mass or enlargement of a viscus adjacent to the large intestine will displace that structure, the direction being dependent on the location of the mass.

i) *Ventral displacement:*
Renal enlargement.
Enlargement of the sub-lumbar nodes.
Sub-lumbar mass - abscess.
Retroperitoneal fluid - haemorrhage, urine etc.

ii) *Dorsal displacement:*
Bladder enlargement.
Uterine enlargement.
Splenic enlargement.
Prostatic enlargement/cyst.

iii) *Right lateral displacement:*
Bladder enlargement.
Uterine enlargement.
Left renal enlargement.

iv) *Left lateral displacement:*
Bladder enlargement.
Mid abdominal mass.

Colitis

Radiography of little value except in severe, advanced, ulcerative colitis. Contrast enema - either barium or double contrast required.

Radiological features (Figure 4.36)

* The normal colon has a very smooth mucosal surface on contrast examination.

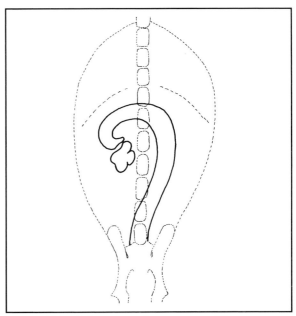

Figure 4.36a: Colitis - normal appearance of Ba enema.

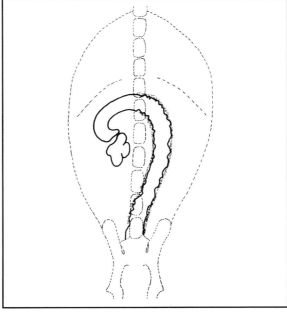

Figure 4.36b: Colitis - appearance of colitis following Ba enema.

Colonic Tumours

More commonly unilateral than annular (unlike small intestinal tumours) and usually involve the distal third of the colon. Again, contrast enemata required for a radiological diagnosis.

Radiological features (Figure 4.37)
- Intraluminal filling defect confluent with the mucosal surface.
- Mucosal irregularity.
- Diffuse neoplasia - lymphosarcoma - will produce an appearance very similar to ulcerative colitis.

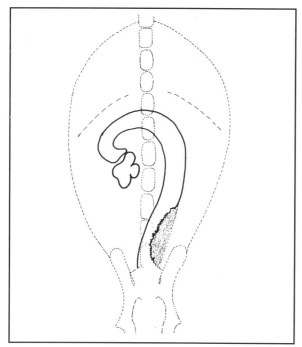

Figure 4.37: Colonic tumour.

IV: THE PARENCHYMATOUS ORGANS

Liver

Radiographic anatomy.
See Figures 4.11, 12 & 13. The liver is normally contained within the costal arch on both the lateral and VD views. The stomach is in contact with the left lateral lobes of the liver.

The cranial pole of the right kidney touches the liver. On lateral views the caudal border appears angular rather than rounded and should not project beyond the costal arch.

Radiographic pitfalls.
- On right lateral abdominal films, the ventral lobes may slide caudally, giving an erroneous impression of hepatomegaly.
- If the animal is obese, the liver may appear enlarged because the pendulous abdomen allows the liver to slide 'downhill'.

Generalised Hepatomegaly

Causes:
i) Secondary neoplasia.
ii) Nodular hyperplasia.
iii) Metabolic diseases - D. mellitus, Cushing's syndrome, Hyperthyroidism etc.
iv) Hepatic cysts.
v) Systemic venous congestion secondary to right heart failure.

Radiological features (Figure 4.38)
- The most important aid to diagnosis is to carefully note the outline of the stomach. This is more easily seen following administration of barium. It is seldom possible to proceed further than the identification of hepatic size and shape on radiological evidence alone.
- Lateral view -
  Projection of the ventral angle of the liver beyond the costal arch.
  Rounding of the ventral angle.
  Caudal displacement of the gastric axis.
- VD view -
  Caudal displacement of the stomach.
  May be possible to identify the caudal margins of the lateral lobes projecting beyond the last rib.

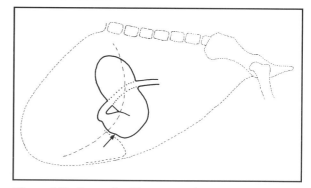

Figure 4.38: Generalised hepatomegaly.

Localised Increase in Hepatic Size

Causes:
i) Primary neoplasia.
ii) Hepatic cyst(s).
iii) Hepatic abscess/haematoma.

Radiological features (Figure 4.39)
- Cranial abdominal mass confluent with hepatic shadow.
- Displacement of either the gastric fundus caudally and/or medially or displacement of the pyloric antrum caudally and/or medially depending on the location of the hepatic mass.
- Primary hepatic tumours more commonly affect the right lobes.

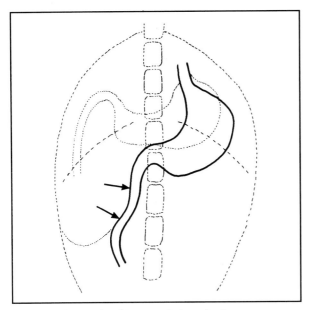

Figure 4.39: Localised increase in hepatic size.

Reduced Liver Size

Causes:
i)   Hepatic cirrhosis/fibrosis.
ii) Congenital porto-systemic shunts.
iii) Herniation of a portion of the liver through a diaphragmatic defect.

Radiological features (Figure 4.40)
- Cranial displacement of the stomach and gastric axis.
- Absence of ventral and lateral margins of the hepatic shadow.

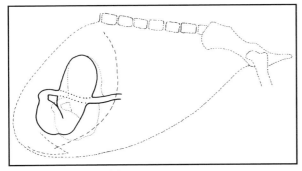

Figure 4.40: Reduced liver size.

Pancreas
Radiographic anatomy. The pancreas will not be identified on plain radiographs.

Pancreatic Neoplasia

Radiological features
- May identify a soft tissue mass in right cranial abdomen displacing duodenum laterally and pyloric antrum/greater curvature of the stomach cranially.
- May be no identifiable radiographic signs.

Pancreatitis

Radiological features (Figure 4.41)
- Mottled increase in radiopacity of right cranial abdomen.
- Lateral displacement of duodenum which may appear dilated.
- Transverse colon may be dilated and displaced caudo-medially.

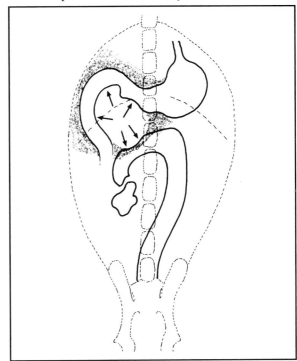

Figure 4.41: Pancreatitis.

Spleen

Radiographic anatomy (Figure 4.42)
On the lateral view the appearance is very variable and the spleen may not be identified at all in some cases particularly in left lateral recumbency. In right lateral recumbency the spleen may be identified as a flattened triangular soft tissue opacity in the ventral abdomen just caudal to the ventral edge of the liver. On occasion it will lie longitudinally along the floor of the abdomen. On the VD view the spleen will normally be seen as a triangular soft tissue mass adjacent to the left abdominal wall just caudal to the fundus of the stomach.

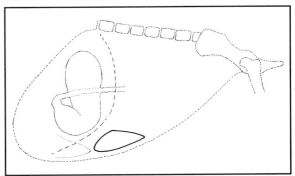

Figure 4.42a: Spleen - radiographic anatomy.

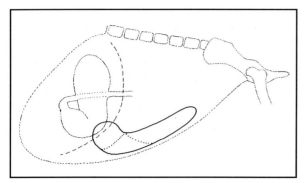

Figure 4.42b: Spleen - radiographic anatomy.

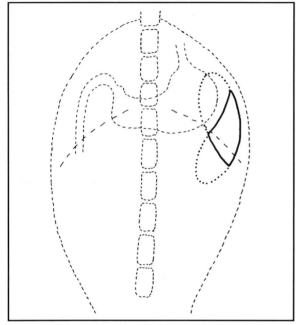

Figure 4.42c: Spleen - radiographic anatomy.

Splenomegaly

Very common and generalised splenomegaly is frequently not significant.

Causes:

i)   Generalised Splenomegaly.
         Idiopathic.
         Anaemia.
         Drugs e.g. barbiturate anaesthetics.
         Neoplasia e.g. lymphosarcoma.
         Splenic torsion.
         Gastric torsion - results in splenic congestion.
ii)   Localised splenomegaly.
         Neoplasia - e.g. haemangiosarcoma, rarely
         haemangioma.
         Abscess.
         Nodular hyperplasia.
         Haematoma.

Splenic Neoplasia

Splenic neoplasia is the commonest cause of a spherical, mid-abdominal mass in the dog.

Splenic neoplasia, especially haemangiosarcoma

may be associated with loss of visceral detail (see page 73) due to spontaneous rupture with resulting intraperitoneal haemorrhage.

Radiological features (Figure 4.43)
*   Soft tissue mass, often very large and spherical in mid abdomen often on the left side.
*   Reduction in visceral detail due to intraperitoneal haemorrhage may mask the outline of the mass which must then be identified by its displacement of other viscera.

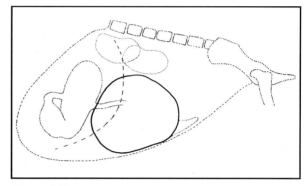

Figure 4.43: Splenic neoplasia.

Splenic Torsion

Radiological features (Figure 4.44)
Splenic torsion is uncommon but is easily diagnosed on VD views when the splenic outline is noted on the right displacing the duodenum rather than on the left adjacent to the stomach.

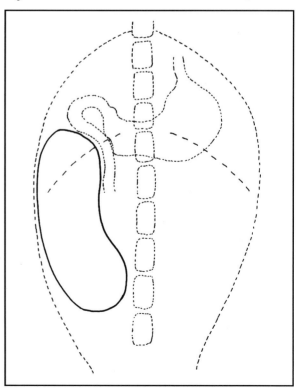

Figure 4.44: Splenic torsion.

V: URINARY TRACT

Kidneys

Radiographic anatomy (Figure 4.45)

Dog:

Normal length	2.5 - 3.5 times the length of the second lumbar vertebra
Right kidney located	T 13 - L 2
Left kidney located	L 2 - L 4

Cat:

Normal length	2.5 - 3.0 times the length of the second lumbar vertebra
Right kidney located	L 1 - L 3
Left kidney located	L 2 - L 5

On lateral abdominal films the two kidneys overlap. This is more pronounced on right lateral films and in the cat. It may not be possible to identify the right kidney on a normal lateral radiograph in the dog. Intravenous urography will be required to demonstrate abnormalities of the renal pelvis, collecting duct system and ureters and to make a crude estimation of renal functions.

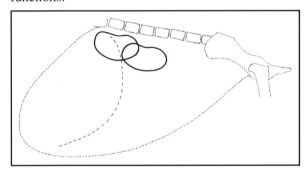

Figure 4.45a: Kidneys - Radiographic anatomy.

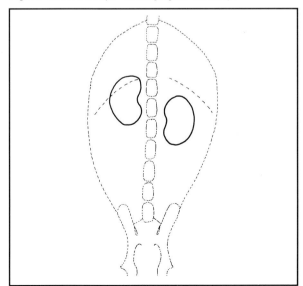

Figure 4.45b: Kidneys - Radiographic anatomy.

Radiographic pitfalls

* In the cat, it is not uncommon to see a radiodense mass cranial to the kidneys on lateral views. This calcification of the adrenals is normal.
* On VD views, beware of diagnosing overlying nipples as renal or cystic calculi.

Renal Enlargement

Causes:

i) Neoplasia.
ii) Acute nephritis.
iii) Cystic Renal Disease.
iv) Hydronephrosis.
v) Feline Infectious Peritonitis.
vi) Porto-vascular anomalies.
vii) Pyelonephritis.
viii) Haematoma.

Radiological features (Figure 4.46)

* *Bilateral:*
  The length of the kidneys is outwith the sizes quoted above.
  The descending duodenum may be deviated ventrally on lateral views.

* *Enlarged right kidney:*
  Ventral displacement of the duodenum on the lateral view.
  Medial displacement of the ascending colon on the VD view.

* *Enlarged left kidney:*
  Ventral displacement of the colon on the lateral view.
  Medial displacement of the colon and SI on the VD view.

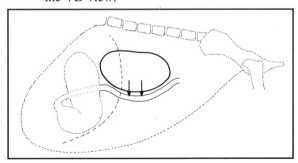

Figure 4.46a: Right renal enlargement.

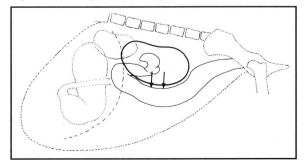

Figure 4.46b: Left renal enlargement.

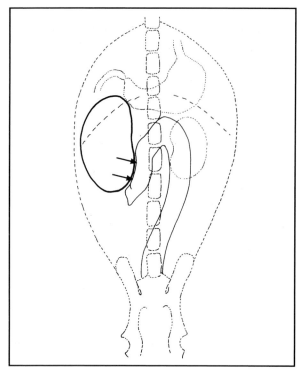

Figure 4.46c: Right renal enlargement.

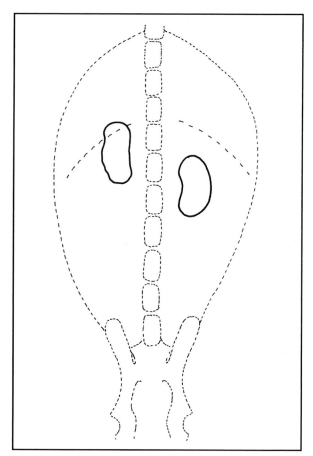

Figure 4.47: Reduced kidney size.

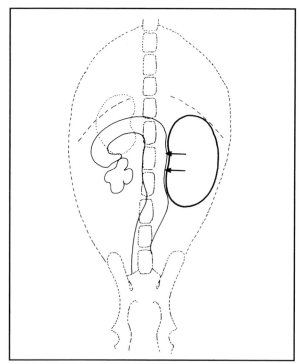

Figure 4.46d: Left renal enlargement.

Reduced Kidney Size

Causes:
  i)   Usually chronic end stage renal disease.
  ii) In young animals congenital nephropathy, renal hypoplasia etc.

Radiological features (Figure 4.47)
  •   The length of one or both kidneys (usually bilateral) is less than the figure quoted above.

Bladder/Ureters

Radiographic anatomy
The bladder is normally seen both lateral and VD views in the ventro-caudal abdomen. The ureters are not seen on plain films.

Radiographic pitfalls
  •   The remnant of the urachus frequently produces a distinct peak on the cranial border of the bladder in lateral projections and this should not be confused with urachal diverticulum. (The latter condition produces thickening of the wall).
  •   On lateral projections, the fabellae may be superimposed on the bladder/urethra and these should not be diagnosed as calculi. If in doubt, position the animal so that the stifles are clear of the area under investigation.
  •   A false impression of thickening of the bladder wall will be obtained if the bladder is insufficiently inflated with air when performing a pneumocystogram.
  •   After performing a pneumocystogram, air will remain in the bladder for a considerable time and if subsequent radiographs are taken, beware of diagnosing this normal finding as emphysematous cystitis.

Enlarged Bladder

Causes:
i) Mechanical:
    Urethral calculi.
    Prostatic lesions.
    Peri-urethral lesions (especially intra-pelvic).
    Urethral neoplasia.
ii) Neurogenic:
    Secondary to spinal lesions.
    Secondary to chronic mechanical
    obstruction.
    Idiopathic 'atonic' bladder.

Radiological features (Figure 4.48)
*   Mass of the small intestine displaced cranially.
*   Colon is displaced dorsally on the lateral view.
*   Colon may be displaced to the right or left on the VD view.

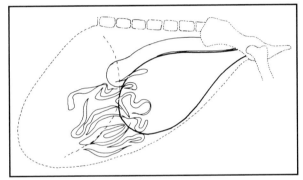

Figure 4.48: Enlarged bladder.

Reduced Bladder Size

Causes:
i)   Animal has just urinated.
ii) Bladder rupture.
iii) Bilateral ectopic ureters with bladder hypoplasia.
iv) Other congenital abnormalities.
v)   Persistent incontinenece.

Radiological features -
*   The bladder is nearly always seen on plain radiographs of the caudal abdomen.
*   If it appears tiny or is absent altogether, why should this be so?

Thickened Bladder Wall

Causes:
i)   Chronic cystitis.
ii) Polypoid cystitis.
iii) Focal haemorrhagic cystitis.
iv) Bladder neoplasia.
v)   Inadequate dilation of bladder with contrast.

Radiological features (Figure 4.49)
*   A positive, negative or double contrast cystogram is required to determine bladder wall thickness.
*   In acute cystitis the changes may be minimal.
*   In chronic cystitis the thickening may be localised, as in focal haemorrhagic cystitis - often at the cranio-ventral aspect, or generalised. There will not normally be any intra-luminal masses except in cases of polypoid cystitis.
*   In bladder neoplasia the changes are most often localised either at the bladder neck or cranial pole.
*   There are often associated intra-luminal soft tissue masses.
*   There is a spectrum of changes and in some cases it may be difficult or impossible to distinguish between focal inflammatory lesions and neoplasia on radiological grounds alone.

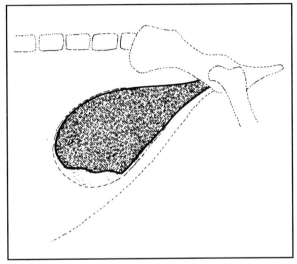

Figure 4.49a: Thickened bladder wall - localised thickening cystisis - pneumocystogram.

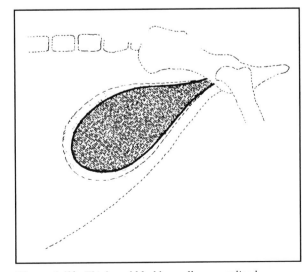

Figure 4.49b: Thickened bladder wall - generalised thickening cystisis - pneumocystogram.

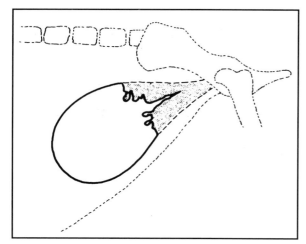

Figure 4.49c: Thickened bladder wall - neoplasis bladder neck - positive contrast.

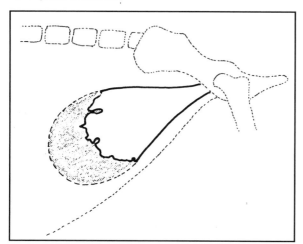

Figure 4.49d: Thickened bladder wall - neoplasis cranial pole - positive contrast.

Cystic Calculi

Radiological features (Figure 4.50)
- Most calculi are radio-opaque but some (especially urates) are radiolucent.
- Radiolucent calculi are best diagnosed using positive contrast techniques where the calculi usually show up in the centre of the pool of contrast medium.
- Vary widely in size and shape.
- Often features of an associated chronic cystitis.

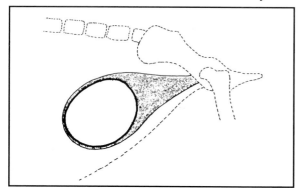

Figure 4.50a: Cystic Calculi - single.

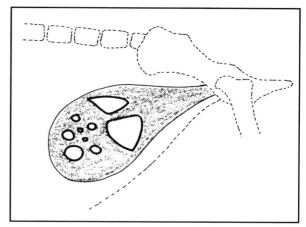

Figure 4.50b: Cystic Calculi - multiple.

Ruptured Bladder

Causes:
Normal sequel to abdominal trauma e.g RTA.

Radiological features
- Loss of bladder outline or bladder size markedly reduced.
- Poor visualisation of abdominal viscera due to free abdominal urine. Best diagnosed by either (Figure 4.51):
  a) **positive contrast cystography**. Look for the tip of the catheter in an unusual position within the abdomen and for free contrast medium distributed around the viscera.
  b) **negative contrast cystography**. Take a horizontal beam decubitus lateral view and look for free gas under the abdominal wall.

It is a misconception that following catheterisation of an animal with a ruptured bladder, little urine will flow from the catheter. The catheter may well pass through the bladder defect and act as an abdominal drain.

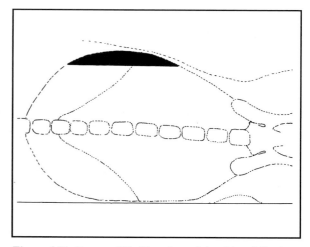

Figure 4.51: Ruptured bladder - lateral decubitus following pneumocystogram.

Ectopic Ureters

Contrast examination of the urinary tract is essential to make a radiological diagnosis of ureteral ectopia.

Two methods can be used -

a) **Intra-venous urography combined with a pneumocystogram.**

b) **Retrograde vagino-urethrography.**

Careful patient preparation is also necessary as faecal shadows may mask the ureters.

Radiological features (Figure 4.52)

- The various combinations of appearance of the distal ureters that may be seen are illustrated.
- Unless the ureters can unequivocally be seen entering the bladder at the trigone, the failure to demonstrate an ectopic ureter on the radiographic study is insufficient evidence on which to eliminate ureteral ectopia as a diagnosis.

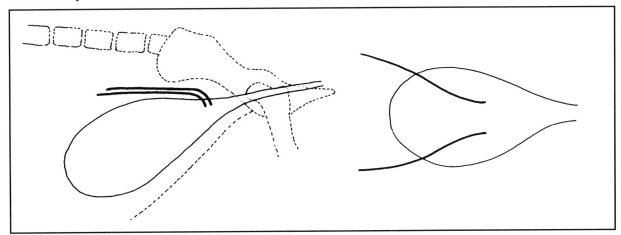

Figure 4.52a: Ectopic ureters - normal.

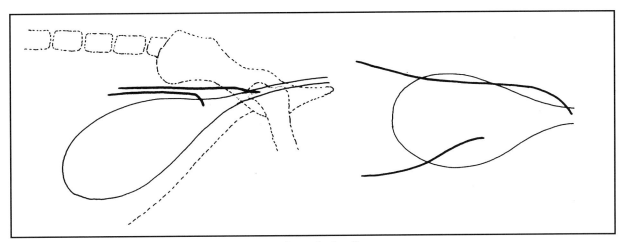

Figure 4.52b: Ectopic ureters - single ectopic ureter outside urethral wall.

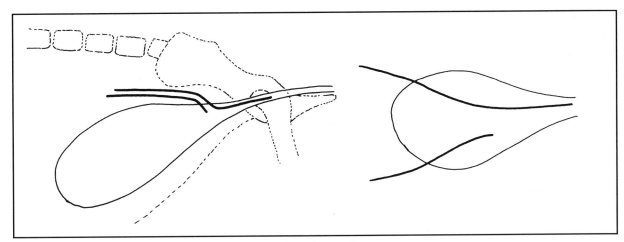

Figure 4.52c: Ectopic ureters - single ectopic ureter running submuscolly.

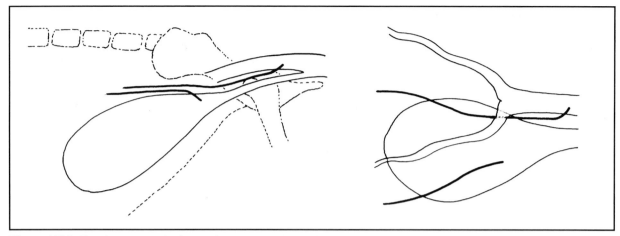

Figure 4.52d: *Ectopic ureters - single ectopic ureter entering vagina.*

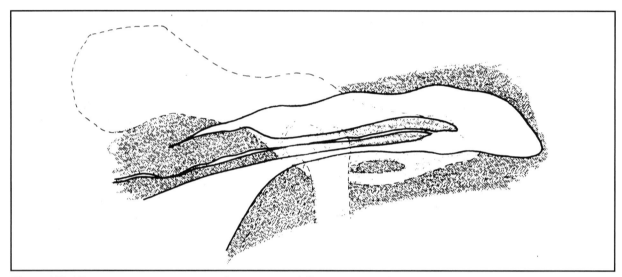

Figure 4.52e: *Ectopic ureters - appearance of ectopic ureter following retrograde vaginourethrogram.*

VI: GENITAL TRACT

Ovaries

Radiographic anatomy
Normal ovaries are not visible on survey radiographs. Ovarian masses are almost always neoplastic. Some ovarian neoplasms are associated with the production of fluid so the radiographic signs may be those of abdominal fluid (see earlier).

Ovarian Mass
If radiologically identifiable, an ovarian mass is most likely to be due to ovarian neoplasia.

Radiological features (Figure 4.53)
*   Soft tissue mass located in mid abdomen - often more dorsally located than splenic masses.
*   Ovarian neoplasia is most commonly unilateral but can be bilateral.
*   Other viscera may be displaced depending on which ovary is affected.

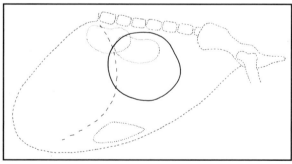

Figure 4.53: *Ovarian mass.*

Uterus

Radiographic anatomy.
The normal, non pregnant uterus is not usually identifiable on plain abdominal radiographs.

Uterine Enlargement

Causes:
   i)   Pregnancy.
   ii) Pyometra/mucometra/endometritis.
   iii) Neoplasia - rare.

Radiological features (Figure 4.54)
*   Increased gap between bladder and descending colon.
*   The mass of the small intestine is displaced cranially.
*   Multiple homogenous fluid filled loops of uterine horn seen in mid and caudal abdomen.

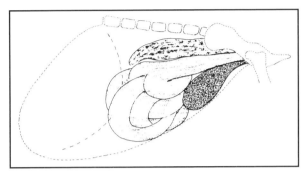
Figure 4.54: Uterine enlargement - Pyometra.

Normal Pregnancy

Radiological features -
*   Until 30 - 35 days may be difficult or impossible to detect uterine enlargement and confidently differentiate it from loops of small intestine.
*   Ossified foetal skeletons are radiographically detectable at 40 days in the cat and 40 - 45 days in the dog.
*   If estimating foetal numbers, count either skulls or spines and remember that the number counted is the minimum number of foetuses to expect!

Abnormal Pregancy

Radiological features (Figure 4.55)
Signs of foetal death include:
*   Overlapping of the bones of the cranial vault.
*   Intra-foetal gas either in the lungs, peritoneal cavity or heart chambers.
*   Intra-uterine gas.
*   Abnormal foetal posture.
*   Loss of uterine fluids resulting in an enhancement of the foetal skeleton.
*   Osteoporosis of the foetal skeleton.

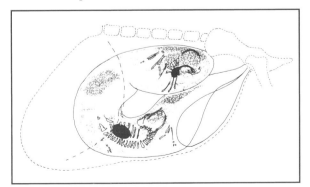
Figure 4.55: Intra-uterine foetal death.

Prostate

Normal radiographic anatomy
Normally located within the pelvis and is rarely seen in young dogs on survey radiographs unless enlarged to some degree. If the prostate has tipped forward into caudal abdomen, may be obvious around the bladder neck.

Radiographic pitfalls
*   The prostate is almost always radiographically visible in the Scottish Terrier.
*   The normal prostate increases in size with age and this should be borne in mind when evaluating for prostatic disease.

Prostatic Enlargement

Causes:
i)   Benign Prostatic Hypertrophy.
ii) Prostatitis
iii) Intra-prostatic cysts/cystic hyperplasia.
iv) Prostatic metaplasia secondary to oestrogen secreting testicular tumours.
v)   Neoplasia.

Radiological features
*   It is often necessary to use contrast techniques - a pneumocystogram is adequate - to differentiate between the bladder, the prostate and other caudal abdominal masses.
*   Positive contrast urethro-cystography is helpful in evaluating the nature of the prostatic disease.
*   Rarely an enlarged prostate will remain intra-pelvic in position in which case the main features will be compression and dorsal deviation of the pelvic descending colon.
*   More commonly the enlarged prostate displaces cranially into the caudal abdomen.
*   The bladder is displaced cranially and the rectum dorsally.

It is difficult to distinguish reliably between the various causes of prostatic enlargement but the following features seen on either the plain film or following cystography may help.

a)   In **benign hypertrophy** the prostatic urethra remains in central and often somewhat dilated. (Figure 4.56)

b)   In **cystic hypertrophy** contrast material may be seen outlining the cysts.(Figure 4.57)

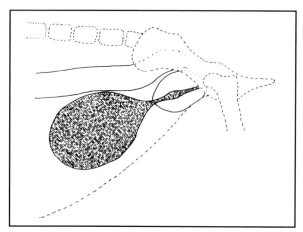

Figure 4.56: Prostatic enlargement - benign hypertrophy.

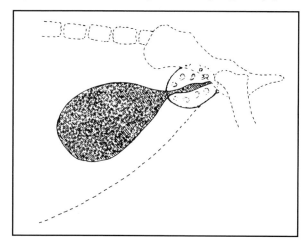

Figure 4.57: Prostatic enlargement - cystic hypertrophy.

c) In **prostatic carcinoma** the prostate may be irregular in shape, the urethra asymmetrically positioned, the clear distinction between bladder neck and prostate indistinct.

There may also be enlargement of the sublumbar lymph nodes and periosteal reaction affecting the bones of the pelvis, sacrum and lumbar spine due to tumour infiltration. (Figure 4.58)

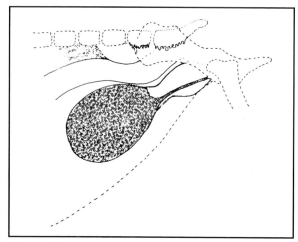

Figure 4.58: Prostatic enlargement - prostatic carcinoma.

d) **Prostatic abscesses** will result in asymmetrical enlargement with deviation of the urethra. Contrast MAY enter the abscess cavity (Figure 4.59)

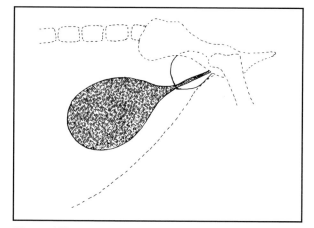

Figure 4.59: Prostatic enlargement - prostatic abscess.

e) In **acute prostatitis** there may be relatively little radiological abnormality.

Paraprostatic Cysts

The clinical signs are more usually those of a large caudal abdominal mass with resultant abdominal enlargement and difficulty in defaecation.

Radiological features (Figure 4.60)
*   Large soft tissue mass in caudal abdomen.
*   May lie dorsal, lateral or ventral to the bladder which is displaced accordingly.
*   Contrast studies often required to identify the bladder from the cyst and vice versa.

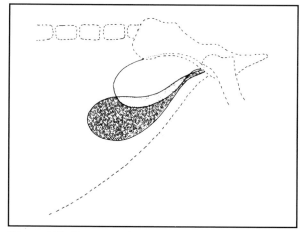

Figure 4.60: Paraprostatic cysts.

CHAPTER FIVE

The Appendicular Skeleton

J. V. Davies and R. Lee

CONTENTS

Each section dealing with a specific region contains details of radiographic technique and positioning.

I. THE EVALUATION OF SKELETAL RADIOGRAPHS

In the past the skeletal system was the major focus of radiographic activity in general veterinary practice. This was perhaps because of two major factors. Firstly, and erroneously, it may have been considered easier to interpret skeletal radiographs than soft tissue films; secondly, the limitations of low output X-ray machines and the speed of traditional film/screen combinations rather limited abdominal and thoracic radiography.

Modern equipment should allow good quality images of both skeletal and soft tissue structures to be achieved. It must be remembered that the evaluation of soft tissue detail is an essential element of skeletal radiography. The fact that bony shadows are visible even on very poor quality films should not be an excuse for substandard radiography.

As with all radiography at least two views at right angles are generally considered to be essential, but there are many situations in which one view will be of major value in reaching a diagnosis. For ease of interpretation these should be taken in the following planes:

a)   Cranio-caudal - Crcd (dorso-palmar or plantar - DP, antero-posterior - AP)

b)   Latero-medial or medio-lateral (Lateral - LAT)

c)   Oblique views at 45 degrees to the standard views are sometimes used. These are described as - Dorsopalmar-lateromedial (DPLMO) or dorsopalmar-mediolateral (DPMLO)

d)   A variety of special views including skyline projections, stressed and weight bearing views and deliberately under or over exposed radiographs may occasionally be indicated.

Note - all views are described in the direction the X-ray beam enters and exits the subject.

The beam should be centred on the area of interest in order to minimise geometric distortion. Radiographs of the whole limb are usually unhelpful except for the assessment of skeletal mineralisation.

Aggressive collimation should always be employed in order to both ensure adequate radiation safety from scattered radiation and also to improve the radiographic image.

On the rare occasions that radiographs of conscious animals are to be taken, full use should be made of restraining devices to minimise the need for manual restraint. At no time should any human anatomy, EVEN PROTECTED BY LEAD CLOTHING, be allowed to enter the primary X-ray beam. The specific radiographic techniques applicable to each region will be discussed later.

Indications

There are a wide variety of clinical indications for radiography of the appendicular skeleton including:

1)   The pre- and post-operative assessment of fractures.

2)   Acute or chronic lameness.

3)   Skeletal pain.

4)   Swelling associated with bones or joints.

5)   Limb deformity.

6)   Metabolic bone disease.

7)   Monitoring of heritable disorders e.g. Hip dysplasia.

8)   Evaluation of systemic disease which may have skeletal manifestations.

The reader is encouraged to follow a step by step approach to the evaluation of skeletal radiograph - an algorithm. In this initial section, such an approach will be outlined and illustrated by examples of specific disease conditions.

1) Evaluation of Soft Tissues

1.1) Increase/decrease in mass

An increase in soft tissue mass will suggest the presence of some space occupying lesion. In the absence of radiographic changes within the bony components such a change may be of great value in indicating the site of an orthopaedic problem e.g. synovial effusion in the early stages of an arthropathy. In order to determine the exact nature of this lesion other techniques may be required e.g. needle aspiration, biopsy etc. (Figure 5.1)

A decrease in mass is indicative of atrophy or, more rarely, dystrophy and may serve to focus the attention on a particular limb. For instance in the early stages of Perthe's disease the bony changes may be marginal but muscle atrophy may well have occurred already and this may be apparent on the film particularly when comparison is made with the contra-lateral limb.

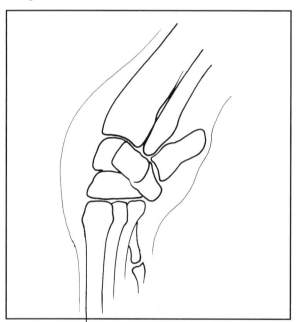

Figure 5.1: *Lateral view of the carpus showing soft tissue swelling round the joint indicative of a synovial effusion.*

1.2) Change in density

An increase in soft tissue density will imply mineralisation of soft tissues. This may be either calcification or ossification. Calcification will generally have a granular amorphous pattern e.g. calcinosis circumscripta, whereas ossification should demonstrate a radiological and histological trabecular pattern e.g. myositis ossificans. (Figure 5.2)

Radiodense foreign bodies will also appear as increases in the normal soft tissue density. Glass often contains significant amounts of lead and may be vis-

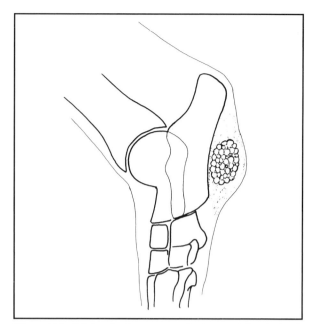

Figure 5.2: *Calcinosis circumscripta lesion caudal to the hock.*

ible on films with adequate detail, but its opacity will vary. If high definition screen films are not available the use of non-screen envelope wrapped film may be considered when attempting to identify possible fragments of glass in an animal's paw.

A decrease in soft tissue density is suggestive of the infiltration of fat and may be indicative of the presence of a lipoma or liposarcoma.

The presence of radiolucent gas densities within soft tissues will arise following surgical intervention and will therefore be evident on post-operative films. However, if such lucencies are present pre-operatively it will be indicative of either an open wound and/or the presence of gas forming bacteria. (Figure 5.3)

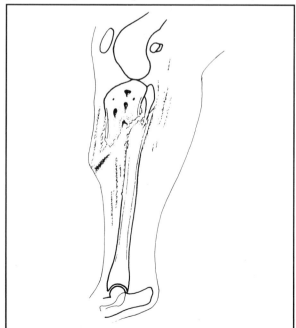

Figure 5.3: *Compound tibial fracture and secondary osteomyelitis with interstitial gas.*

1.3) Shift in fascial planes

Many fascial planes contain small quantities of fat the inherent contrast of which helps to delineate soft tissue structures.

Swelling of tissues may shift or obscure these fascial planes e.g. identification of joint effusion in the stifle. (Figure 5.4)

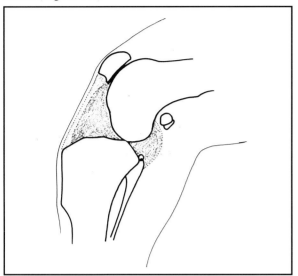

Figure 5.4: *Lateral view of the stifle.*
The infra patellar fat pad has been compressed/infiltrated by the increased synovial fluid. The normal fascial planes that run caudal to the joint have been displaced. These changes are indicative of an effusion

1.4) Soft tissue masses

Accumulation of fluid within soft tissue structures will not be visible unless bordered by a contrasting density. Subcutaneous swellings will alter the contour of the limb. However, deeper swellings will only be apparent if structures of contrasting density are displaced. As mentioned above there may be displacement or loss of normal fascial planes. The popliteal lymph node is often embedded in fat and so visible within the surrounding soft tissues, as a result enlargement of the node may occasionally be identifiable.

1.5) Foreign bodies

Radiodense foreign bodies will be more or less readily identified as described above. Radiolucent foreign bodies will not be seen unless highlighted by gas lucencies resulting from either gas forming organisms or direct communication to the atmosphere through a wound.

2) Evaluation of the Joints

2.1) Alignment

The alignment of the components of a joint should be assessed to determine whether luxation or subluxation has occurred. When the small bones of the carpus or tarsus are involved it is often helpful to make comparisons with the contra-lateral limb or to refer to an atlas of radiographic anatomy.

Malalignment is most likely to be traumatic in origin but a variety of congenital and developmental anomalies are also seen e.g. congenital dislocation of the shoulder and subluxation of the elbow following premature physeal closure. (Figure 5.5)

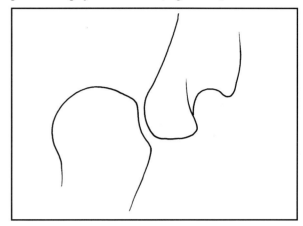

Figure 5.5: *Congenital luxation of the shoulder.*

2.2) Bony structures

The bony components of the joint should be examined individually. Remodelling of the bones concerned may have occurred because of congenital or developmental anomalies or as a result of longstanding misalignment following either an unreduced fracture or dislocation.

The subchondral bone should be evaluated for the presence of increased lucency. Degenerative joint disease and developmental diseases, such as osteochondrosis and Perthes disease, may be associated with subchondral lucency. (Figure 5.6)

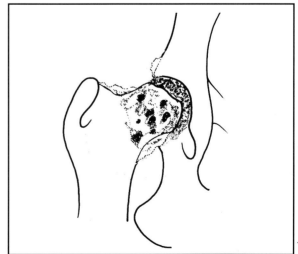

Figure 5.6: *Perthes disease showing subchondral lucencies.*

Cystic subchondral lucencies occasionally occur but are rare in small animals.

Periarticular deposits of new bone are usually indicators of degenerative joint disease. These bony spurs are usually referred to as osteophytes, although when associated with the origins or insertions of soft tissue elements are more correctly called enthesiophytes.

Trauma. especially when associated with joint instability, infectious and non-infectious arthroses may all result in the formation of periarticular bony deposits. (Figure 5.7)

A number of sesamoid bones are identified in association with joints. These, and the normal variations in their appearance, must not be mistaken for pathological lesions. In cases of doubt a comparison with the contralateral limb will usually resolve the dilemma.

A small sesamoid is occasionally found on the lateral aspect of the elbow joint in larger breed dogs. It lies within the ulnaris lateralis tendon and is a normal structure. (Figure 5.8, page 146)

The sesamoids in the manus and pes may appear 'fragmented'. Fracture of these bones has been reported, however, congenital anomalies where the bones are bipartite or multipartite are not uncommon.

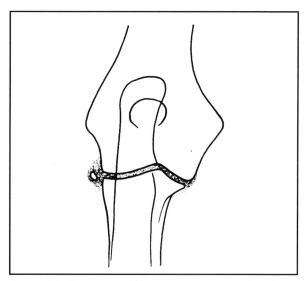

Figure 5.8: The normal ulnaris lateralis sesamoid found lateral to the elbow joint in some larger breeds of dogs.

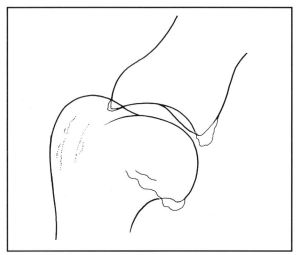

Figure 5.7: Osteoarthritis of the shoulder.
New bone with sharp and ragged or smooth margins may be present at the periphery of the component bones of a joint. The smoother and more well defined the osteophytes are, the more established and inactive the condition.

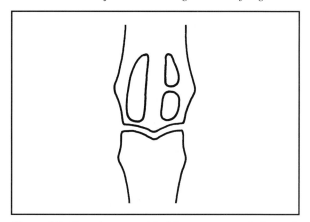

Figure 5.9: Bipartite sesamoid of the metacarpo-phalangeal joint.

The second and seventh sesamoid are those most often affected i.e. the abaxial sesamoids of the second and seventh digits. The clinical significance of these changes is dependant on the symmetry of the changes and the presence of pain on palpation of the region. (Figure 5.9)

The patella may fracture but can occasionally be bipartite. Again, a clinical assessment and comparison with the opposite limb will help to resolve the dilemma.

Two fabellae are always present caudal to the distal femur and may be displaced if the gastrocnemius muscle is damaged. A small sesamoid is usually present caudo-lateral to the stifle in the head of the popliteus muscle but variations in projection mean that it is not always identified.

Clavicular remnants, whilst not a true sesamoid, are present in the muscles at the base of the neck in the cat and rarely in the dog and should be recognised as normal.

2.3) Joint space

Capsular distension will be evident in distal limb joints such as the carpus and tarsus by virtue of the displacement of the skin contour. In the stifle displacement of the caudal fascial planes and obliteration or reduction of the infra-patellar fat pad will be indicative of a synovial effusion. Similar but more subtle displacement of fascial planes and fat pads may be of value in the assessment of capsular distension in the canine elbow. Synovial distension of the shoulder or hip joint cannot be assessed radiographically. (Figure 5.10)

Intra-capsular gas may be evident in compound wounds or septic arthritides where gas forming organisms are present.

The width of the joint space can only be evaluated critically if weight bearing films have been taken. However gross increases in the width of the joint space may be evident if a space occupying lesion is present within the joint e.g. synovial cell tumour. A decrease in the width of the joint space is indicative of loss of articular cartilage and if severe enough to be identifiable radiographically must be a significant finding. (Figure 5.11)

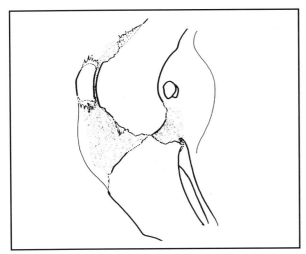

Figure 5.10: Distension of the joint capsule and erosion of the subchondral bone is seen in this example of septic arthritis.

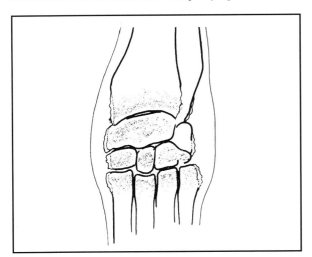

Figure 5.11: Osteoarthritis of the carpus with narrowing of the joint space.

Radio-dense bodies free within the joint space may be visible and can be interpreted as small fracture fragments, mineralised cartilage resulting from osteochondrosis, or the result of soft tissue mineralisation within the joint. In young dogs a small separate ossification centre may be seen just caudal to the glenoid cavity of the scapula and is a normal variant thought to be a seperate ossification centre. (Figure 5.12)

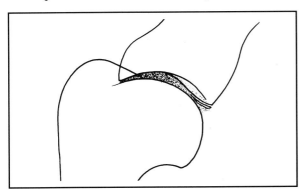

Figure 5.12: Separate ossification centre of the glenoid rim in a young dog.

2.4) Number of joints involved

The number of joints affected may give some evidence regarding the aetiology of the condition. Single damaged joints are most likely to result from trauma, infection or neoplasia. If the changes are bilaterally symmetrical then congenital or developmental disease must be suspected although trauma cannot be ruled out. Multiple joint involvement suggests that the aetiology is related to a systemic problem in which infective, degenerative or autoimmune factors may be suspected.

2.5) Categorisation of the type of joint disease

Once the above steps have been completed it may be possible to categorise the nature of the arthrosis. This may only allow a list of differentials in order of probability to be drawn up. The definitive diagnosis will only be possible when the radiological features are viewed in conjunction with the clinical and laboratory findings.

3)   Evaluation of Bone Architecture

Bones are only able to react to disease in a limited number of ways and it is the combination and distribution of these changes together with the progression over a period of time which will lead to the radiograph indicating the most likely diagnosis.

Altered size and shape
   Decreased size with normal conformation
   Decreased size with altered conformation

Decreased bone density
   Generalised
   Polyostotic
   Monostotic with multiple lesions
   Monostotic with a solitary lesion

Increased bone density
   Generalised
   Polyostotic
   Monostotic with multiple lesions
   Monostotic with a solitary lesion

Changes to the bone cortex
   Cortical thinning
   Cortical thickening
   Focal destruction of the cortex
   Subchondral destruction

Changes to the trabecular bone
   Trabecular thickening/thinning

Endosteal new bone

Periosteal new bone
   Parallel - 'onion skin'
   Smooth - well defined
   Irregular
   Radiating - 'sunburst'

3.1) Altered size and shape

Decreased size with normal conformation - This is seen in an individual where there is no structural deformity, merely a reduction in growth potential. The bones will be of normal proportion and mineralisation but reduced in size e.g. stunting due to congenital cardiovascular defects, hypothyroidism or pituitary dwarfism.

Decreased size with altered conformation - This occurs in those situations where there is either an alteration in overall skeletal proportions e.g. chondrodystrophy or an alteration in size and shape of a portion of the skeleton e.g. secondary to premature physeal closure.

3.2) Decreased bone density

A decrease in radiopacity of the skeleton may be very obvious on the radiograph or it may be necessary to compare the affected bone with another part of the skeleton, the radiopacity of the soft tissues or with an animal of similar size and age where similar exposure factors have been used.

Decrease in bone density may be due to osteopaenia - decreased bone mass due to failure of osteoblasts to lay down bone matrix - or to osteomalacia - insuffient or abnormal mineralisation of an otherwise adequate amount of osteoid tissue. It will not be possible to differentiate between these radiologically.

Generalised: Either primary (rare) or secondary (common) hyperparathyroidism will result in generalised reduced bone density with cortical thinning and often pathological fractures. The nutritional form is seen in young growing animals where there is a high phosphorus: low calcium ratio in the diet. In animals with chronic renal disease retention of phosphorus, a more selective form, primarily affecting the bones of the skull and mandible is seen.

Generalised reduction in bone mineralisation will occur in persistently high levels of circulating corticosteroids. This may be secondary to hyperadrenocorticism or iatrogenic.

Chronic protein deprivation or loss will also result in generalised demineralisation of the skeleton.

Polyostotic: The reduced bone density may affect several bones, e.g. one limb, but not be generalised to the whole skeleton. Chronic disuse of a limb will lead to bone atrophy and demineralisation - this is reversible once limb function is regained.

Metastatic neoplasia or multicentric primary bone neoplasms such as multiple myeloma will result in focal reductions in density in several bones throughout the skeleton.

Retained cartilage cores are often seen in the distal ulnar metaphyses of young large breed dogs. They are sometimes incidental findings but may be associated with angular limb deformities. Their significance is not well understood. (Figure 5.13)

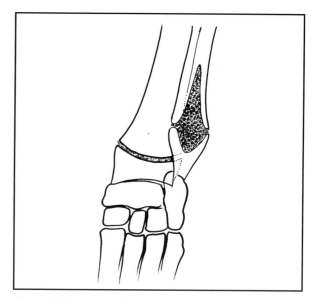

Figure 5.13: A retained core of cartilage in the distal metaphysis of the ulnar resulting in a characteristic shaped lucency.

Monostotic with multiple lesions: This is an uncommon finding but conditions to be considered would include haematogenous osteomyelitis or possibly neoplasia.

Monostotic with a solitary lesion: Osteomyelitis either haematogenous or resulting from penetrating wounds will cause in focal bone destruction. (Figure 5.14)

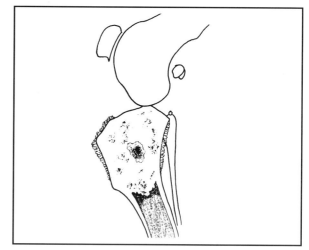

Figure 5.14: Haematogenous osteomyelitis of the tibia showing a central focal lucency and surrounding metaphysea sclerosis and periosteal new bone.

Primary and metastatic neoplasia will regularly result in bone lysis. The metaphyses are the most likely sites to be affected.

3.3) Increased bone density

Generalised: This is rare. Osteopetrosis resulting from hypervitaminosis D and myelofibrosis have both been reported and an hereditary anaemia reported in Basenjis will cause a generalised increase in bone density.

Polyostotic: Panosteitis is an enigmatic disease affecting primarily young German Shepherd dogs, although it must not be overlooked in other breeds. It is manifested by patchy increases in density of the medulla of long bones - humerus, femur, radius/ulna, tibia - progressing to an even opacification of the medulla. Periosteal reaction will be seen in a proportion of the cases.

Although more than one bone is often affected the changes are rarely bilaterally symmetrical. (Figure 5.15)

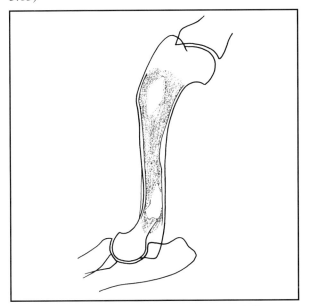

Figure 5.15: Amorphous, pathcy increases in medullary density typical of panosteitis.

Metastatic bone tumours are more frequently sclerotic than lytic. Fungal osteomyelitis is rare in this country and focal increase in bone density is one of the characteristic radiological signs and should be considered in imported animals.

Metaphyseal osteopathy affecting the metaphyses of young large breed dogs is characterised by metaphyseal lucency in the early stages. However, in the later and healing phases there will be increased metaphyseal density and the deposition of periosteal bone. (Figure 5.16)

Lead poisoning is reported to cause increase in metaphyseal density in a banded pattern but such changes are rarely seen.

Monostotic with multiple lesions - Rarely seen although a sclerotic metastatic neoplasm could have several deposits in a single bone.

Monostotic with a solitary lesion - Primary bone tumours will not infrequently be more osteogenic than osteolytic and so result in increased density. Metastatic neoplasms will also be frequently sclerotic in appearance. (Figure 5.17)

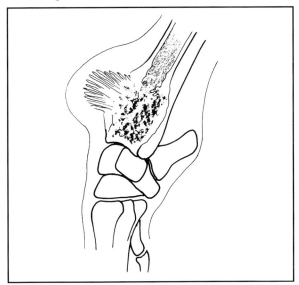

Figure 5.17: Amorphous lucencies admixed with marked bony proliferation in the metaphysis of the radius characteristic of a bony tumour.

Healing and healed fractures and fresh impacted fractures will produce areas of increased density within a bone. Sequestrae and area of bone necrosis are often claimed to show an increased radiopacity but this is not the case. There is, however, usually hyperaemia and demineralisation of the surrounding bone which results in an apparent increase in opacity of the dead bone.

Haematogenous and iatrogenic osteomyelitis although containing single or multiple areas of lucency

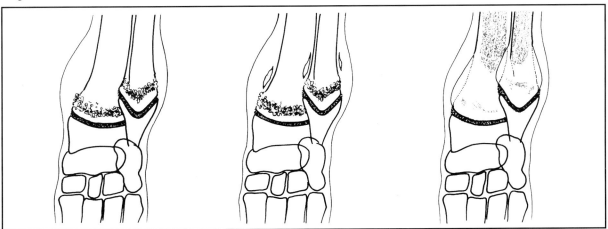

Figure 5.16: Metaphyseal deposits of new bone in metaphyseal osteopathy will result in increased density in several bones.

will usually be surrounded by a zone of proliferating sclerotic bone resulting in marked increase in radio-pacity.

Traumatic or septic periostitis will give a bone an increased radiodensity as the collar of periosteal new bone will be superimposed on the cortex and medulla in most planes.

3.4) Changes to the bone cortex.

Cortical thinning: Cortical thinning will occur in osteoporosis resulting from either nutritional factors or disuse. (Figure 5.18)

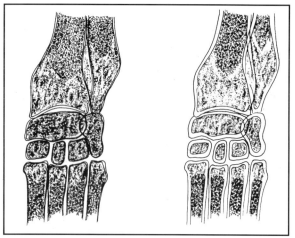

Figure 5.18: Thinning of the cortices and generalised increased radiolucency of the bones in disuse osteoporosis.

Physeal abnormalities resulting in angular limb deformities will have a thinned cortex on the non-weight bearing aspect of the limb. (Figure 5.19)

Expansile intra-osseous lesions such as bone cysts and slowly growing cystic neoplasms will result in cortical thinning from the medullary aspect whilst expanding soft tissue lesions adjacent to the bone can result in cortical thinning from the periosteal aspect.

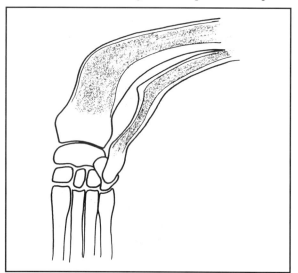

Figure 5.19: The angular deformity in this limb resulting from a malunion fracture repair has led to a discrepancy in cortical thickness.

Cortical thickening: May be difficult to differentiate from the deposition of periosteal new bone. e.g.

Hypertrophic osteopathy   Periostitis
Metaphyseal osteopathy   Angular limb deformities
Chronic osteomyelitis   Panosteitis
Healing fractures

Focal lesions of the cortex: are not common but greenstick or impacted fractures may result in focal cortical thickening whilst benign tumours and bone cysts may result in focal cortical thinning. (Figure 5.20)

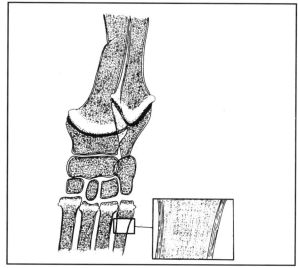

Figure 5.20: Folding or 'greenstick' fracture associated with nutritional osteoporosis.

Subchondral destruction: May be single or multiple focal lucencies or defects. Osteochondritis dissecans of the humeral head, medial distal humeral condyle, femoral condyles and medial ridge of the tibial tarsal bone are all associated with subchondral defects. (Figure 5.21)

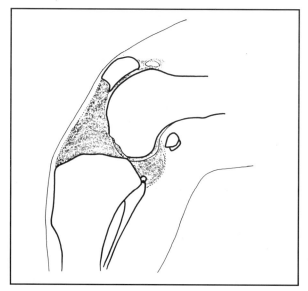

Figure 5.21: Subchondral bone destruction seen in an osteochondritis dissecans lesion of the femoral condyle.

Avascular necrosis of the femoral head - Perthes disease - will result in subchondral collapse and irregularity. Septic arthritis will frequently extend into the subchondral bone which becomes irregular and pitted. Similar erosive changes will be seen in the erosive inflammatory arthritides such as rheumatoid arthritis.

In degenerative joint disease the margins of the articular bone will become irregular due to the deposition of posteophytes whilst the subchondral bone may become irregular and sclerotic. (Figure 5.22)

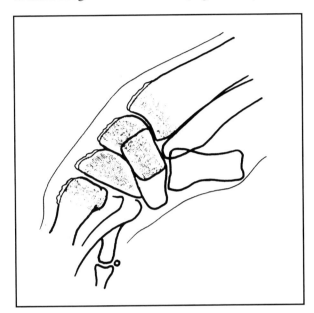

Figure 5.22: Degenerative joint disease of the carpus with margina osteophytes and subchondral sclerosis.

3.5) Changes to the trabecular bone

Trabecular thickening: The trabecular pattern of bone should be evaluated carefully. Good quality radiographs are essential and the exposure factors must be appropriate.

Both primary and metastatic bone tumours will disrupt the trabecular pattern and may lead to thickening and coarsening of the trabeculation.

Any area of bone sclerosis such as that seen in osteomyelitis will also have associated trabecular thickening.

The late stages of panosteitis may show a resolution of the medullary densities but leave a subtle coarsening of trabecular detail.

3.6) Endosteal new bone

Endosteal deposition of bone will occur in panosteitis and in the region of a fracture callus.

3.7) Periosteal new bone

The deposition of periosteal new bone is a frequent finding, the significance and appearance of which is highly variable. The pattern of the periosteal new bone may be of value in indicating the aetiology of a bone lesion.

The types of periosteal responses seen are -

Parallel - 'onion skin' - associated with slowly growing progressive relatively non-aggressive lesions, e.g. trauma, infection, slowly growing benign tumours. (Figure 5.23)

Smooth - well defined - associated with chronic non-aggressive lesions, e.g. healed fractures, chronic infection etc. (Figure 5.24)

Irregular - associated with active aggressive lesions e.g. osteomyelitis, neoplasia, hypertrophic osteopathy etc. (Figure 5.25)

Radiating - 'sunburst' - associated with very active aggressive often malignant lesion e.g. osteosarcoma. (Figure 5.26)

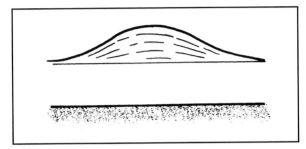

Figure 5.23: Periosteal new bone - 'onion skin' type.

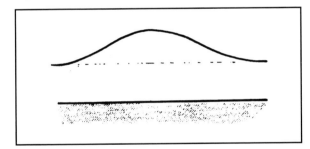

Figure 5.24: Periosteal new bone - Smooth well defined.

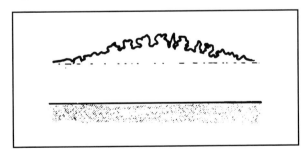

Figure 5.25: Periosteal new bone - Irregular.

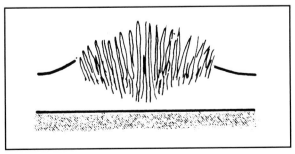

Figure 5.26: Periosteal new bone - Radiating/'sunburst'.

	Benign/non-aggressive		Malignant/aggressive
Margin	Sharp	→	Indistinct
Border	Well defined	→	Ill defined
Cortex	Intact	→	Broken
Periosteum	Intact	→	Interrupted
Periosteal bone	Well structured	→	Irregular
Rate of change	Slow	→	Rapid
Zone of transition	Short, well defined	→	Long, ill defined

Table 5.1: Aggressiveness and/or malignancy of a lesion.

4) Identification of the Part of the Bone Involved

The part of the bone involved may give some indication of the aetiology of the changes observed. Long bones are divided into the epiphysis, physis, metaphysis and diaphysis.

4.1) The epiphysis
This may be the site of haematogenous osteomyelitis and occasionally primary bone tumours may arise in this region. Multiple epiphyseal dysplasia has been described in certain breeds and results in irregular epiphyseal shape with mixed punctate lucencies and densities due to irregular ossification. (Figure 5.27)

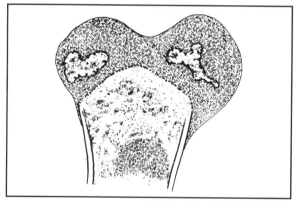

Figure 5.27: Irregular epiphyseal mineralisation seen in epiphyseal dysplasia.

4.2) The physis
Because of the rich blood supply this may be the site of infection in the growing animal. Damage to the physis may result in premature closure and angular limb deformities.

4.3) The metaphysis
Primary bone tumours, particularly osteosarcomas regularly arise in the metaphyses. Similarly, skeletal metastases although rare in the dog and cat are most often deposited in the cancellous bone of the metaphysis. In the growing large breed dog metaphyseal osteopathy, as its name suggests, is located at this site.

4.4) The diaphysis
This is the region frequently affected by injury resulting in fractures.

5) Assessing the Agressiveness and/or Malignancy of a Lesion

The final radiological diagnosis may depend on monitoring the rate of change over a period of time by obtaining sequential films. Mixed osteo-destructive and osteo-productive lesions may be difficult to categorise initially as infective or neoplastic but assessment of the rate of progression will give evidence as to their aetiology. (Table 5.1)

II: INTERPRETATION BONES - GENERAL

Fractures
It is not proposed to deal with the wide variety of fractures that can occur in the dog and cat. A full evaluation of any fracture prior to surgical repair will include at least two views taken at right angles to each other and in some cases additional radiographs will also be required. The features of fresh fractures will include:

- Discontinuity of the affected bone or bones, with two more fragments.
- The fracture surfaces will normally be sharply defined.
- The fragments may be either minimally displaced or grossly out of position.
- If adjacent fragments overlap, instead of a lucent line there may be a linear increase in opacity in one plane whereas the radiograph taken in the other plane will clearly demonstrate the degree of displacement and overlap.
- There will usually be soft tissue swelling and loss of soft tissue detail such as fascial planes.
- The presence of abnormal lucencies may indicate that the fracture is compound with either entrapped air or infection with gas forming organisms present.
- In fractures involving joints there may be associated subluxation of the joint.

If the fracture is not fresh - ie. one week or more since the original injury - the radiographic appearance will be slightly different:

- The fracture surfaces will have resorbed to some degree and may be less clearly defined.
- The fracture line may appear slightly widened.
- There may be evidence of early periosteal reaction both immediately adjacent to the fracture site and also in some cases extending some way along the adjacent cortical bone surface.

The signs of normal fracture healing after either internal or external fixation include:

- The production of well mineralised callous.
- The amount of callous produced depends on the location and type of fracture as well as the means of stabilisation.
- There will be less callous produced following stable internal fixation than after external methods of fracture support.
- There will also tend to be less callous associated with the healing of small bones of the carpus, hock and spine than in long bones such as the femur and humerus.
- The fracture line will initially widen and become less distinct and then will become mineralised after the fracture has been bridged by callous eventually disappearing.
- The callous will initially be composed of mottled, randomly structured bone but will gradually mature into well trabeculated cancellous bone with a smooth periosteal surface.

It is important to distinguish from this normal pattern of fracture healing and the two main complications of fracture repair - Non union, which may be either hypertrophic or atrophic, and Osteomyelitis.

Non-Union

Hypertrophic: usually a sequel to either inadequate stabilisation of the original fracture or infection.

Atrophic; seen more commonly in the distal radius and ulna of miniature breeds.

Radiological features (Figure 5.28)
- Lucent line at site of fracture still evident.
- Fracture ends smooth.
- Sclerosis of the opposing fracture margins.
- Sealing of the medullary cavity with endosteal bone.
- Any callus on the bone adjacent to the fracture site fails to bridge the fracture.
- There may be clear evidence of a psuedo-arthrosis with one fracture surface convex and the opposing surface concave.
- In the atrophic type there is little or no periosteal bone reaction.

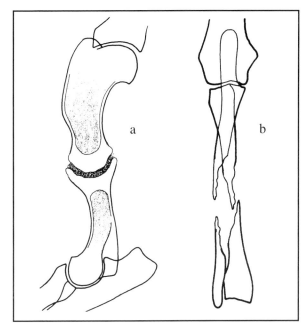

Figure 5.28a and b: *Fracture non-union.*
a: Hypertrophic non-union. b: Atrophic non-union.

Osteomyelitis

Most commonly a sequel to surgical fracture repair. Less commonly a sequel to an open fracture or an open/puncture wound. Occasionally may be haematogeneous.

Radiological features (Figure 5.29)

Acute:
- Moderately aggressive periosteal reaction.
- May be some lysis of cortical and trabeculabone.
- Swelling of adjacent soft tissue.
- If associated with fracture repair the periosteal reaction will be more extensive and irregular than normal callus.

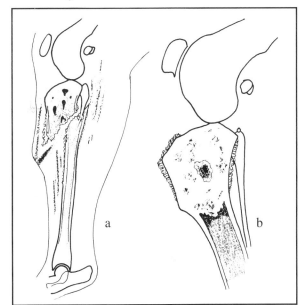

Figure 5.29a and b: *a: Acute osteomyelitis secondary to a compound fracture with interstitiak gas. b: Haematogenous osteomyelitis.*

Chronic:
- Sclerotic bony proliferation round margin of lesion.
- May be mature irregular periosteal reaction.
- Central area of bone lysis - cortical and trabecular.
- Minimal soft tissue swelling.

    N.B. Acute or chronic osteomyelitis of haematogenous origin may be very difficult to differentiate from a primary bone tumour on purely radiological evidence.

Osteomyelitis - Sequestra
Usually secondary to repair of a comminuted fracture with or without secondary osteomyelitis.

Radiological features (Figure 5.30)
- Exuberant periosteal reaction.
- Sequestrum identified as a more or less well delineated fragment of bone with no surface periosteal reaction.
- Surrounded by a radiolucent halo, the involucrum, outside which is sclerotic bone.
- Sequestrum may appear radiodense due to the surrounding lucency.

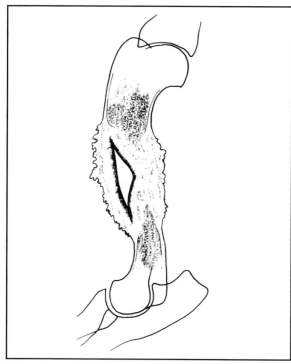

Figure 5.30: Osteomylitis - sequestrae.

Panosteitis
Synonyms - enostosis, eosinophilic panosteitis. Most commonly seen in juvenile German Shepherd dogs 6-18 months old, predominantly males. Must also be considered in other large breed dogs. Acute or shifting lameness. Pain on pressure of the affected bone or bones. Aetiology unknown, usually self limiting as dog matures.

Radiological features (Figure 5.31)
- May be seen in one or more sites.
- Most commonly affects femur, humerus, radius/ulna and tibia.
- Rarely bilaterally symmetrical.
- Areas of increased medullary opacity either patchy or diffuse - 'thumbprint' opacity.
- Endosteal thickening of the cortical bone often close to the nutrient foramen.
- Occasionally a smooth periosteal reaction will be seen.

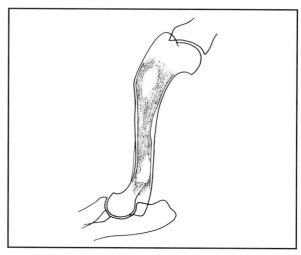

Figure 5.31: Panosteitis.

Osteopaenia/Osteoporosis
Nutritional secondary hyper-parathyroidism. Seen in young rapidly growing dogs more commonly of the larger breeds fed on a mainly meat diet with inadequate calcium supplementation. May also be seen in kittens and exotic animals also fed a diet with an incorrect cacium/phosphorus ratio.

Radiological features (Figure 5.32)
- Decreased radiopacity of bone.
- Cortical thinning.
- Cortical bone may become lamellated.
- Relative increase in radiopacity of the metaphyseal bone.
- Flaring of the metaphyseal bone.
- Physis of normal width.
- May be folding or collapse fractures.

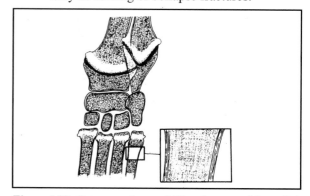

Figure 5.32: Osteoporosis note folding fracture of the radial diaphysis.

Generalised Osteopaenia due to other Causes

Most other causes are more likely to be encountered in adult animals. Associated with longstanding hyperadrenocorticism (Cushing's syndrome) or prolonged steroid therapy. May be sequel to primary hyperparathyroidism. May be associated with disseminated neoplasia such as lymphoma.

Radiological features (Figure 5.33)
*   Reduced radiopacity of bone most easily appreciated in the spine.
*   Has to be very severe and longstanding before changes apparent in the appendicular skeleton.

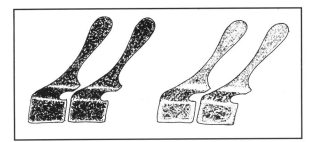

Figure 5.33: Generalised osteoporosis due to other causes.

Disuse Osteoporosis

Will be seen as a sequel to disuse oimmobilisation of a limb.

Radiological features (Figure 5.34)
*   Changes restricted to the affected limb.
*   Reduced radiopacity and cortical thinning.
*   Often most apparent in the bones of the carpus/tarsus and foot.

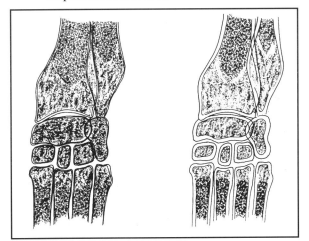

Figure 5.34: Disuse osteoporosis.

Metaphyseal Osteopathy

Synonyms - Hypertrophic osteodystrophy, Skeletal scurvy, Barlow's disease, Avitaminosis C. Aetiology unclear - often associated with nutritional over supplementation. Most commonly seen in large breed young dogs 3-6 months old. Lameness usually affecting all four limbs. Metaphyseal swelling and pain. Pyrexia.

Radiological features (Figure 5.35)
*   Physes normal width with zone of provisional calcification of cartilage visible.
*   All metaphyses have irregular bands of radiolucency most obvious in distal radius and ulna.
*   Changes bilaterally symmetrical.
*   Initially soft tissue swelling round metaphyses.
*   Latterly para-periosteal deposition of new bone eventually forming a collar of bone around the metaphysis and subsequent bone deformity.

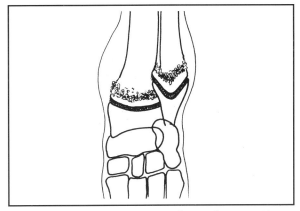

Figure 5.35a: Metaphyseal osteopathy - early stage with metaphyseal lucencies.

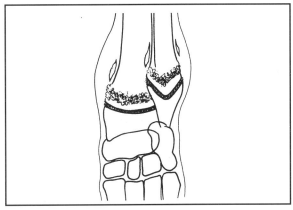

Figure 5.35b: Metaphyseal osteopathy - later stage with para-periosteal new bone deposition.

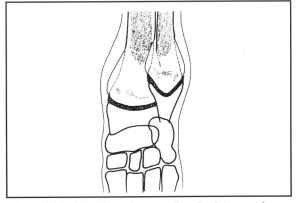

Figure 5.35c: Metaphyseal osteopathy - final stage with metaphyseal thickening sclerosis.

Rickets

Very RARE as naturally occurring condition in dog and cat. Associated with combination of inadequate mineral supplementation and vitamin D deficiency. A possible genetic defect resulting in disturbed vitamin D metabolism has recently been reported.

Radiological features (Figure 5.36)
- Marked widening of all physes.
- Cupping or 'mushrooming' of the metaphyses.
- In addition usually evidence of nutritional osteoporosis as described above.

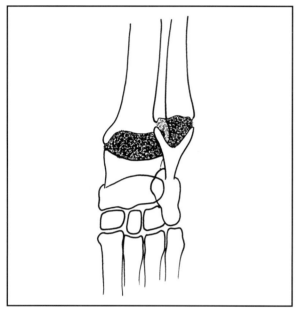

Figure 5.36: Rickets.

Muco-Polysaccharidoses

Inherited metabolic defect in the metabolism of polysaccharides. Seen in cats primarily Siamese. Results in epiphyseal dysplasia.

Radiological features (Figure 5.37)
- Mottled irregular epiphyses to long bones and vertebral end plates.

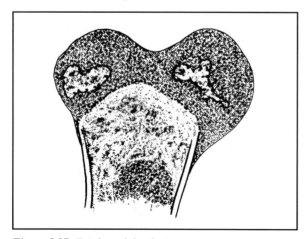

Figure 5.37: Epiphyseal dysplasia seen in muco-polysaccharidoses.

Cranio-Mandibular Osteopathy

Seen mainly in the West Highland White Terrier and related breeds. Pain and swelling round mandibular rami and temporal regions. May be difficulty in opening mouth.

Radiological features (Figure 5.38)
- Active periosteal reaction on ventral aspect of mandibular rami and/or petrous temporal bones.
- Changes may affect one or both sites and be uni- or bi-lateral.
- May progress to produce large bony swellings and osteo-sclerosis.
- Reactive new bone may encroach onto the margins of the temporo-mandibular joint and restrict range of movement.

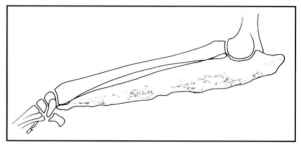

Figure 5.38: Cranio-mandibular osteopathy (for skull changes see Fig. 2.10). This diagram illustrates the changes occasionally affecting the long bones.

Renal Secondary Hyperparathyroidism

Synonyms - Rubber jaw, Renal osteodystrophy. Associated with clinical signs of chronic renal disease. Most common in adult and elderly dogs with chronic nephritis. Also seen in young animals with familial nephropathies.

Radiological features (Figure 5.39)
- Demineralisation of the mandibles and fascial bones.
- In the early stages may only be loss of the lamina dura and radiolucent halos round the tooth roots.
- The mineralised tissue of the teeth remains unaffected so that they stand out against the osteoporotic fascial and mandibular bones.
- May be dystrophic calcification of soft tissues in advanced cases e.g. mesenteric vessels and aorta.

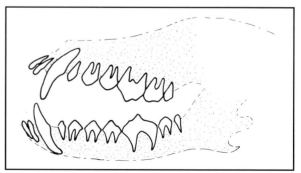

Figure 5.39: Renal secondary hyperparathyroidism.

Calcinosis Circumscripta

Seen mainly in larger breeds of dog, mainly German Shepherd dogs. Subcutaneous fibrous nodules associated with the carpus, tarsus and feet. May also occur in the cervical muscle adjacent to the transverse processes of the vertebrae. Often asymptomatic.

Radiological features (Figure 5.40)

- Nodular soft tissue mass with amorphous mineralisation.
- No lysis or periosteal reaction of adjacent bones although the lesion may be closely associated with them.
- Occasionally seen associated with the dorsal spinous process when there may be pressure erosion of the bone and spinal cord compression.

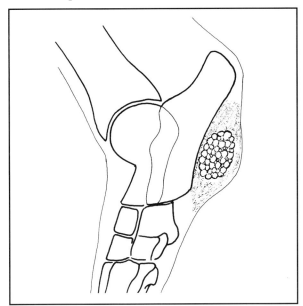

Figure 5.40: Calcinosis circumscripta.

Hypertrophic Osteopathy

Synonyms - Hypertrophic pulmonary osteo- arthropathy (HPOA), Maries disease. Most commonly associated with chronic or space occupying lesion of the thoracic or, rarely, the abdominal cavity. All four limbs become swollen but pain free. Increasing stiffness and lameness.

Radiological features (Figure 5.41)

- Marked soft tissue swelling of all four limbs.
- Well structured pallisade or plaque like periosteal reaction.
- Initially affects metapodial bones and extends progressively more proximally to involve carpal/tarsal bones, radius/ulna/tibia, eventually femur/humerus.
- No underlying bone destruction.
- Articular surfaces unaffected.
- Radiographic examination of thorax for the underlying causative lesion indicated.

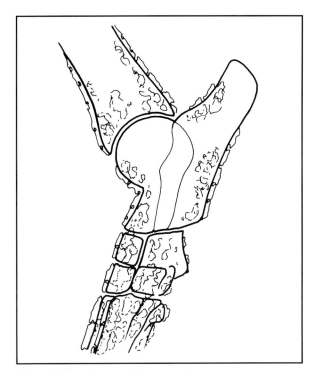

Figure 5.41a: Hypertrophic osteopathy.

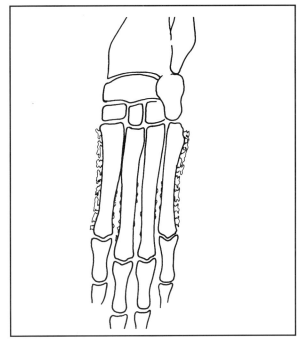

Figure 5.41b: Hypertrophic osteopathy.

Osteosarcoma

Most common primary tumour of bone. Seen mainly in large breed dogs and sporadically in other breeds and in cats. Clinical evidence of acute lameness, pain, swelling and often heat in the affected bone. Classical sites are - (Figure 5.42)

i) Proximal humerus
ii) Distal radius
iii) Distal femuir
iv) Proximal tibia
v) Also seen sporadically in the axial skeleton- skull, ribs and pelvis.

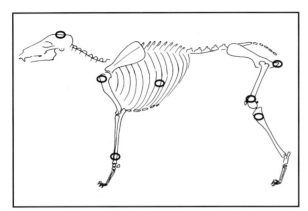

Figure 5.42: Classical sites of osteosarcoma in the dog.

Radiological features (Figure 5.43)
- Lysis of cortical and trabecular bone.
- Proliferation of variable amount of tumour bone in the form of irregular structured and spiculated bone.
- Most commonly arise in the metaphyseal region of long bones.
- Poorly marginated.
- May be marginal periosteal reaction forming a so called 'Codman's triangle'.
- Usually marked soft tissue swelling.
- Rarely invade adjacent bones or cross joint spaces.
- Ratio of bone lysis: bone proliferation varies from one extreme to the other.
- Osteosarcomas affecting skull and pelvis frequently very osteo-proliferative whereas those affecting ribs often mainly lytic.
- In the cat much less common and usually very lytic and aggressive in appearance.

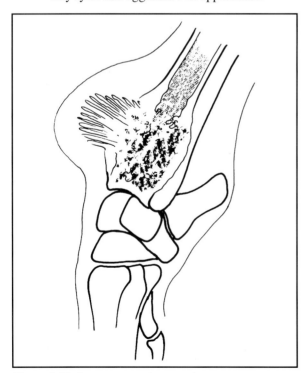

Figure 5.43: Osteosarcoma.

Enchondroma
Uncommon tumour of bone seen mainly associated with the skull.

Radiological features (Figure 5.44)
- Spiculated proliferation of periosteal bone inter-mixed with lucencies.
- No underlying cortical destruction.

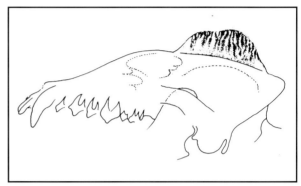

Figure 5.44: Enchondroma.

Osteoma
Uncommon benign tumour of bone most commonly affecting the skull.

Radiological features (Figure 5.45)
- Very dense accumulation of bone tissue forming a more or less spherical bony mass.
- No underlying bone destruction although original architecture may be masked.

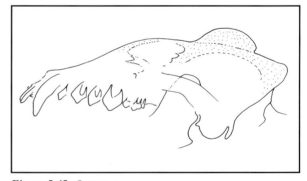

Figure 5.45: Osteoma.

Other Primary Bone Neoplasms
Much less common than osteosarcoma. May affect a wide variety of breeds and no particular site predilection.

Radiological features (Figure 5.46)
- Will usually be predominantly lytic although there may be some marginal periosteal reaction.
- May extend to involve adjacent bones.
- May cross joint spaces.
- Usually very extensive soft tissue swelling.

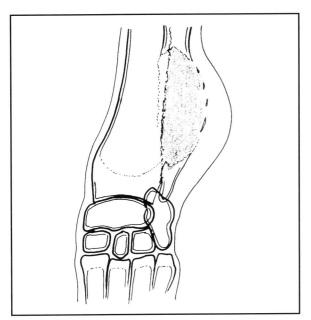

Figure 5.46: Primary bone neoplasms other than osteosarcomas.

Bone Cysts

Rare in small animals. Most often seen in the larger breeds of dog.

Radiological features (Figure 5.47)
- Smooth walled lucencies often septate.
- Sharply demarcated from the surrounding bone.
- May result in cortical thinning but with no accompanying periosteal reaction.

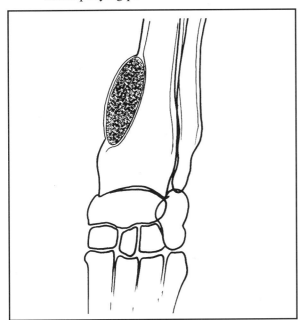

Figure 5.47: Bone cysts.

Multiple Cartilaginous Exostoses

Occasionally seen in both dogs and cats. Occur in the young growing animal and stop developing as the skeleton matures. Neurological signs may develop when the vertebral column is affected.

Radiological features (Figure 5.48)
- Expansile bony protrusion from the periosteal surface of the growing bones.
- May affect both the appendicular and axial skeleton.
- Usually multiple bones involved.
- Usually well defined thin cortical shell with coarse bone trabeculations.
- May result in skeletal and soft tissue deformity due to the expansile nature of the lesions.

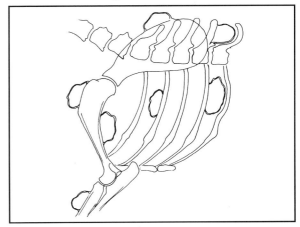

Figure 5.48: Multiple cartilagenous exostoses.

Metastatic Bone "Disease"

Uncommon in the dog and rare in the cat. Metastatic spread from bronchial, mammary, thyroid, tonsillar and prostatic carcinomas have all been recorded.

Radiological features (Figure 5.49)
- For lesions in the axial skeleton see the appropriate section.
- Lesions in the appendicular skeleton most frequently seen in the metaphyses.
- May be either lytic or sclerotic in appearance.
- Differentiation from primary bone neoplasia based mainly on identification of the soft tissue primary and the usually polyostotic distribution of the metastases.

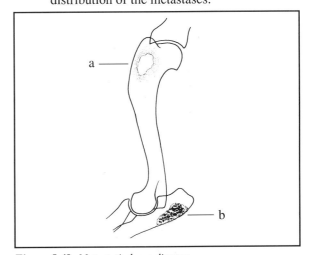

Figure 5.49: Metastatic bone disease
a: ostesclerotic type. b: osteolytic type

Premature Growth Plate Closure - Ulna

Seen in young growing dogs. Often secondary to known trauma to the distal limb. May occur apparently unrelated to injury. Often associated with angular limb deformities.

Radiological features (Figure 5.50)
- Lateral angulation of the distal radius, carpus and foot.
- Proximal distraction of the styloid process.
- Dorsal bowing of the radius with alterations in cortical thickness.
- Humero-ulnar subluxation with distal distraction of the semilunar notch and coronoid processes may be seen in a proportion of cases.

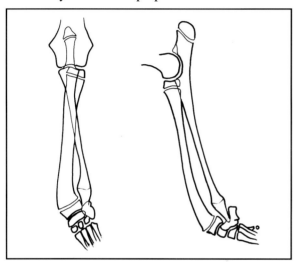

Figure 5.50a and b: Premature growth closure - ulna.

Premature Growth Plate Closure - Radius

Seen in young growing dogs. Often secondary to known trauma to the distal limb. May occur apparently unrelated to injury. Rarely associated with angular limb deformities. Less common than premature closure of the distal ulna growth plate.

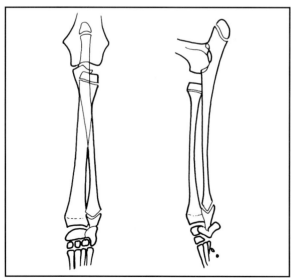

Figure 5.51a and b: Premature growth closure - radius.

Radiological features (Figure 5.51)
- Shortened radius when compared with contralateral limb.
- Widening of the humero-radial and radio-carpal joint spaces.

Retained Cartilage Core in the Distal Ulnar Metaphysis

Seen in large breed young dogs. Clinical significance uncertain. May be associated with angular limb deformities.

Radiological features (Figure 5.52)
- Elongated lucency extending from the physis into the metaphysis of the ulna.

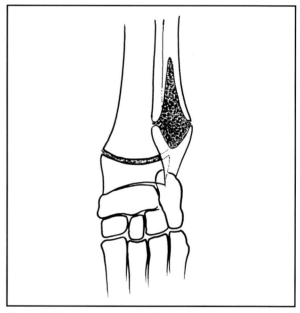

Figure 5.52: Retained core in the distal ulna metaphysis.

III: JOINTS - GENERAL

The changes described in this first section are general comments that apply to whichever joint may be affected. Some joints may be more likely to be involved in a particular type of pathological change and the precise response may vary from joint to joint. Where relevant these variations will be indicated in the next sections dealing with individual joints.

Arthritis

Primary Osteoarthritis
Rare in the dog and cat.

Radiological features (Figure 5.53)
- Soft tissue swelling round the affected joint.
- Periarticular osteophytic reaction.
- Narrowing of the joint space.
- True primary osteoarthritis is likely to affect several joints simultaneously.

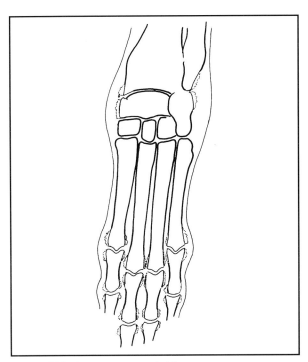

Figure 5.53: Primary osteoarthritis.

Secondary Osteoarthritis

May affect any joint. Usually a sequel to either:
a)   injury.
b)   joint instability.
c)   developmental or acquired joint deformity.

Characterised by lameness, stiffness, joint swelling and crepitus on manipulation.

Radiological features (Figure 5.54)
- Soft tissue swelling round the affected joint.
- Synovial hypertrophy and joint effusion where this can be detected radiologically.
- Periarticular osteophytic proliferation.
- In the late stages narrowing of the joint space indicative of articular cartilage erosion may be detected.

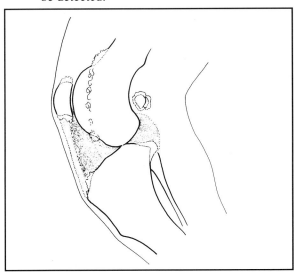

Figure 5.54: Secondary osteoarthritis of the stifle.

Inflammatory Non-Erosive Polyarthritis

May occur in any breed of dog and also in cats. Can occur in animals of all ages. May be associated with other signs of systemic illness. Usually results in a shifting lameness with involvement of more than one joint.

Radiological features (Figure 5.55)
- Soft tissue swelling of the affected joint(s).
- Synovial effusion may be seen where this can be detected radiologically.
- Usually no other abnormalities observed.

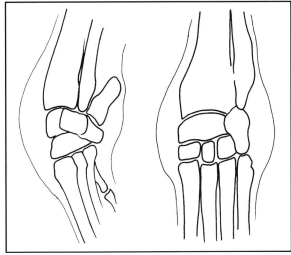

Figure 5.55a and b: Inflammatory non-erosive polyarthritis.

Inflammatory Erosive Polyarthritis

Much less common than the non- erosive type. Can affect dogs and cats (usually male neutered).

Radiological features (Figure 5.56)
- Soft tissue swelling of the affected joint(s).
- Synovial effusion may be seen where this can be detected radiologically.
- Erosion of articular cartilage, subchondral bone and articular margins may be seen.
- Often associated aggressive peri- articular periosteal reaction.

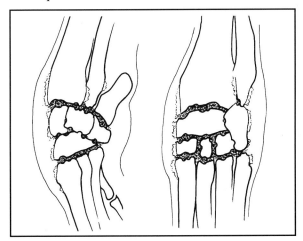

Figure 5.56a and b: Inflammatory erosive polyarthritis.

Septic Arthritis

Can affect any joint. May be sequel to a penetrating wound. Infection may be primary in young animals. May get secondary joint infection superimposed on a pre-existing osteoarthritis.

Radiological features (Figure 5.57)
- Soft tissue swelling around the joint - usually very marked.
- Synovial effusion where this can be detected radiologically.
- Erosion of subchondral bone may occur in severe or persistent infections.
- Peri-articular osteophytic reaction often more marked and aggressive looking than that seen in osteoarthritis.

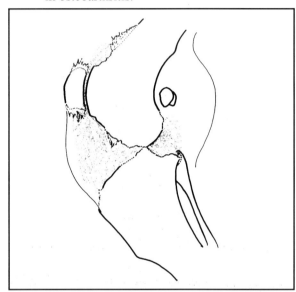

Figure 5.57: Septic arthritis.

Joint Neoplasia

Uncommon. Both benign and malignant synovial tumours can occur. Lameness and joint swelling usually develop gradually in the majority of cases.

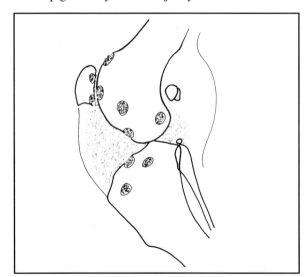

Figure 5.58: Synovial neoplasia.

Radiological features (Figure 5.58)
- Marked soft tissue swelling within and around the affected joint.
- Joint space will often appear widened due to the soft tissue proliferation.
- Usually no periarticular osteophytic reaction.
- Erosion of articular margins and subchondral bone with clearly marginated area of bone lysis.

THE FORELIMB

The standard radiographic positions for the examination of the joints will be described and illustrated. These views are adapted for the examination of the long bones by the appropriate centring of the X-ray beam.

Scapula: position as for shoulder but centre midway along the blade of the scapula.

Humerus: position as for shoulder or elbow but centre midway between the shoulder and the elbow.

Radius/ulna: position as for elbow or carpus but centre midway between the elbow and the carpus.

IV: THE SHOULDER

Positioning

Lateral view (Figure 5.59)
  i)   The animal should be in lateral recumbency with limb to be radiographed adjacent to the table.
  ii) The head and neck should be extended and held with sandbags.
  iii) The upper limb should be retracted caudally and secured with either ties or sandbags.
  iv) The limb under examination should be drawn forward and ventrally to ensure that the shoulder is not overlaid by either the pectoral muscle or the cervical spine.
  v) The beam should be centred on the shoulder which can be located by palpating the lateral tuberosity and centring the beam level with and caudal to it.

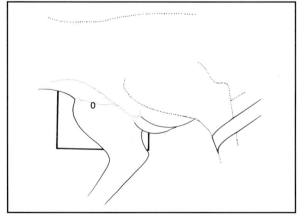

Figure 5.59: Shoulder positioning - lateral view.

Caudo-cranial view (Figure 5.60)

i)   This is the best position for imaging either the scapula or shoulder.

ii)   The animal is positioned on its back supported by sandbags or a radiolucent trough.

iii) The affected limb is drawn cranially, fully extended and secured with a tie.

iv)   The thorax may need to be rotated slightly away from the limb to be radiographed in order to prevent it being overlaid by the thoracic wall.

v)   For the shoulder joint the beam should be centred level with the acromion process, for the scapula it should be centred midway between the acromion and the caudal level of the scapula blade.

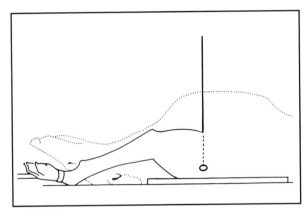

Figure 5.60: Shoulder positioning - caudo-cranial view.

Osteochondrosis/Osteochondritis Dissecans (O.C.D.)

Seen mainly in giant breeds and also in the Border Collie. Young animals 5-9 months of age.

Forelimb lameness with pain on extension of the shoulder.

Radiological features (Figure 5.61)

• Lateral view is the most useful projection - occasionally arthrography may be of value in demonstrating the lesion.

• Lateral views with the shoulder rotated either medially or laterally have been advocated but are rarely necessary.

• Lucent defect of the subchondral bone of the caudal third of the humeral articular surface.

• May see flap of cartilage and subchondral bone overlying the defect.

• In later stages a separated, mineralised joint mouse may be seen in the caudal compartment of the joint capsule.

• If the plain films are equivocal or non diagnostic a positive contrast or double contrast arthrogram may provide valuable radiological information.

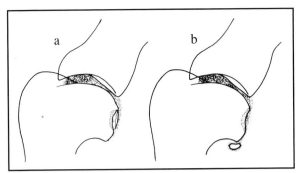

Figure 5.61a and b: Osteochondritis dissecans - a: Osteochondral flap in situ and defect in the articular surface. b: Free body in the joint and a subchondral defect.

Traumatic Luxation

Uncommon lesion. Lameness and assymmetry of the shoulders. Acromion process relatively more prominent and the shoulder joint increased in width with restricted mobility.

Radiological features (Figure 5.62)

• On the lateral view the humeral head will be seen overlying the glenoid.

• The joint space will be lost.

• On the Cdcr view the humeral head will be identified lying medial to the glenoid cavity.

• Radiographs should be examined for the presence of marginal fractures of the glenoid rim or scapular tuberosity.

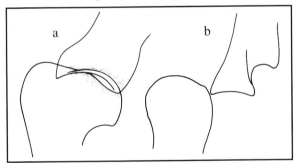

Figure 5.62a and b: Traumatic luxation of the shoulder. Note the overlap of the articular surfaces on the lateral film.

Congenital Dislocation

This is seen mainly in miniature and toy breeds of dog. May be associated with lameness or may be bilateral and identified because of abnormal conformation with wide bow-legged stance.

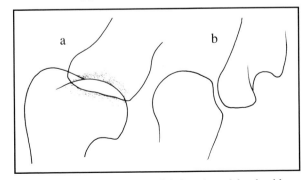

Figure 5.63a and b: Congenital dislocation of the shoulder.

Radiological features (Figure 5.63)
- On the lateral view there will be no normal joint space or glenoid identifiable.
- The humeral head will overlay the distal scapula.
- On the Cdcr view the humeral head will be displaced medially.
- The glenoid cavity is usually undeveloped so that the distal end of the scapula has a convex shape lateral to the humerus.

Separation of the Scapular Tuberosity
Uncommon injury seen in the dog. Forelimb lameness with pain and possible instability of the shoulder. May be associated with traumatic luxation of the shoulder.

Radiological features (Figure 5.64)
- Lateral view of most value.
- Lucent defect separating the scapular tuberosity from the cranial aspect of the scapula - in animals less than seven months old there may be a physeal line visible as a normal feature.
- Displacement of the free bone fragment due to the traction of the biceps tendon.

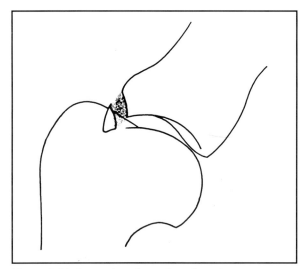

Figure 5.64: Separation of scapular tuberosity.

Bicipital Bursitis
Cause of vague forelimb lameness in mature dogs. May be very difficult to confirm clinically other than by the demonstration of mild shoulder discomfort.

Radiological features (Figure 5.65)
- Often no abnormalities are identified - this is of value in eliminating other possible causes of shoulder discomfort.
- May occasionally be mottled increased radiopacity of the bicipital groove with slight roughening of the bony margins.

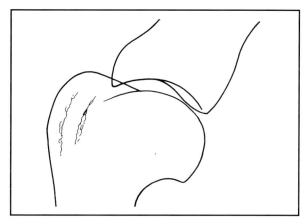

Figure 5.65: Bicipital bursitis.

Calcifying Tendinopathy of the Shoulder
Infrequent cause of mild and/or intermittent forelimb lameness in large breed dogs. Usually mature animals. Pain on manipulation of the affected joint.

Radiological features
- Linear or focal areas of mineralisation in the affected tendon.
- Supraspinatus and Biceps brachii tendons most frequently affected.
- In the case of mineralisation on the biceps brachii multiple filling defects may be seen in the tendon sheath following contrast arthrography of the shoulder.

Osteoarthritis
Seen as a cause of forelimb lameness in mature and elderly animals. May be a sequel to previous lesions such as OCD, trauma etc.

Radiological features (Figure 5.66)
- Osteophytic reaction on the caudal margins of the humeral head and glenoid rim will be seen on the lateral view.
- Less commonly osteophytes will be apparent in this view superimposed on the humeral head at the articular margin.
- On the Cdcr view margin osteophytes will be seen on the medial and lateral aspects of the humeral and glenoid articular surfaces.

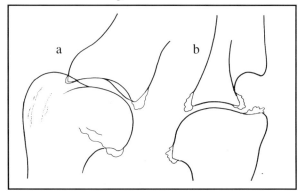

Figure 5.66a and b: Osteoarthritis of the shoulder.

Ossification of the Glenoid Rim in Juvenile

Seen as normal feature in some immature dogs. No clinical signs.

Radiological features (Figure 5.67)
- Linear lucency parallel and adjacent to the caudal rim of the glenoid.
- Do NOT mistake for an osteochondrosis lesion. This will fuse to the scapula as the animal matures.

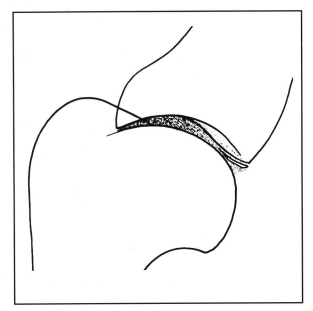

Figure 5.67: Ossification of the glenoid rim in juvenile.

V: ELBOW

Positioning

Medio-lateral view (Figure 5.68)
The elbow may be radiographed either in flexion or extension.

A flexed view is of value in demonstrating the anconal process and humeral epicondyles whilst the extended view is necessary to fully evaluate the cranial aspect of the radial head and humero-radial joint space

i) The animal is placed in lateral recumbency with the upper leg drawn caudally and secured.

ii) For an extended view the beam is then centred over the medial aspect of the elbow - it may be necessary to place a foam support under the olecranon to prevent rotation.

iii) For a flexed view the elbow is flexed as far as possible, care being taken not to push the elbow under the pectoral muscles or sternum. Again, a foam support may be required under the olecranon to prevent rotation.

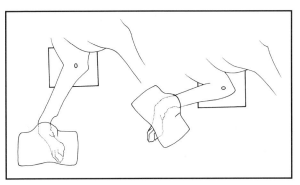

Figure 5.68: Elbow - positioning - medio-lateral view.

Cranio-caudal view

i) There are three methods of obtaining this view and each requires careful positioning to ensure there is no rotation.

a) The animal may be positioned in sternal recumbency with the limb extended and held with ties. The thorax may need to be slightly rotated towards the limb being radiographed and supported. The beam is centred on the radio-humeral joint and angled approximately 15° cranio-caudally (Figure 5.69).

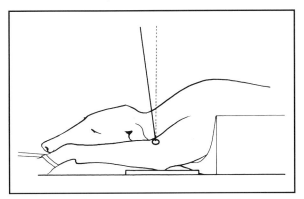

Figure 5.69: Elbow - positioning - cranio-caudal view - sternal recumbency.

b) The animal is placed in dorsal recumbency with the trunk and thorax supported. The limb is extended caudally and the X-ray beam centred vertically over the radio-humeral joint. (Figure 5.70)

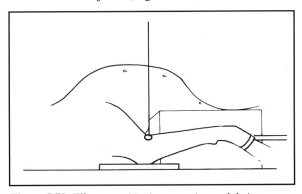

Figure 5.70: Elbow - positioning - cranio-caudal view - dorsal recumbency.

c) The animal is placed in lateral recumbency, the upper fore limb extended and the cassette supported behind the elbow. A horizontally positioned X-ray beam is then centred perpendicularly to the elbow. The usual comments about attention to radiation safety when using a horizontal X-ray beam apply (Figure 5.71).

On occasion oblique views may be required but the indications for these views are very limited

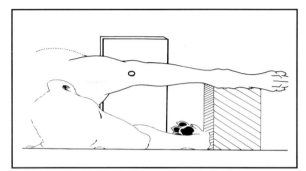

Figure 5.71: Elbow - positioning - cranio-caudal view - lateral recumbency using a horizontal beam.

Classical Fractures
e.g. lateral condyle, Monteggia. Sequel to trauma. Lateral condylar fractures more common in young dogs especially spaniel types.

Radiological features (Figure 5.72)

Fractures of the lateral condyle
- May be identified on the lateral view.
- Superimposition of the medial humeral articular surface on the proximal radial articular surface.
- More easily seen on Crcd view.
- Lucent defect through lateral epicondyle.
- Lateral condyle normally remains *in situ* on radial head.
- Lateral condyle and radius/ulna displaced proximally.
- Humeral shaft and medial condyle displaces medially.

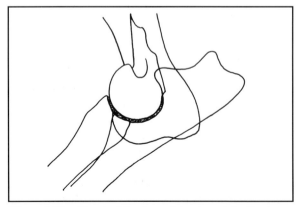

Figure 5.72a: Classical fracture - lateral condylar fracture.

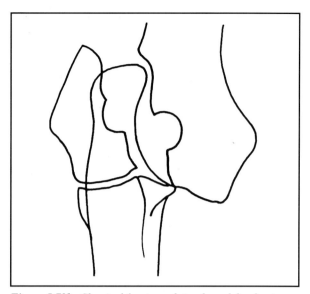

Figure 5.72b: Classical fracture - lateral condylar fracture.

Monteggia Fracture
- Seen most readily in lateral view.
- Fracture line through ulna at base of semilunar notch.
- Cranial luxation of radial head from humeral articular surface.

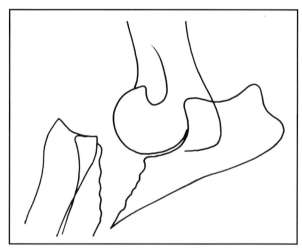

Figure 5.72c: Classical fracture - Monteggia fracture.

Traumatic Dislocation
Severe post traumatic lameness. Increased width of elbow. Marked reduced mobility.

Radiological features (Figure 5.73)
- On lateral view superimposon of humeral articular surface on radial/ulnar articular surfaces.
- Soft tissue swelling.
- On Crcd view radius and ulna usually displaced laterally.
- In chronic dislocation there will be evidence of secondary joint disease with periarticular osteophytic reaction and remodelling of the articular surfaces.

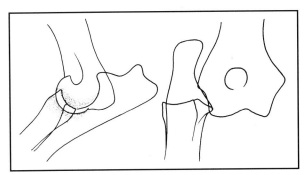

*Figure 5.73a and b: Traumatic dislocation of the elbow
Note the overlap of the joint surfaces on the lateral view.*

Congenital Dislocation - I

Seen most commonly in small breeds of dog but can occur sporadically in larger breeds.

Radiological features (Figure 5.74)
- Humero-ulnar articulation relatively normal.
- Head of radius subluxated laterally and caudally.
- Shaft of radius and ulna 'splayed' apart proximally.
- May be remodelling of articular surfaces.

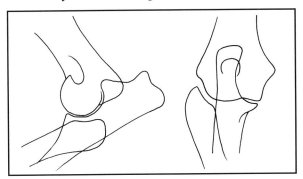

Figure 5.74a and b: Congenital dislocation - I.

Congenital Dislocation - II

Seen mainly in miniature and toy breeds.

Radiological features (Figure 5.75)
- Humero-radial joint appears relatively normal.
- Proximal ulna appears to be rotated through 90 degrees.
- On lateral view no semilunar notch can be seen whilst on the Crcd the semilunar notch is directed medially.

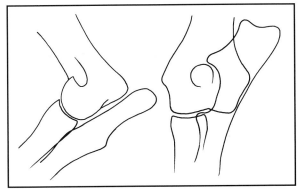

Figure 5.75a and b: Congenital dislocation - II.

Subluxation Due to Short Radius/Ulna

Seen in young dogs following trauma to the distal limb but occasionally apparently spontaneously.

Radiological features

Short radius syndrome (Figure 5.76a)
- Widening of the humero-radial joint.
- Displacement of the semilunar notch proximally.
- Interference between the humeral articular surfaces and the coronoid processes of the ulna.

Short ulna syndrome (Figure 5.76b)
- Widening of the distal joint space of the humero- ulna articulation.
- Distal displacement of the coronoid processes of the ulna.
- Interference between the anconeal process and the caudal aspect of the humeral articular surface.

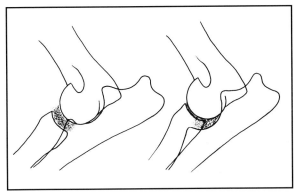

Figure 5.76 a and b: Subluxation due to: a. Short radius syndrome. b. Short ulna syndrome.

Osteochondrosis of the Elbow

1) Fragmented coronoid process
Seen in young large breed dogs 5-10 months of age. Usually Labrador/Retriever and Rottweiler most commonly affected but seen occasionally in other large breeds, e.g. German Shepherd dog, Bernese Mountain dog etc. Forelimb lameness often bilateral resulting in shortened stilted gait. Pain on manipulation of the elbow especially extension.

Radiological features (Figure 5.77)
- Lesion per se not usually seen but the secondary changes can be identified.
- On the lateral view periosteal reaction on the proximal aspect of the anconeus and sometimes on the dorsal aspect of the radial head.
- On the Crcd view roughening of the medial aspect of the humeral condyle.
- Spur formation on the medial aspect of the ulna articular surface.
- Occasionally a separated fragment of bone may be identified medially.
- Loss of clarity of the medial joint space (humero-ulnar) with associated humero-radial incongruity.

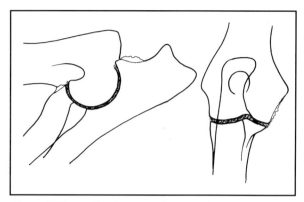

Figure 5.77a and b: Fragmented coronoid process.

2) Osteochondritis dissecans
Seen mainly in Labradors/Retrievers. Clinical features identical to those seen in fragmented coronoid process.

Radiological features (Figure 5.78)
- As with fragmented coronoid process periarticular osteophytic proliferation.
- May see lucent defect in medial humeral condylar articular surface.
- Occasionally may identify a separated osteo-chondral flap overlying the humeral defect.

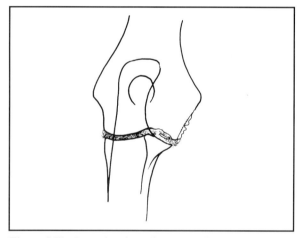

Figure 5.78: Osteochondritis dissecans. The changes on the lateral projection would be identical to 5.77a.

3) Un-united anconeal process
Occurs in German Shepherd dog, Bassett Hound and rarely in other breeds.

Forelimb lameness with pain on elbow extension and thickening of the caudal aspect. May be bi-lateral.

Radiological features (Figure 5.79)
- Lucent defect separating triangular anconeal process from proximal ulna usually periosteal reaction of the adjacent bony surfaces.
- Soft tissue swelling due to caudal capsular distension.
- May be a growth plate seen in the normal animal but this closes at about four months and is rarely identified.

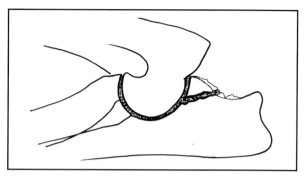

Figure 5.79: Un-united anconeal process.

4) Un-united medial humeral epicondyle
Seen uncommonly in young dogs of the breeds associated with the other forms of elbow osteochondrosis.

Often associated with a much milder lameness than other forms of osteochondrosis.

Radiological features (Figure 5.80)
- Separated fragment of bone on the caudal or distal aspect of the epicondyle on the lateral view and distal and medially displaced on the Crcd view.
- May be a defect in the epicondyle.
- Usually little or no secondary arthritic changes within the joint.

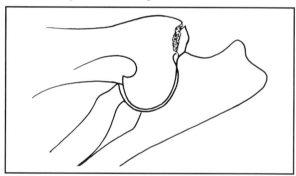

Figure 5.80: Un-united medial humeral epicondyle.

Lateral Sesamoid
Incidental finding in large breed dogs. No clinical signs attributable to it.

Radiological features (Figure 5.81)
- Small, smooth circular opacity adjacent to the lateral aspect of the elbow joint on the Crcd view.

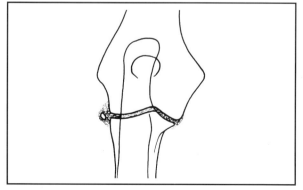

Figure 5.81: Lateral sesamoid of the elbow.

VI: CARPUS

Medio-lateral view (Figure 5.82)

i)   The animal is positioned in lateral recumbency with the upper limb retracted caudally and secured with ties.

ii) The X-ray beam is centred on the carpus which is normally in the extended position.

iii) Flexed views may be indicated on occasion to check for articular fractures. The carpus should be held in the flexed position either by sandbags or with a tie round the foot and mid radius. (Figure 5.83)

iv) Stressed views with the carpus held in the weight bearing position are sometimes of value in the assessment of ligamentous injuries. If these require to be held then attention must be paid to radiation protection and to ensure that they are kept as far from the primary beam as possible. (Figure 5.84)

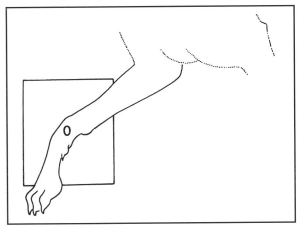

Figure 5.82: Carpus - positioning - mediolateral view.

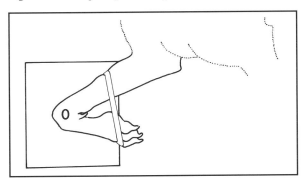

Figure 5.83: Carpus - positioning - flexed mediolateral view.

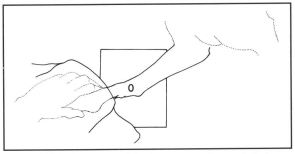

Figure 5.84: Carpus - positioning - stressed extended view.

Cranio-caudal view (Figure 5.85)

i)   The animal is placed in sternal recumbency with the forelimb extended.

ii) It is generally unsatisfactory to attempt to radiograph both left and right carpi simultaneously as there will almost certainly be outward rotation.

iii) To ensure there is no rotation it is often necessary to rotate the supporting trunk slightly towards the limb being examined.

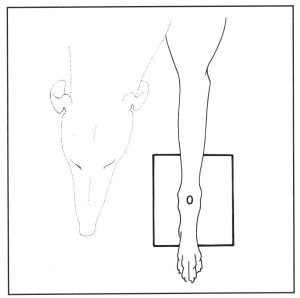

Figure 5.85: Carpus - positioning - craniocaudal view.

Oblique views

i)   These are occasionally indicated for the assessment of carpal fractures.

ii) The caudo-medial cranio-lateral view is best taken with the animal positioned as for the lateral view but with the elbow supported by a foam support in order to rotate the carpus. (Figure 5.86)

iii) The cranio-medial caudo-lateral view is best obtained with the animal positioned as for the cranio- caudal view but with the carpus rotated laterally (Figure 5.87).

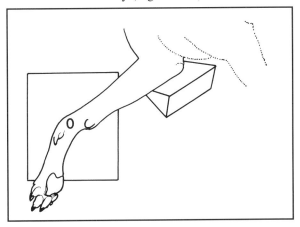

Figure 5 86: Carpus - positioning - Caudo-medial cranio-lateral oblique view.

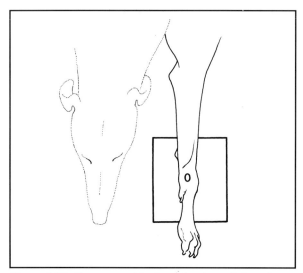

Figure 5.87: Carpus - positioning - Cranio medial caudo-lateral oblique view.

Osteoarthritis

Mainly results from previous trauma to the carpus or may occur as part of a polyarthritis.

Lameness associated with pain on manipulation of the carpus and usually marked restriction to the normal range of movement, especially flexion.

Radiological features (Figure 5.88)

* Osteophytic reaction on the articular margins of the radius, radio-carpal and distal carpal bones and proximal metacarpus on both lateral and Crcd views. Degree of osteophytic reaction often much less than the clinical signs would suggest.
* Soft tissue swelling of the affected carpus.

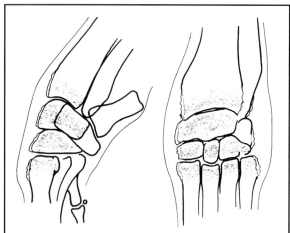

Figure 5.88a and b: Carpus - osteoarthritis.

Fracture of the Accessory Carpal Bone

Almost entirely associated with the racing greyhound. Forelimb lameness, usually of the right limb, during or immediately after racing. Pain on flexion of the carpus and deep pressure on distal aspect of accessory carpal bone. Lameness may settle with kennel rest but recur when next trialled or raced.

Radiological features (Figure 5.89)

* Lateral view of main value occasionally slightly oblique views may be required.
* Linear bone fragment adjacent to the ventral aspect of the accessory carpal bone which may appear slightly roughened.
* Occasionally several smaller fragments may be seen.
* May also be comminuted fracture with several major fragments.

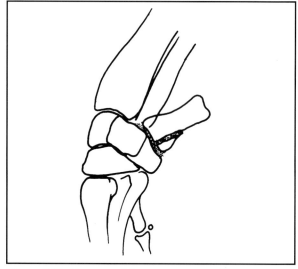

Figure 5.89: Fracture of the accessory carpal bone.

Palmar Ligament Collapse

Sequel to trauma or may develop insidiously in some dogs e.g. Rough Collie and related breeds. Forelimb lameness and hyper-extension of the carpus when weight bearing or when stressed.

Radiological features (Figure 5.90)

* On non-manipulated lateral and Crcd views there may be either no abnormality or evidence of OA.
* Stressed film will demonstrate the hyper-extension of the carpus.
* The hyper-extension may occur at differing levels - radio carpal, inter carpal or carpo-metacarpal.

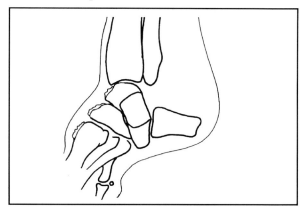

Figure 5.90: Palmar ligament collapse.

Collateral Ligament Damage

Sequel to trauma. Forelimb lameness.

Radiological features

- As with palmar ligament collapse there may be little or no plan film abnormally but stressed films will demonstrate degree and level of the joint instability.

VII: FEET

Positioning

Lateral view

i) As for the carpus but with the beam centred on the metacarpo-phalangeal joints.

Cranio-caudal view

i) As for carpus but with the beam centred on the metacarpo-phalangeal joints.
ii) For the hind foot the animal should be supported in dorsal recumbency and rotated away from the limb under investigation which is extended and held by either sandbags or ties. (Figure 5.91)

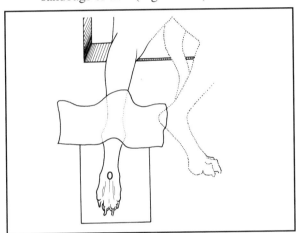

Figure 5.91: Feet - positioning - craniocaudal view.

Lateral views with the toes separated

i) This view may be required for the localisation of foreign bodies in the pads.
ii) The animal is positioned as for a lateral view of the foot but with the toes held spread apart with tape. (Figure 5.92)

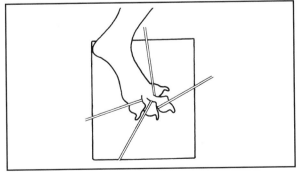

Figure 5.92: Feet - positioning - Lateral view with toes separated.

Bipartite/Multipartite Sesamoids

Seen as an incidental finding in many breeds. No clinical signs normally associated with this developmental variant.

Radiological features (Figure 5.93)

- Sesamoid in two or more smooth fragments with little or no periosteal reaction.
- Must be differentiated from a fractured sesamoid.

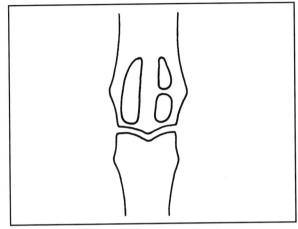

Figure 5.93: Bipartite/multipartite sesamoids.

Fractured Sesamoid

Lameness with pain on deep palpation over the affected sesamoid. (Figure 5.94). Opposing surfaces sharply defined and angular.

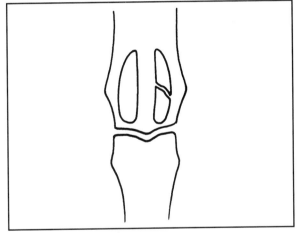

Figure 5.94: Fractured sesamoid.

Fragmented Sesamoids

Seen commonly in Rottweilers where they may be of doubtful clinical significance unless associated with lameness and pain on pressure over affected bone.

Radiological features (Figure 5.95)

- Lateral (axial) sesamoid of digits II and medial (axial) of V most commonly affected.
- Sesamoid usually in several fragments often with an irregular outline and some bony proliferation.

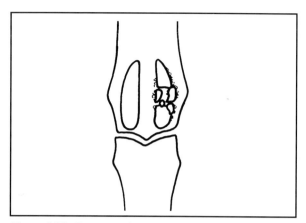

Figure 5.95: Fragmented sesamoid.

HINDLIMB

The standard radiographic positions for the examination of the joints will be described and illustrated. These views are adapted for the examination of the long bones by the appropriate centring of the X-ray beam.

Femur - position as for stifle but centre midway between the hip and stifle.

Tibia - position as for stifle or hock but centre midway between the stifle and hock.

VIII: HIPS PELVIS

Positioning

Lateral view (Figure 5.96)
i)   Animal placed in lateral recumbency.
ii) Ensure that the pelvis is not rotated by placing padding between the hindlimbs.
iii) Centre the beam over the greater trochanter.

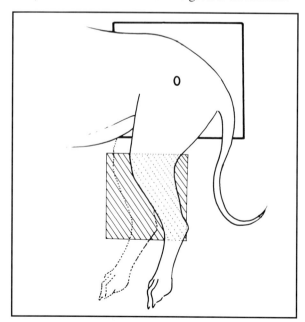

Figure 5.96: Hips/pelvis - positioning - lateral view.

Ventro-dorsal view (Figure 5.97)
i)   This is the standard view for the assessment of the pelvis and hips.
ii) The animal is supported in dorsal recumbency ensuring that there is no rotation about the longitudinal axis.
iii) The hindlimbs are extended so that the femora are parallel and rotated medially. When correctly positioned the hind feet will be slightly turned medially.
iv) For the assessment of pelvic fractures the legs may be left in the resting abducted position.

Various other views such as the flexed ventro-dorsal, the stressed ventro-dorsal used to demonstrate the degree of hip joint laxity and the dorsal acetabular rim view have been described but are not used routinely.

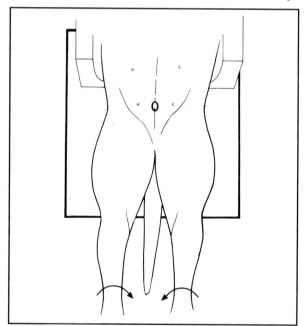

Figure 5.97: Hips/pelvis - positioning - ventro-dorsal view.

Hip Dysplasia
Very common congenital defect of the hips. Much more prevelant in certain breeds. May be associated with clinical problems of hind leg lameness, stiffness etc. in young animals, adults or elderly animals. Also occurs in small breeds but less often associated with clinical problems. Does occur sporadically in the cat.

Radiological features (Figure 5.98)
•   The radiological features vary greatly in severity and the range of changes which may be encountered are illustrated.
•   Progressive degrees of shallowness of the acetabulum manifest as flattening and cranial sloping of the cranial acetabular edge.
•   Subluxation of the femoral head manifest by widening of the medial joint space and reduction in cover of the femoral head by the dorsal acetabular edge.

- Subluxation of the femoral head manifest by widening of the medial joint space and reduction in cover of the femoral head by the dorsal acetabular edge.
- Recontouring of the acetabular articular surface with widening of the lateral joint space.
- Remodelling of the femoral head and neck.

- Proliferation of periarticular osteophytes on the acetabular rim and femoral neck and the development of secondary osteoarthritis.
- Infilling of the acetabular fossa with new bone.
- Abnormalities in the Norberg-Olsson angle.

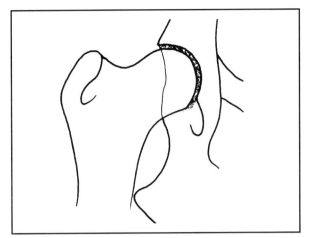

Figure 5.98a: Hip dysplasia - Normal hip.

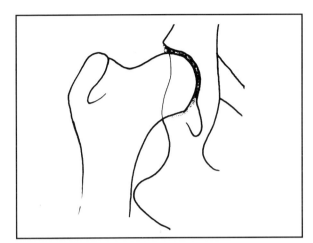

Figure 5.98b: Hip dysplasia - Flattening of the cranial acetabular edge and widening of the joint space laterally.

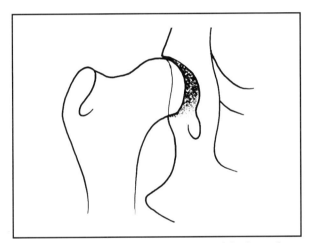

Figure 5.98c: Hip dysplasia - Subluxation of the femoral head with widening of the medial joint space and reduced cover by the dorsal acetabular edge.

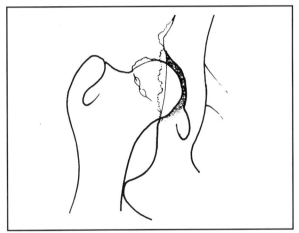

Figure 5.98d: Flattening and cranial sloping of cranial acetabular edge and secondary osteophytic proliferation on the acetabular margins and femoral neck.

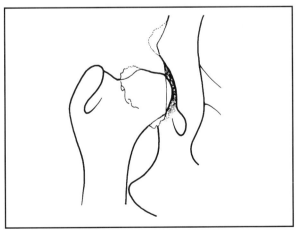

Figure 5.98e: Hip dysplasia - Gross recontouring of the femoral head and acetabulum.

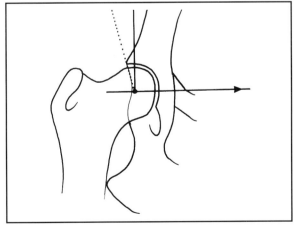

Figure 5.98f: Hip dysplasia - Normal hip showing the method of measuring the Norberg angle. The arrowed horizontal line joins the centres of the two femoral heads.

Perthes Disease

Seen in young small breed dogs 5-10 months of age. A number of breeds affected but most common in West Highland White Terriers, Cairn Terriers, Miniature Poodles and Yorkshire Terriers. Insidious onset hind limb lameness. Pain on manipulation of the affected hip. Muscle atrophy.

Radiological features (Figure 5.99)
- Deformity of the femoral head with flattening of the articular surface.
- Mixed radiolucency and radiodensity of the femoral head.
- Increase in width of the joint space.
- Secondary periarticular osteophytic proliferation round the acetabular rim and femoral neck.

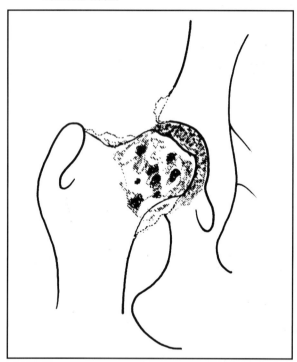

Figure 5.99: Perthes disease.

Dorso-Cranial Dislocation

Traumatic - usually RTA. Occasionally follows trivial trauma in an animal with hip dysplasia. Restricted mobility of the hip and shortening of the limb.

Radiological features (Figure 5.100)
- Lateral view - the femoral head will usually be seen displaced dorso-cranially.
- VD view - femoral head seen displaced cranially lying adjacent to the ilial shaft.
- This view should always be taken and examined carefully for evidence of fractures of the femoral head - avulsed with round ligament - or acetabular rim. (Figure 5.101).
- If chronic a pseudo-arthrosis may have formed between the femoral head and the ilial shaft.

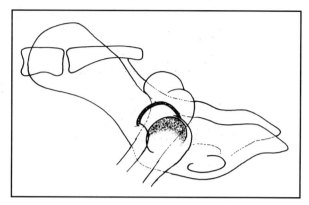

Figure 5.100a: Dorso-cranial dislocation of the hip.

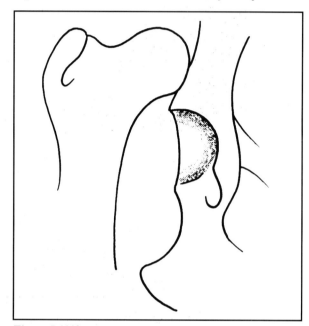

Figure 5.100b: Dorso-cranial dislocation of the hip.

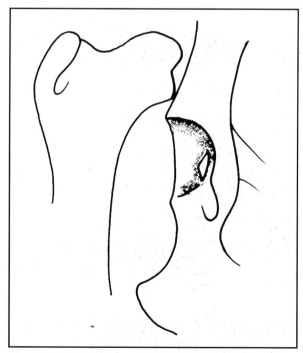

Figure 5.101: Dislocation of the hip with an associated chip fracture of the femoral head.

Ventral Dislocation
As for dorsal dislocation except limb length increased on affected leg.

Radiological features (Figure 5.102)
- Femoral head seen ventral to the pelvis on the lateral view.
- Femoral head usually superimposed on obturator foramen in VD view.
- Again the acetabulum should be checked for fractures.

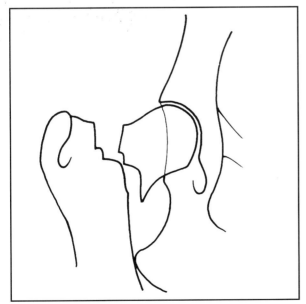

Figure 5.102: Ventral dislocation of the hip.

Femoral Neck Fractures
Trauma most commonly RTA. Clinical signs may be indistinguishable from dislocated hip.

Radiological features (Figure 5.103)
- Lucent fracture line crossing the femoral neck.
- If femoral head displaced this is usually distally.

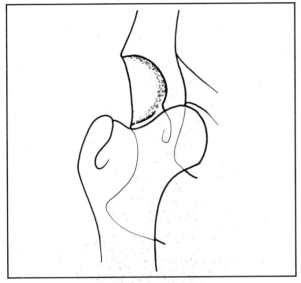

Figure 5.103: Femoral neck fracture.

Pelvic Fractures
Traumatic most commonly RTA.

Radiological features (Figure 5.104)
- Can vary widely but there is usually more than one fracture present and frequently multiple fractures affecting any part of the pelvis.

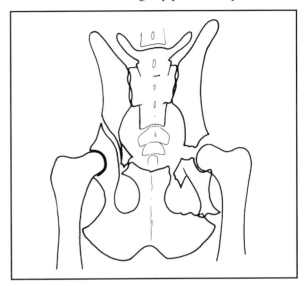

Figure 5.104: Multiple pelvic fractures.

Sacro-Iliac Subluxation
As for pelvic fractures.

Radiological features (Figure 5.105)
- Displacement of the ilium relative to the sacrum assessed by examining the surface of the medial cortex of the ilium with the caudal edge of the sacral wing.
- May be widening of the sacro-iliac joint space.
- May be associated with pelvic fractures.
- If present there could be associated neurological problems to tail, bladder and rectum.

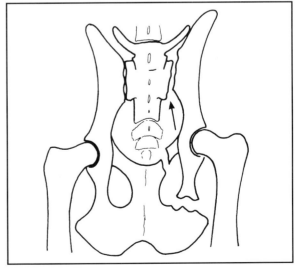

Figure 5.105: Sacro-iliac subluxation. Note the step at the junction of the medial cortex of the ilium and caudal edge of the sacral wing (arrow).

IX: THE STIFLE

Positioning

Medio-lateral view (Figure 5.106)
  i)   The animal is placed in lateral recumbency with the limb to be radiographed down.
  ii)   Either abduct the upper limb and secure with ties so that it does not overlay the stifle being radiographed, or draw the upper limb cranially and secure with ties.
  iii) The stifle should be in a neutral position i.e. neither flexed nor extended.
  iv)   Any tendency to rotate should be corrected by placing a foam support under the caudal aspect of the hock.
  v)   Centre the beam over the distal femoral condyle.

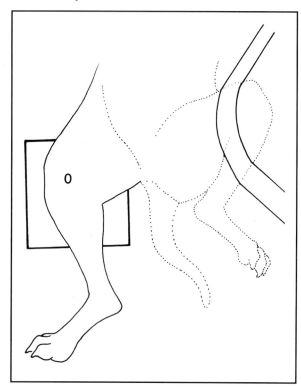

Figure 5.106: Stifle - positioning - mediolateral view.

Cranio-caudal view (Figure 5.107)
  i)   Position the animal in dorsal recumbency rotated slightly away from the side under examination.
  ii)   Extend the limb caudally and secure.
  iii) Centre the beam over the patella.
  iv)   For the assessment of collateral ligament damage stressed films may be required. Positioning is as for the routine Crcd view but with the joint stressed either medially or laterally. This almost always requires manipulation of the joint by hand during radiography and attention should be paid to the attendant radiation hazards.

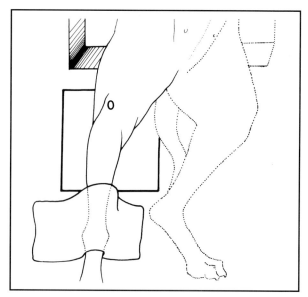

Figure 5.107: Stifle - positioning - cranio-caudal view.

Osteoarthritis
Most commonly seen as a secondary feature of traumatic rupture of the cranial cruciate ligament. Also secondary to other developmental lesions such as OCD and patellar instability.

Radiological features (Figure 5.108)
  •   Soft tissue proliferation with reduction in the size of the infra-patellar fat pad and caudal displacement of the fascial planes caudal to the joint.
  •   Proliferation of peri-articular osteophytes seen on both lateral and Crcd views.
     i)   At the proximal end of the trochlear groove.
     ii)   Lateral/medial aspects of the trochlea.
     iii) Proximal and distal ends of the patella.
     iv)   Margins of the tibial articular surface.
     v)   Dorsal aspect of the tibia cranial to the tibiacrest and in the inter-condylar notch.

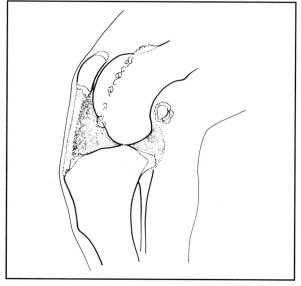

Figure 5.108: Osteoarthritis of the stifle.

- It may be possible to see cranial displacement of the tibia - normally the tibial spine lies at the mid point of the femoral condylar articular surface.

Idiopathic Effusive Athritis

Seen in certain breeds, e.g. Rottweiller and Boxer, as an apparently idiopathic arthropathy with subsequent cruciate rupture. Young animals 1-3 years old. Hind limb lameness, joint swelling and pain. May be joint instability latterly. Often bilateral stifle involvement.

Radiological features (Figure 5.109)
- Initially soft tissue swelling may be the only abnormality.
- Later similar changes to those described above for osteoarthritis.

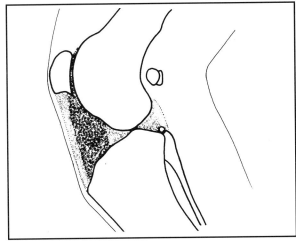

Figure 109a: Idiopathic effusive arthritis - Normal stifle.

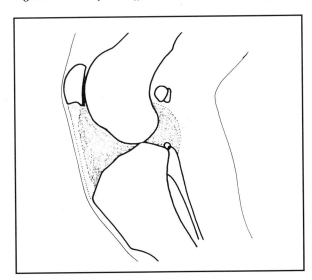

Figure 109b: Idiopathic effusive arthritis - Stifle with soft tissue swelling indicative of an effusive arthritis.

Synovial Osteochondromatosis

Affected mainly medium to large dogs. Affected animals mature or elderly. Joints affected are the stifle (most commonly), shoulder and hock. Lameness and swelling of the affected joint.

Radiological features (Figure 5.110)
- Multiple mineralised foci both within the joint space and the associated soft tissues.
- May or may not be periarticular osteophytes unconnected with the mineralised.

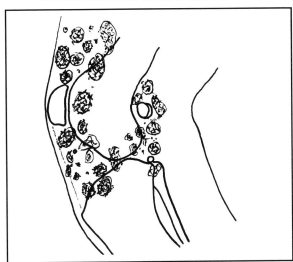

Figure 5.110.

Cranial Cruciate Ruture

May be traumatic and affect any breed of dog. Uncommon but does occur in the cat. Lameness accompanied with instability of the femoro-tibial joint in a cranio-caudal direction.

Radiological features (Figure 5.111)
- In the acute stage -
    Soft tissue swelling with or without evidence of cranial displacement of the proximal tibia.
    The presence or absence of cranial displacement must not be interpreted as evidence of joint instability/stability.
- In the chronic stages -
    As described for osteoarthritis of the stifle.

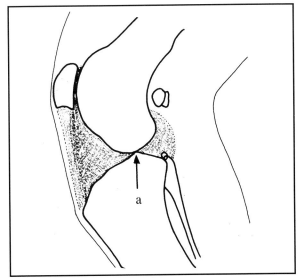

Figure 5.111a: Cranial cruciate rupture - No cranial displacement of the tibia but soft tissue swelling.

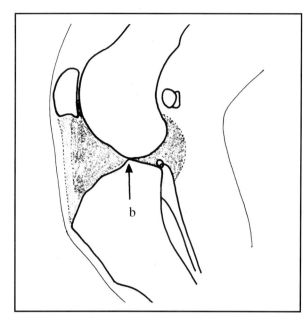

Figure 5.111b: *Cranial cruciate rupture - Cranial displacement of the tibia evident.*

Collateral Ligament Damage

Traumatic in origin - often due to leg being caught on fence etc. Medio-lateral instability of the joint. May be associated with other ligament injuries.

Radiological features (Figure 5.112)
*   Lateral view of little help.
*   Non stressed Crcd view may show no abnormality.
*   Medially and/or laterally stressed Crcd view will demonstrate subluxation with widening of the joint space on the affected side.
    NB. Great care must be taken with regard to radiation safety when obtaining stressed views of joints.

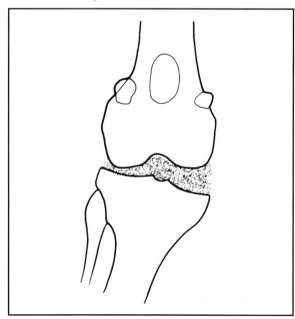

Figure 5.112: *Collateral ligament damage. Stressed Crcd view.*

Osteochondrosis / Itis Dissecans of the Stifle

One of the less common sites for OCD. Occurs mainly in the giant breeds but also seen sporadically in Labrador/Retriever. Young animals 6-10 months old. Lameness with pain and crepitus on manipulation of the stifle. May be bilateral.

Radiological features (Figure 5.113)
*   Soft tissue swelling.
*   Radiolucent defect in femoral condylar articular surface with flattening and irregularity often seen on the lateral view.
*   Either medial or lateral condyle may be affected - lateral more common.
*   May identify mineralised intra-articular bodies - may be located in the supra-patella pouch or caudal to the joint.
*   In late stages there may be secondary degenerative joint disease.

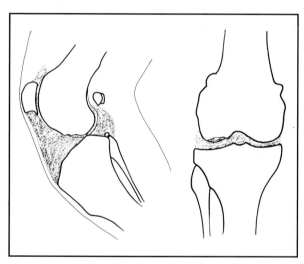

Figure 5.113 a and b: *Osteochondritis dissecans of the stifle. Note the loose body in the supra-patella pouch. Loose bodies may not always be identified on the plain film*

Patella Subluxation - Small Breeds

May be congenital or aquired. Normally medial subluxation or luxation. Clinical problem varies from an incidental finding to severe lameness and secondary limb deformity.

Radiological features (Figure 5.114)
*   If only intermittent luxation radiological findings may be minimal.
*   If patella luxated seen superimposed on trochlea on lateral view and adjacent to medial aspect on Crcd.
*   Trochlear ridge may appear flattened.
*   If permanent luxation may be secondary femoral shaft bowing and tibial rotation.
*   Secondary OA of the femoro-patella joint in longstanding cases.

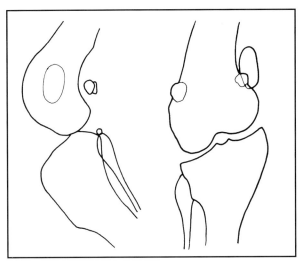

Figure 5.114 a and b: Congenital patella subluxation - small breeds.

Tibial Tuberosity Avulsion

Traumatic. Young animals less than 8-10 months old.

Radiological features (Figure 5.115)
- Important to appreciate normal pattern of closure of the physis of the tibial tuberosity.
- Joins to proximal tibial epiphysis at 6-8 months.
- Completely fuses to tibial shaft 8-12 months.
- Soft tissue swelling cranially.
- Increased width of physeal plate often with irregularity of opposing bone surfaces.
- Displacement of the tibial tuberosity either cranially or proximally.
- May also be occasional displacement of the proximal tibial epiphysis.

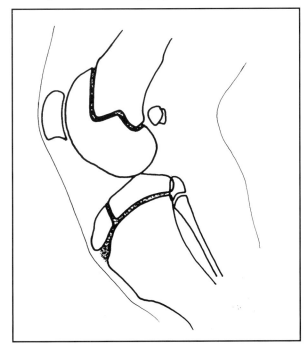

Figure 5.115a: Tibial tuberosity avulsion - Normal appearance of the growth plates in the young dog.

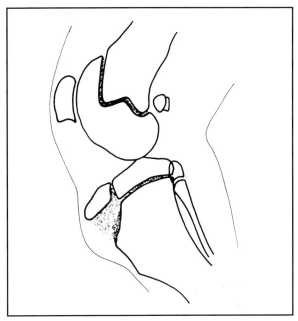

Figure 5.115b: Tibial tuberosity avulsion - one variation in the way the tibial tuberosity displaces.

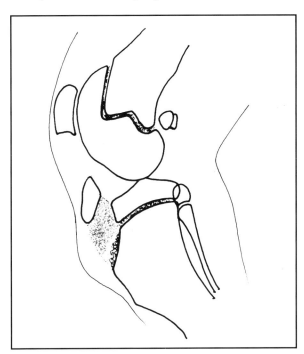

Figure 5.115c: Tibial tuberosity avulsion - one variation in the way the tibial tuberosity displaces.

Avulsion of Long Digital Extensor Tendon

Uncommon sequel to trauma to the stifle. Seen occasionally in young large breed dogs.

Radiological features (Figure 5.116)
- Soft tissue swelling.
- Avulsed fragment of bone on the proximal end of the tendon may be seen lateral to the lateral condyle on a Crcd view.
- A lucent defect may be seen at the cranial margin on the lateral condylar articular surface of the lateral view.

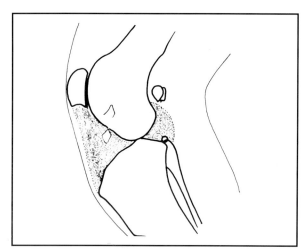

Figure 5.116a: Avulsion of the long digitaextensor tendon.

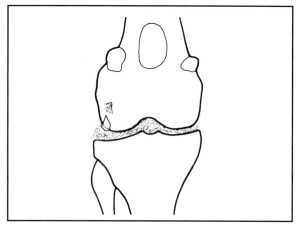

Figure 5.116b: Avulsion of the long digitaextensor tendon.

Rupture of the Straight Patella Ligament

Traumatic - often results from blow to the cranial aspect of the stifle.

Radiological features (Figure 5.117)
- Proximal displacement of the patella in the trochlear groove.
- Soft tissue swelling of the patella ligament with compression of the infra-patella fat pad.

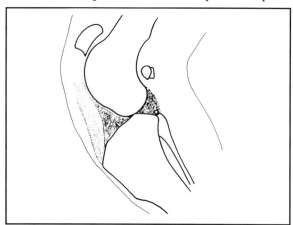

Figure 5.117: Rupture of the straight patella ligament. Note the proximal displacement of the patella and the soft tissue swelling of the patella ligament.

Patella Fractures

Uncommon - similar aetiology to rupture of the straight patella ligament.

Radiological features (Figure 5.118)
- Sharply delineated fracture line with patella in two or more fragments.
- More proximal fragment(s) may be displaced proximally above level of the trochlear groove.
- Bipartite patellae have been reported but the pieces would be rounded and not displaced.

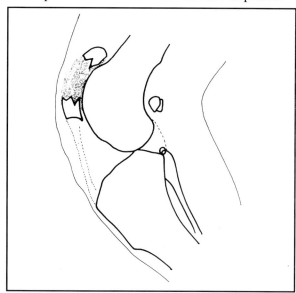

Figure 5.118: Patella fracture.

X: HOCK

Positioning

Lateral view (Figure 5.119)
i) Animal is placed in lateral recumbency with the limb being radiographed down.
ii) The upper limb is either abducted or drawn caudally or cranially and secured.
iii) The beam is centred on the tibio-tarsal joint.

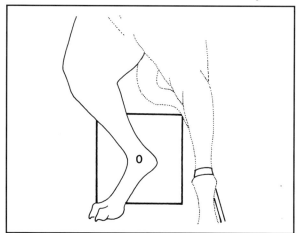

Figure 5.119: Hock - positioning - lateral view.

Cranio-caudal (dorso-plantar) view (Figure 5.120)
i) The animal should be supported in dorsal recumbency and rotated away from the limb under investigation which is extended and held by either sandbags or ties.
ii) The beam is centred over the tibio-tarsal joint.

Occasionally a flexed cranio-dorsal view may be of value in demonstrating defects in the trochlear ridges of the tibio tarsal bone.

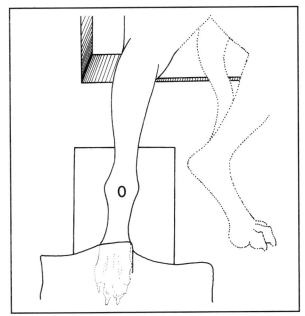

Figure 5.120: Hock - positioning - craniocaudal view.

Osteoarthritis
As a sequel to trauma involving dislocation, fracture odevelopmental defects such as OCD. May be a late stage of inflammatory joint disease.

Radiological features (Figure 5.121)
• Periarticular osteophytic proliferation round the articulamargins of the tibia, tarsal bones and proximal metatarsus.
• As in the carpus the severity ootherwise of the radiologicachanges may correlate poorly with the clinical severity of the lameness.

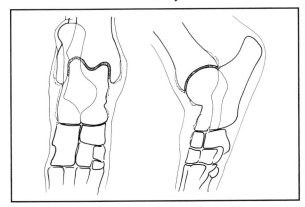

Figure 5.121a and b: Osteoarthritis of the hock.

Malleolar Fractures
Traumatic - usually RTA.

Radiological features (Figure 5.122)
• Crcd view essential for accurate evaluation.
• Stressed views may also be required to demonstrate joint laxity.
• Separated malleolus seen either medially or laterally.

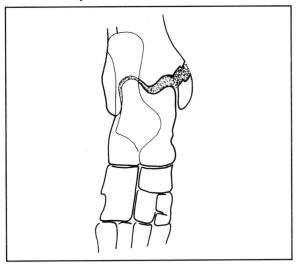

Figure 5.122: Fracture of the medial malleolus.

Fractures of the Central, Third and Fourth Tarsal Bones
Injury of racing Greyhound. Almost always the right tarsus. Acute onset severe lameness while racing. Hock swollen and painful

Radiological features (Figure 5.123)
• Both lateral and Crcd views essential for full evaluation.
• Disruption of the trabecular pattern of the central tarsal bone.
• Displacement of one or more fragments cranially and/or medially.
• May be collapse of the medial aspect of the hock with angular deformity.
• Central tarsal is the most commonly affected.

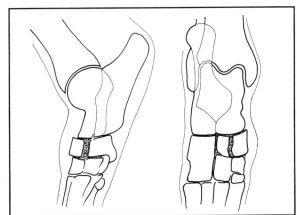

Figure 5.123a and b: Fracture of the central tarsal bone.

Osteochondrosis / Itis Dissecans

Seen in any of the breeds susceptible to osteochondrosis lesions mainly encountered in Labradors/Retrievers and Rottweillers. Hind limb lameness. Hock often appears hyper-extended. Swelling and crepitus - degree of discomfort variable.

Radiological features (Figure 5.124)
- Lateral and Crcd views required but the Crcd view is the most valuable.
- Increase in the width of the medial joint space.
- Reduced height of medial trochlear ridge of tibio- tarsal bone.
- May see osteochondral fragment.
- Secondary changes in chronic cases with osteophytes on the articular margins of the tibio- tarsal joint.

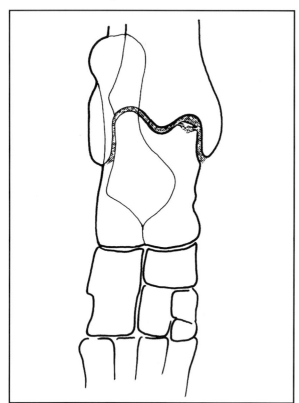

Figure 5.124: Osteochondritis dissecans of the tibiotarsal joint.

Inter-Tarsal Subluxation

May be traumatic in any breed but can develop insidiously in Shetland Sheepdogs and related breeds. Pain free lameness with hyper-extension of the hock.

Radiological features (Figure 5.125)
- Subluxation at the proximal intertarsal joint.
- A step will be seen on the cranial aspect of the tibio-tarsal and central tarsal bones.
- Periosteal reaction on the caudal aspect of the fibular tarsal and distal tarsal bones.
- Soft tissue swelling of the plantar ligament.

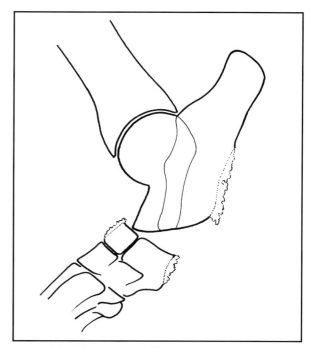

Figure 5.125: Inter-tarsal subluxation.

Tarso-Metatarsal Subluxation

Traumatic - any breed. Hindlimb lameness with hyper-extension of the hock plus pain and swelling.

Radiological features (Figure 5.126)
- Hyper-extension at the tarso-metatarsal joint seen on the lateral view.
- May be associated fractures of the proximal metatarsal bone(s).
- Crcd view will allow full evaluation of the tarso-metatarsal joint.
- Stressed views may be required if damage to the collateral ligaments suspected.

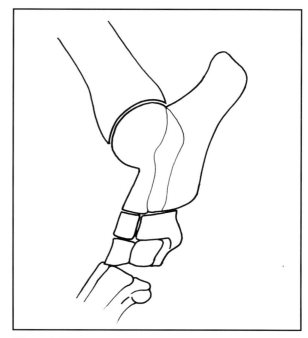

Figure 5.126: Tarso-metatarsal subluxation.

Avulsion of the Calcaneal Tuberosity

Uncommon result of trauma.

Radiological features (Figure 5.127)
- Separated fragment of bone from proximal aspect of the Os calcis.
- Soft tissue swelling around Os calcis and distal end of Achilles tendon.

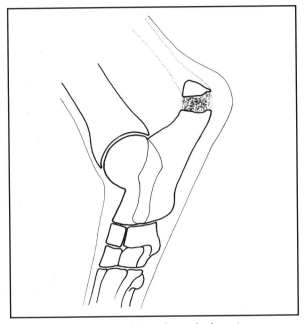

Figure 5.127: *Avulsion of the calcaneal tuberosity.*

Rupture of the Achilles Tendon

Usually traumatic. Occasionally may be sequel to inflammatory tendonitis.

Radiological features (Figure 5.128)
- Soft tissue swelling of Achilles tendon.
- May be an avulsion of the tendinous attachment to the calcaneal tuberosity without any bone injury.

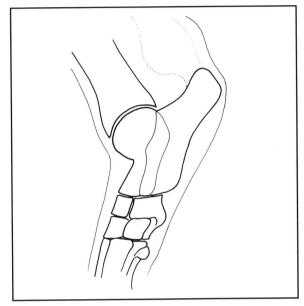

Figure 5.128: *Rupture of the achilles tendon.*

CHAPTER SIX

The Vertebral Column

R. Lee

CONTENTS

I: INDICATIONS

The main indications for radiography of the spine are for the radiological assessment of the following clinical presentations.

1) Mono-, para-, and quadri-plegia
2) Fore and hind limb paresis or paraparesis
3) Incoordination
4) Pain referable to a spinal lesion
5) Stiffness
6) The evaluation of vertebral deformities

Radiography of the spine should be preceded by a detailed clinical examination including the full evaluation of any identified neurological deficits. This is important as it will provide valuable information about the approximate location of the suspected lesion so that the appropriate radiographic examination can be performed. It will also be of value in eliminating those conditions which may mimic the clinical appearance of spinal lesions e.g. orthopaedic problems such as bilateral rupture of the anterior cruciate ligaments of the stifle and medical or metabolic conditions such as hypoglycaemia or myasthenia gravis.

Technique

Screen films should always be used and in all but the smallest of subjects a grid will be of value. In the larger breeds and when using low powered X-ray equipment, fast film screen combinations and, where available, rare earth screens will provide considerable advantages.

The problems of accurate positioning and radiation safety mean that anaesthesia is mandatory for radiography of the vertebral column. In addition, the results of a plain film study may indicate the need for myelography.

It is important to remember that protective muscle reflex tone is abolished under anaesthesia and there-fore particular care must be exercised when positioning an anaesthetised animal with a suspected spinal lesion. This is particularly true when there is possible instability of the spine. Initial survey films should be taken with the animal in lateral recumbency. This view may provide sufficient diagnostic information in itself or may indicate the need for further views.

The ventro-dorsal rather than dorso-ventral projection should be used in order to minimise any loss of image quality due to increased subject-film distance. Further projections may be required depending on the level of the column being examined and the nature of the lesion suspected.

Positioning

Lateral view (Figure 6.1)
i)   The spine must be parallel to the table top. If necessary foam supports should be positioned under the neck and lumbar spine.
ii) It is important to prevent rotation by the use of supports between the limbs and, if necessary, under the sternum.
iii) For the examination of the cervical spine a foam wedge can be used to support the nose and prevent rotation of the head.
iv) For examination of the lower cervical spine the forelegs should be drawn caudally taking care not to cause rotation of the spine.
v)   The X-ray beam must be centred over the level of the suspected lesion as indicated by the clinical features. If this initial film fails to demonstrate any abnormality then further films taken both cranial and caudal to the initial film should be obtained.
vi) If no localising signs are present, or if a complete survey of the vertebral column is required, then the beam should be centred at the levels indicated below.
  a) Upper cervical - C2/3
  b) Lower cervical - C5/6
  c) Mid thoracic - T8
  d) Thoraco-lumbar junction - T13/L1
  e) Mid-lumbar - L4/5
  f) Sacrum.

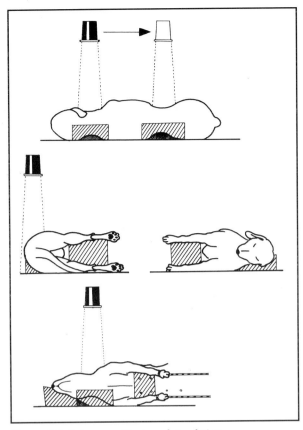

Figure 6.1: Spine - positioning - lateral view.

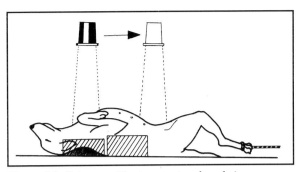

Figure 6.2: Spine - positioning - ventro-dorsal view.

Fewer films may suffice in smaller dogs and cats.

vii) Flexed and extended views of the cervical spine may be of value in demonstrating vertebral instability and cord compression in cases of cervical spondylopathy. It may be hazardous to the animal to use this technique in atlanto-axial instability or fractures.

viii) In order to demonstrate suspicious features more clearly it is often helpful to adjust the collimation so that only the area of interest is covered by the X-ray field. This will significantly improve radiographic contrast and definition.

ix) If no lesions are identified on these initial projections then it is most unlikely that a ventro-dorsal view will contribute any more information. However, VD views should be taken to enable full evaluation of reactive or destructive changes of the vertebrae, fractures and dislocations and in the full assessment of myelographic abnormalities.

Ventro-dorsal view (Figure 6.2)

i) Position the animal on its back, preferably supported either in a radiolucent trough or by firm pads placed on either side of the thorax. It is important to ensure that there is no rotation about the longitudinal axis of the spine. This is particularly difficult in deep chested dogs.

ii) In order to prevent flexion of the lumbar spine the hind legs should normally be tied in the extended position.

iii) The neck should be extended and held by either tape or a sandbag overlay. A foam support under the neck may be of assistance.

iv) The X-ray beam must be centred over the level of the suspected lesion as indicated by the clinical features. If this initial film fails to demonstrate any abnormality then further films taken both cranial and caudal to the initial film should be obtained.

v) If no localising signs are present, or if a complete survey of the vertebral column is required, then the beam should be centred at the levels indicated below.

   a) Upper cervical - C2/3
   b) Lower cervical -C5/6
   c) Mid thoracic -T8
   d) Thoraco-lumbar junction - T13/L1
   e) Mid lumbar - L4/5
   f) Sacrum.

Fewer films may suffice in smaller dogs and cats.

Rostro-cranial 'open mouth' view (Figure 6.3)

This projection is used for the demonstration of C1 and C2 and the atlanto-axial articulation. By slightly modi-

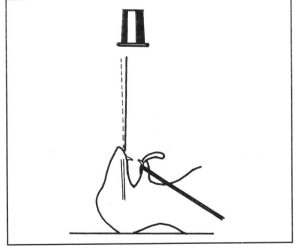

Figure 6.3: Positioning. Rostro-cranial 'open-mouth' view.

fying the angle of projection it can also be used to demonstrate the size and shape of the foramen magnum.

i)   The subject is positioned in dorsal recumbency as for the VD view but with the atlanto-axial joint fully flexed so that the saggital plane of the skull is perpendicular to the film.

ii) The tongue must be pulled forward between the lower canines and the mandible secured with a loop of bandage so that the mouth is secured in the fully opened position. Tape should be secured to the table alongside the shoulders.

iii) The palate should be tilted approximately 5 degrees rostrally and the X-ray beam centred on the back of the soft palate.

iv) In order to eliminate superimposed shadows it is desirable to temporarily extubate the animal whilst the exposure is made.

v)   As there is the potential for causing respiratory obstruction the endotracheal tube should not be removed until immediately prior to making the exposure. The mandible should be released and the tube repositioned as soon as possible.

Evaluation of The Radiograph

It will NOT be possible to identify the following lesions on a plain film.

i)   Tumours of the soft tissue contents of the vertebral canal unless these have extended into the bony components of the spine and are causing bone lysis or proliferation, or unless there has been pressure erosion of adjacent vertebral structures.

ii) Inflammatory disease of the spinal cord and meninges.

iii) Degenerative conditions of the spinal cord and nerve roots. Mineralised dural plaques are not diagnostic of chronic degenerative radiculo-myelopathy (CDRM) and may be seen in unaffected dogs.

iv) Vascular lesions of the spinal cord such as infarcts and spinal arteritis.

In a good quality spinal study it should be possible at each level to identify the anatomical features illustrated. (Figure 6.4).

Figure 6.4: Vertebral column - radiographic anatomy.

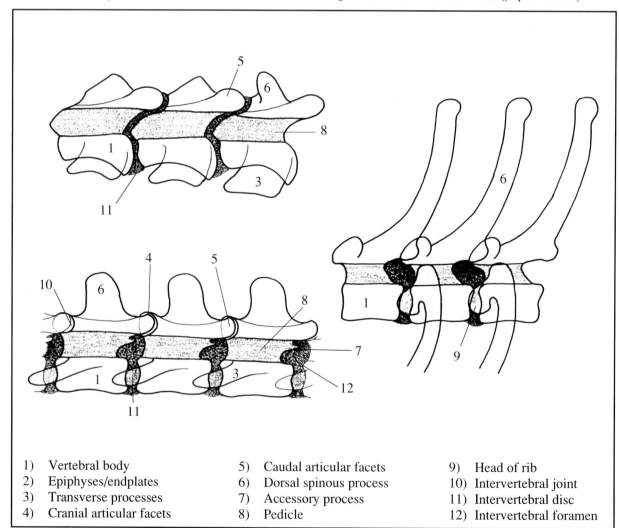

1)	Vertebral body	5)	Caudal articular facets
2)	Epiphyses/endplates	6)	Dorsal spinous process
3)	Transverse processes	7)	Accessory process
4)	Cranial articular facets	8)	Pedicle

9)	Head of rib
10)	Intervertebral joint
11)	Intervertebral disc
12)	Intervertebral foramen

There are a number of radiological findings which may be identified but which are unlikely to be of any clinical significance. These include the following:

a) Anomalies of the spine such as variations in the number of vertebrae, transitional vertebrae, block vertebrae and hemi-vertebrae. (see next section)

b) Scoliosis or lordosis unless it is extreme and associated with cord compression on myelographic examination.

c) Ventral spondylosis unless it is very severe and providing there is no evidence of erosive changes within the vertebral endplates.

d) Fine linear opacities due to mineralisation of the dura mater provided there is no other evidence of abnormality.

Each region of the vertebral column should be systematically assessed for abnormalites. The major elements of each vertebra should be identified and compared with the same features in those immediately neighbouring.

With the exception of the first two cervical vertebrae and at the junctions of the major levels of the vertebral column most of the changes in vertebral conformation occur gradually.

In a systematic evaluation of the spine the following features should be checked.

1) The width of the intervertebral disc spaces. Beware of the false impression of disc narrowing due to an oblique projection of the vertebral end plate. This may be caused either by inaccurate centering of the beam or by inadequate positioning of the subject.

2) The presence of mineralisation of the disc and the shape of any mineralised annulus.

3) The alignment of the floor of the vertebral canal. There should be no abrupt changes in level or angulation.

4) The length and shape of the vertebral centra. As with all changes this should be gradual.

5) The presence of normal cortical and trabecular architecture in all parts of the vertebra. The cortices are thin but should be intact, the density even and similar to adjacent vertebrae. There should be no periosteal reaction evident.

6) Sclerosis, erosion or irregularity of the vertebral endplates.

7) The size, shape and lucency of the intervertebral foramina. In the thoraco-lumbar area they are usually lucent and likened in shape to a 'donkey's' head. In the cervical region the articular processes are superimposed on the I/V foramina except for that between C2 and C3. In the thoracic region they are obscured by the dorsal part of the ribs.

8) The presence of opacities within the vertebral canal which may be diffuse, nodular or linear and either soft tissue density or mineralised. These are most easily appreciated over the intervertebral foramina but mineralised densities may be seen at any level but the precise location should be confirmed on a second view. Soft tissue densities may be recognised because they displace or replace the predominantly fatty contents of the spinal canal.

If no abnormalities are identified on the plain films then myelography in conjunction with a laboratory evaluation of the cerebro-spinal fluid should be considered. However, it must be understood that myelographic examination will only produce positive diagnostic information in those cases resulting in compression of the spinal cord and subarachnoid space. A negative result may, of course, be of value in ruling out such a lesion.

For a description of the techniques and media which should be used for myelography refer to the section dealing with contrast media and techniques.

Interpretation

Variations in Vertebral Number

Normal formula	C7 T13 L7 S3 Cy 6-14
May be	C7 T13 L8 S2 Cy 6-14
or	C7 T12 L8 S3 Cy 6-14
or	C7 T13 L6 S4 Cy 6-14

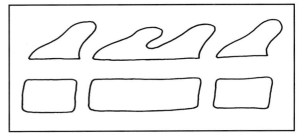

Figure 6.5: Block vertebrae.

Block Vertebrae
Adjacent vertebral bodies may be fused.

Most frequently seen in the cervicaor lumbar regions (Figure 6.5)

Hemivertebrae
Most common in thoracic and coccygeal regions. Mainly Pugs, English Bulldogs, Boston Terriers and related breeds. May cause spinal curvature but infrequent cause of spinal cord compression.

Radiological features
*   Two main types of hemivertebrae -
a) Partial ossification resulting in a wedge shaped deformity seen on the lateral view (Figure 6.6)

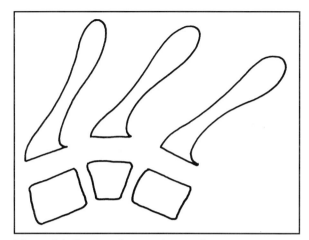

Figure 6.6: Hemivertebra - wedge vertebra.

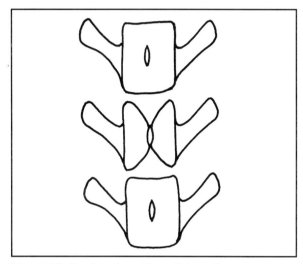

Figure 6.7: Hemivertebra - 'butterfly' vertebra.

b)   Failure of ossification sites to fuse. This
     results in a bi-partite 'butterfly' vertebra best
     seen on the VD view (Figure 6.7)
•   In both types the adjacent vertebrae and
     associated structures may be secondarily
     altered in shape.
•   May be solitary or multiple hemivertebra in
     an individual.

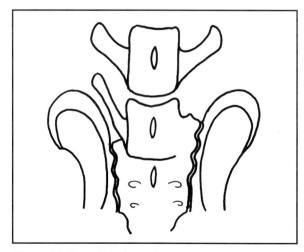

Figure 6.8: Transitional vertebrae.

Transitional Vertebrae

Mainly seen on the lumbo-sacral junction. Best seen
on VD view. Transverse process present on one side
but on the other the vertebra is incorporated into the
sacro- iliac articulation.

Radiological features (Figure 6.8)
•   May result in pelvic assymetry.
•   Can result in problems in assessing hips for
     hip dysplasia.
•   May also be occasionally seen at the thoraco-
     lumbar junction with only a single thirteenth
     rib. This is rarely of any significance.

Atlanto-Axial Subluxation

Congenital anomaly of young small and toy breed
dogs. Can result in varying degrees of spinal cord
compression. Clinical signs produced, which may be
intermittent, range from mild paresis and ataxia to
quadriplegia. Requires care when positioning for radiography to prevent cord damage.

Radiological features (Figure 6.9)
•   Abnormal widening of the space between the arch
     of C1 (atlas) and the dorsal spine of C2 (axis).
•   Marked angulation of floor of vertebral canal
     at atlanto-axial junction.
•   Odontoid process may be hyperplastic or absent.
•   May be associated with other radiological
     features of occipital dysplasia qv.

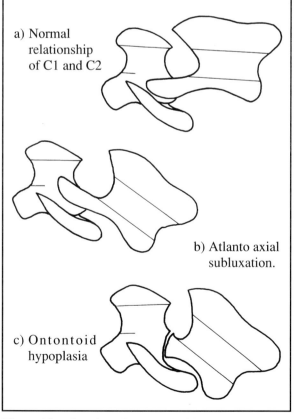

a) Normal
   relationship
   of C1 and C2

b) Atlanto axial
   subluxation.

c) Ontontoid
   hypoplasia

Figure 6.9: a, b and c. Atlanto axial subluxation.

Cervical Spondylopathy (Wobbler Syndrome)

Affected breeds are:

a) Juvenile Great Danes usually under 1 year.
b) Mature Doberman Pinschers 3-8 years.
c) Bassett Hounds.

Results in ataxia and fore and/or hind limb paresis.

Radiological features (Figure 6.10)
- Tilting or subluxation of the vertebral bodies - this may be accentuated on flexion of the neck.
- Normally affects the lower cervical spine.
- Abnormal conformation of the vertebral bodies.
- Stenosis of the spinal canal at the cranial end of the vertebral canal which may be funnel shaped.
- Narrowing of the disc space(s).
- Soft tissue mass dorsal to disc space resulting in marked spinal cord compression (*this requires myelographic examination).
- May also be dorsal compression due to hypertrophy of the ligamentum flavum.

- The abnormalities in the Bassett Hound are usually at the C2/3 junction.
- Abnormal angulation of the vertebral bodies.
- Stenosis of the spinal canal.
- Compression of the contrast columns on myelography (Figure 6.11)

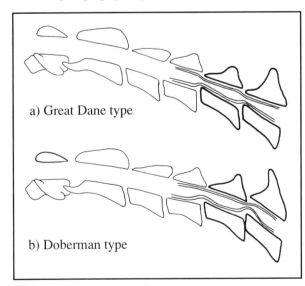

Figure 6.10: Cervical spondylopathy.

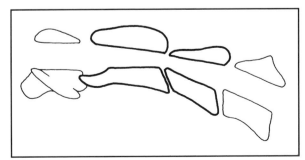

Figure 6.11: Cervical spondylopathy - Bassett type.

Lumbo-Sacral Instability

Possible cause of clinical signs seen in cauda equina syndrome. Pain, hindlimb paresis, neurological involvement of bladder and/or anus. Mainly seen in mature German shepherd dogs.

Radiological features (Figure 6.12)
- 'Step' in floor of vertebral canal at lumbo-sacral junction.
- This may be accentuated by flexion of the l/s spine.
- Narrowing of the sacral canal.
- May be associated ventral spondylosis.

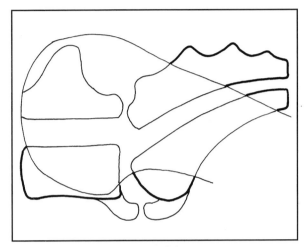

Figure 6.12: Lumbo-sacral instability.

Degenerative Disc Disease

Seen in a wide variety of breeds. More common in chondrodystrophoid types.
Clinical signs depend on level of lesion.

a) Cervical disc prolapse.
    Pain, forelimb paresis, occasionally quadriplegia.
b) Thoraco-lumbar disc prolapse.
    Pain, hind limb paresis, paraplegia.

Radiological features (Figure 6.13)
- Calcification of the nucleus pulposus. Not by itself diagnostic of disc prolapse but indicative of degenerative disc disease.
- Narrowing of the affected disc space.
- Mineralised prolapse disc material in spinal canal.
- Non-mineralised prolapsed disc material seen as soft tissue opacification of the intervertebral foramen.
- Extension of mineralised disc material through dorsal annulus.
- Evidence of ventral or ventro-lateral extra-dural mass within spinal canal on myelographic examination.

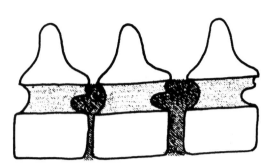

Figure 6.13a: Narrowed disc space.

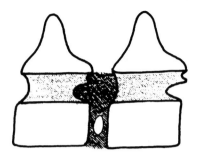

Figure 6.13b: Mineralised nucleus pulposus.

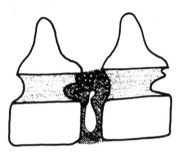

Figure 6.13c: Extension of mineralised nucleus through dorsal annulus.

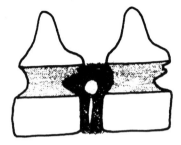

Figure 6.13d: Calcification protrusion.

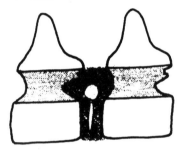

Figure 6.13e: Collapsed disc and opacity of the intervertebral foramen.

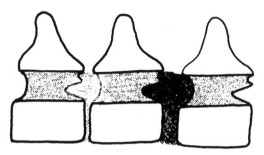

Figure 6.13f: Protruded disc materiaonly demonstrated on myelography.

Figure 6.13: a – f Degenerative disc disease.

Disco-Spondylitis

Any breed may be affected but more commonly large breeds. Common sites are lower cervical, mid thoracic and lumbo-sacral regions. Clinical signs include pain and stiffness. May be neurological deficits. May be associated pyrexia and malaise. May be history of previous infection possibly urinary.

Radiological features (Figure 6.14)
- Initial increase in width of disc space.
- Lysis and irregularity of vertebral end plates.
- Irregular periosteal reaction on adjacent vertebrae ventrally and laterally.
- Latterly decrease in width of disc space.
- Marked sclerosis of end plates and adjacent vertebral bodies.
- Periosteal reaction results in marked irregular spondylosis and in some cases vertebral fusion.

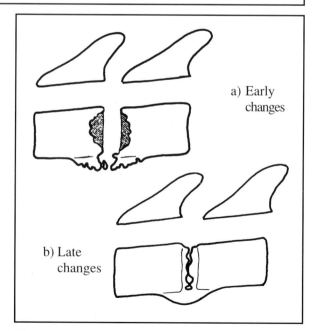

a) Early changes

b) Late changes

Figure 6.14: Disco-spondylitis.

Spondylosis

Very common in adult and elderly dogs of all breeds. Particularly common and usually very extensive in boxers. Can affect any level of the column. Uncommon in cervical spine.

Radiological features (Figure 6.15)
- Usually smooth bony spurs on the ventral aspects of the vertebral end plates.
- Progressively enlarge and may fuse.
- May also be lateral in location in which case there may appear to be sclerosis of the end plates and narrowing of the disc space.

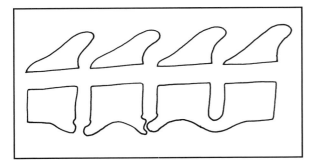

Figure 6.15: Spondylosi.

Primary Vertebral Neoplasia

Wide range of breeds affected. Variety of tumour types may be identified histologically. The clinical signs depend on the level of the column affected and the degree of spinal cord compression.

Radiological features (Figure 6.16)
- Usually a mixed pattern of bone lysis and periosteal proliferation.
- May occasionally be predominantly lytic or proliferative.(see multiple myeloma below)
- Any part of the vertebra may be involved.
- Adjacent vertebrae are not ususally involved.
- If the bone lysis is severe vertebral collapse may occur.

Multiple myelomas are often multifocal.
- Discrete lytic foci in vertebral body and processes.
- Usually no periosteal reaction.
- Often lesion elsewhere throughout the skeleton including ribs and limb bones.
- Clinical features often unassociated with the vertebral changes.

Secondary Vertebral Neoplasia

Clinical features as for primary vertebral tumours but possibly also associated with the features of the primary tumour. Skeletal metastases are uncommon but the spine is a predilection site. Primary tumours which may metastasise to the spine include bronchial and prostatic carcinomas.

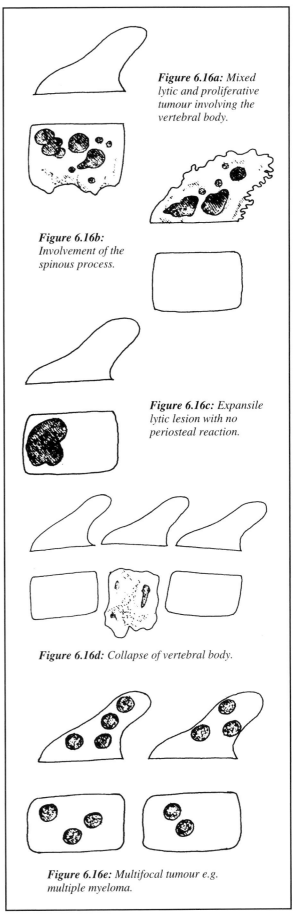

Figure 6.16a: Mixed lytic and proliferative tumour involving the vertebral body.

Figure 6.16b: Involvement of the spinous process.

Figure 6.16c: Expansile lytic lesion with no periosteal reaction.

Figure 6.16d: Collapse of vertebral body.

Figure 6.16e: Multifocal tumour e.g. multiple myeloma.

Figure 6.16: Primary vertebral neoplasia.

Radiological features (Figure 6.17)

- As for primary vertebral tumours but may be more than one site affected.

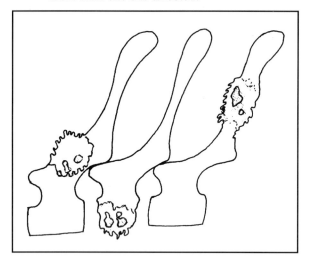

Figure 6.17: Secondary vertebral neoplasia.

Vertebral Osteomyelitis

Any breed or age of animal. Much less common than neoplasia. May be associated with either a penetrating wound or a migrating foreign body. Rarely haematogenous.

Radiological features (Figure 6.18)

- Mainly periosteal proliferation but can sometimes see evidence of bone lysis.
- May involve several adjacent vertebrae.
- Possibly associated soft tissue mass and gas.
- May be an associated disco-spondylitis.

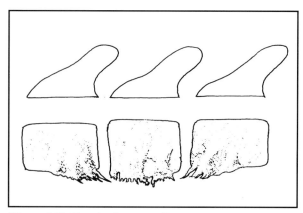

Figure 6.18: Vertebral osteomyelitis.

Neoplasia of the Spinal Cord and Meninges

As with vertebral tumours there may be a variety of tumour types and the clinical signs are dependent on the location of the tumour and the degree of cord compression. Plain radiographs are almost always normal. Myelography is required to diagnose and evaluate these tumours.

Radiological features seen on myelography.

Extra-dural masses (Figure 6.19)

- Partial or complete obstruction to the flow of contrast. (NOTE)
- Displacement or deviation of the contrast column(s).
- If laterally positioned there may be apparent widening of the columns on the lateral view.
- An annular mass will result in narrowing on both views.

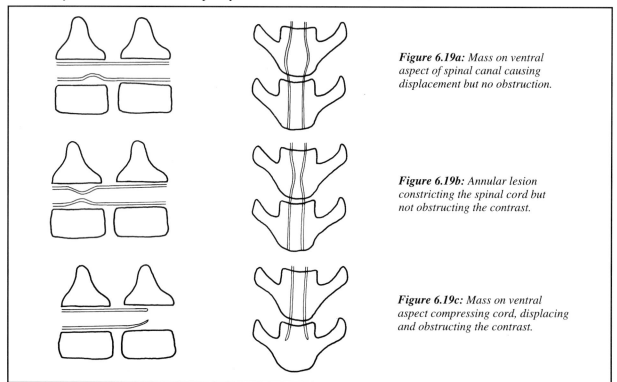

Figure 6.19a: Mass on ventral aspect of spinal canal causing displacement but no obstruction.

Figure 6.19b: Annular lesion constricting the spinal cord but not obstructing the contrast.

Figure 6.19c: Mass on ventral aspect compressing cord, displacing and obstructing the contrast.

Figure 6.19: Neoplasia of the spinal cord and meninges extra-dural masses

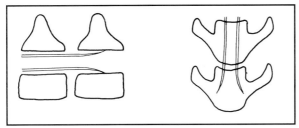

Figure 6.20: Neoplasia of the spinal cord and meninges - intra-dural masses.

Intra-dural masses (Figure 6.20)
- These may be either extra-medullary (within the meninges but outside the cord) or intra-medullary (within the cord).
- Result in partial or complete obstruction.*
- Usually expansion and thinning of the contrast columns.

NOTE: Although a cisternal myelogram will be adequate in many cases, if there is a complete block then a lumbar myelogram will be more likely to demonstrate the full extent of the lesion.

Vertebral Fractures and Dislocations.
May present with a wide variety of neurological signs depending on the degree of cord damage. The clinical signs may bear little correlation with the severity of the radiological features.

Radiological features (Figure 6.21)
A wide variety of appearances may be observed but the main features to look for include -
- Marked narrowing of a disc space.
- Separation of the articular facets.
- Reduced length of the vertebral body.
- Abrupt changes in the angulation of the vertebral canal.
- 'Stepping' of the floor of the vertebral canal.
- Displacement of adjacent vertebral segments. This may require two views and great care must be taken when positioning for the VD to avoid further spinal injury.
- For subtle changes a careful comparison with adjacent vertebral segments will be necessary.

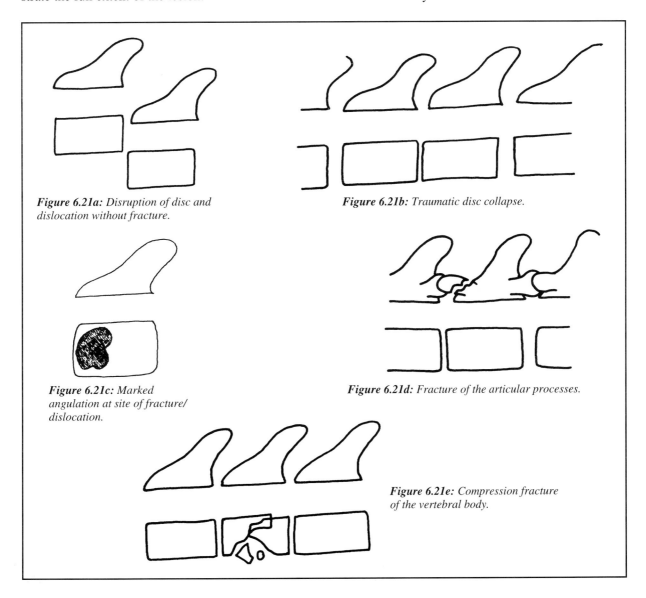

Figure 6.21a: Disruption of disc and dislocation without fracture.

Figure 6.21b: Traumatic disc collapse.

Figure 6.21c: Marked angulation at site of fracture/ dislocation.

Figure 6.21d: Fracture of the articular processes.

Figure 6.21e: Compression fracture of the vertebral body.

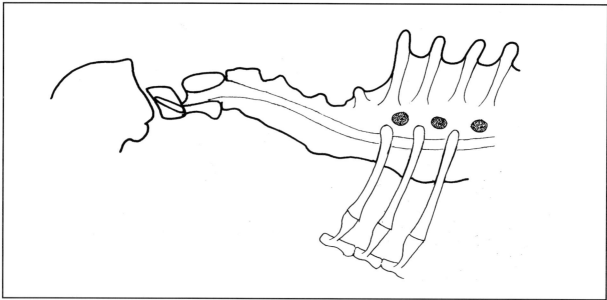

Figure 6.22: Hypervitaminosis A.

Hypervitaminosis A

Seen in cats fed a diet containing a high proportion of liver. Usually adult to elderly. Vertebral changes have not been described in the dog.

Clinical features include stiffness, inability to groom, lethargy etc. May be lameness associated with limb lesions.

Radiological features (Figure 6.22)
- Marked periosteal reaction on the ventral and/or dorsal aspects of the cervical and cranial thoracic vertebrae.
- When advanced there will be complete bony fusion of several vertebrae.
- May be mild generalised osteoporosis.

CHECKLIST FOR THE EXAMINATION OF SPINAL RADIOGRAPHS

CHANGE IN SHAPE OF VERTEBRAE
    Congenital anomalies
    Fractures
    Osteomyelitis
    Neoplasia

VARIATION IN VERTEBRAL NUMBER
    Congenital anomalies

INCREASE IN DENSITY
    Osteomyelitis
    Neoplasia
    Hypervitaminosis A

DECREASE IN DENSITY
    Juvenile secondary hyperparathyroidism
    Osteoporosis associated with Cushing's syndrome
    Neoplasia - Iy and IIy
    Osteomyelitis

DECREASE IN WIDTH OF DISC SPACE
    Disc prolapse
    Chronic discospondylitis
    Fracture/luxation
    Lateralised spondylosis
    Poor positioning/centring.

INCREASE IN WIDTH OF DISC SPACE
    Acute discospondylitis
    Fracture/luxation

REACTIVE OSTEOPHYTES ON ARTICULAR FACETS
    Degenerative joint disease (spondylitis)
    Neoplasia

CHAPTER SEVEN

Contrast Media and Techniques

M.E. Herrtage and R. Dennis

CONTENTS

Due to the inherent limitations of plain films, special radiographic procedures may be required to supplement or confirm the information obtained from survey radiographs. These special techniques, which involve the use of contrast media, can be used to identify or enhance soft tissue structures or organs that might be difficult or impossible to visualise clearly due to their lack of inherent contrast with the surrounding tissues and structures.

These structures or organs can then be more effectively evaluated for size, shape and position. In addition, contrast techniques can be used to gain valuable information about the mucosal surface of a hollow viscus or its contents which would not be apparent on the plain radiograph. In some instances contrast techniques may also be used to evaluate organ function.

I: CONTRAST MEDIA

The contrast media used for these examinations usually contain elements of high atomic number, either barium or iodine, since they absorb a high proportion of the incident X-ray beam and are thus relatively opaque to X-rays. They provide positive contrast with the soft tissues.

Gases may also be used as contrast agents, not because of their atomic number, but because they have a very low specific gravity and therefore are more radiolucent to X-rays, providing negative contrast relative to other tissues. Double contrast techniques combine both types of media whereby a small quantity of positive contrast is introduced into a viscus followed by a larger volume of negative contrast medium. This procedure produces optimum mucosal detail and avoids the complete obliteration of small filling defects, such as small calculi or foreign bodies, by a large volume of dense positive contrast agent.

1) Barium Sulphate Preparations

These agents are used almost exclusively for the investigation of the alimentary tract. The advantage of barium is that it is completely insoluble and is neither acted on by alimentary secretions nor absorbed through the intestine.

Barium sulphate suitable for radiological use is prepared as a fine micropulverised salt which can form a colloidal suspension providing excellent mucosal detail.

It is available commercially (Table 7.1) in three forms:-
i)   A ready prepared stabilised colloidal suspension.
ii) A dry powder suitable for either preparing a liquid suspension or adding to food.
iii) A thick, viscous paste specially formulated for outlining the pharynx and oesophagus.

The main disadvantage of barium sulphate is that being non-absorbable it may result in granulomatous reactions or adhesions if it leaks into the peritoneal cavity through a perforated bowel. If inhaled accidentally during administration it may cause aspiration pneumonia.

2) Water-Soluble Iodine Containing Preparations

These form the largest group of contrast agents (Table 7.2). They are all derivatives of tri-iodinated benzoic acid and being water-soluble can be injected directly into the vascular system and used for angiographic studies. Following injection they are rapidly excreted almost entirely by the urinary system and so will opacify the kidneys and urinary tract. Certain formulations are intended for use in the alimentary tract following oral administration in cases where perforation of the tract is suspected, as they are rapidly absorbed from the peritoneal cavity. However, being bitter to the taste, they are not tolerated well and produce poorer contrast than

Table 7.1: Barium Sulphate Preparations.

Presentation	Proprietary name	Manufacture
Suspension	Micropaque standard Baritop 100	Nicholas Bioglan
Powder	Micropaque HD Baritop Plus E-Z-Paque E-Z-Paque HD	Nicholas Bioglan Henleys Henleys
Paste*	Microtrast	Nicholas

* Not currently available in the U.K.

Table 7.2: Water-Soluble Iodine Containing Preparations.

Presentation	Proprietary name	Concentration mg I/ml	Manufacture
Ionic media - For intra-vascular use			
Na/Meglumine iothalamate	Conray 280	280	Mallinckrodt
Sodium iothalamate	Conray 420	420	Mallinckrodt
Sodium diatrizoate	Hypaque 25%	150	Sanofi Winthrop
	Hypaque 45%	270	Sanofi Winthrop
Na/Meglumine diatrozoate	Urografin 150	146	Schering
	Urografin 325	325	Schering
	Urografin 370	370	Schering
Na/meglumine metrizoate Ca & Mg	Isopaque 350	350	Nycomed
	Isopaque 440	440	Nycomed
Na/meglumine iodamide	Uromiro 300	300	E Merck
	Uromiro 340	380	E Merck
Ionic media - For alimentary tract studies			
Na iothalamate	Gastro-Conray	360	Mallinckrodt
Na/meglumine diatrizoate	Gastrografin	370	Schering
Low osmolar non-ionic media			
Metrizamide	Amipaque	170-300*	Nycomed
Iopamidol	Niopam 200	200	E Merck
	Niopam 300	300	E Merck
	Niopam 370	370	E Merck
Iohexol	Omnipaque 240	240	Nycomed
	Omnipaque 300	300	Nycomed
	Omnipaque 350	350	Nycomed
Iotrolan	Isovist 240	240	Schering
	Isovist 300	300	Schering
Low osmolar ionic media - Not suitable for myelography			
Na/meglumine ioxaglate	Hexabrix	320	Mallinckrodt

*Supplied as a freeze dried powder with solvent to prepare required iodine concentration.

barium and so their application is very limited.

Although relatively safe in domestic animals the intra-vascular use of water-soluble contrast media can produce side effects such as vomiting or, more rarely, anaphylactic or idiosyncratic reactions. These side effects are related to their high osmotic pressure, which is five to eight times that of normal body fluids, their ionic charge and their chemical toxicity.

The low osmolar contrast media were introduced to reduce the adverse effects due to hyperosmolality. The non-ionic group, metrizamide, iopamidol and iohexol, are suitable for myelography as well as intravascular studies. The low osmolar ionic compound, ioxaglate, is not suitable for myelography but shares the same advantages as the non-ionic low osmolar contrast media in reducing the side effects for intravascular studies and for excretion urography.

3)   Negative Contrast Agents

A number of gases have been used as contrast agents but air, oxygen, carbon dioxide and nitrous oxide are the most frequently employed. They provide negative contrast with the tissues of the body but there is less radiographic contrast and much poorer mucosal detail than is obtained with positive contrast agents. However, they can be used to advantage in conjunction with positive contrast media in double contrast studies.

For some of the techniques listed at the end of this section more specialised contrast agents may be required and this is indicated where appropriate.

Techniques

General considerations

Contrast studies should not be used to enhance, or as a substitute for, poor quality radiographs. They are intended to provide information additional to that on the plain radiograph. Plain films should routinely be taken prior to any contrast examination and examined for -

i)   Adequate technical quality
ii)   Radiological features indicative of a
        diagnosis
iii) Adequate patient preparation where necessary
iv)   Suitability of the chosen contrast technique
        and agent
v)   An assessment of the amount of contrast
        medium required
vi)   Comparison with subsequent radiographs

II: CONTRAST RADIOGRAPHY OF THE ALIMENTARY TRACT

Whilst bearing in mind the necessary requirements of radiation safety it must be pointed out that, with the exception of barium enemas, anaesthesia should not be used for contrast studies of the alimentary tract as it will not only interfere with normal physiological activity but there will be serious risk of regurgitation and inhalation of contrast into the lungs. Certain sedatives may delay gastric and intestinal transit times.

The Oesophagus

Indications:
   • Regurgitation
   • Retching
   • Dysphagia
   • Vomition of undigested food soon after eating.

Technique

Little preparation of the subject is necessary if the examination is to be confined to the oesophagus. Plain films should always be taken initially otherwise significant findings such as foreign material may be masked by the contrast. Unless gross lesions or abnormal function is present liquid barium suspension will pass rapidly down the oesophagus into the stomach before radiographs can be obtained. It is therefore preferable for such cases to use thick barium sulphate paste which adheres well to the oesophageal mucosal surface. The paste is placed on the back of the patient's tongue and/or hard palate and will remain coating the surfaces of the pharynx and oesophagus for several minutes whilst the necessary radiographs are taken.

If a dilated oesophagus is suspected from the plain films, a more satisfactory technique is to encourage the subject to eat a mixture of soft tinned food to which has been added about 20-30 ml of 100% w/v barium sulphate suspension. This technique will reliably demonstrate the degree and extent of any dilation and indicate the level of any oesophageal constriction. Liquid barium will usually fail to demonstrate these features adequately. However, it must be remembered that administration of a barium/meal mixture it is not suitable for the subsequent evaluation of the stomach and small intestine as part of the same study.

Lateral views of the cervical and thoracic oesophagus, which are described elsewhere, are the most informative, although occasionally additional information may be gained from a dorsoventral view of the thoracic oesophagus.

The evaluation of functional disorders resulting in dysphagia such as cricopharyngeal achalasia or pharyngeal incoordination may prove difficult or impossible without access to image-intensified fluoroscopy and such cases would be better referred to a centre with these facilities. In addition, particular care should be taken when administering barium to animals with swallowing disorders so as to minimise the risk of aspiration of contrast and subsequent inhalation pneumonia.

The Stomach and Small Intestine

Indications:
   • Persistent vomiting
   • Haematemesis
   • Displacement of the GI tract associated with
      diaphragmatic rupture
   • Assessment of GI tract displacement by
      changes in size or position of adjacent organs
   • Unexplained dilation of the small intestine.

NB. A barium study is often unrewarding in the investigation of cases of vomiting associated with diarrhoea.

Technique

In an elective examination an empty alimentary tract should be ensured by withholding food for 24 hours and, if necessary, by the administration of an enema. As stated above wherever possible the subject should be unsedated, although if sedation is necessary acepromazine has been found to have the least effect on gastrointestinal motility and will assist restraint and accurate positioning.

Plain radiographs should precede the contrast examination. As a general guide 20-100ml of 100% w/v barium sulphate suspension, depending on the size of the subject, should be adequate. This may be administered by a syringe or small plastic bottle fitted with a nozzle or alternatively by stomach tube in a co-operative patient.

For a full evaluation of the stomach, four views should be taken immediately following the administration of contrast - right and left lateral views, ventrodorsal and dorsoventral views, in each case centred over the cranial abdomen at the level of the last rib.

For a reliable diagnosis lesions should be demonstrable on more than one film. Due to gravity the barium collects in the dependent portion, of the stomach and the gastric gas bubble in the non-dependent portion thus the radiological appearance of these four views will vary and can aid the clinician in detecting lesions.

This effect can be further optimised by performing a double contrast gastrogram to provide enhanced detail of the mucosal pattern. Some proprietary brands of barium sulphate suspension are formulated to be slightly effervescent to produce this effect.

Radiographs of the stomach should be repeated 5-10 minutes after the initial films to verify the presence of any observed lesions and to assess normal onset of gastric emptying. Further films at 10-15 minute intervals may be required in some cases.

A full assessment of gastric motility and the assessment of lesions seen only transiently will require the use of image-intensified fluoroscopy.

Evaluation of the small intestine should follow the gastric examination with lateral and ventrodorsal views taken at regular intervals, depending on the rate of passage in the individual case, until either a diagnosis has been reached or the barium has entered the large intestine. Films taken at random may miss the outlining of significant lesions or may show artefactual 'lesions' resulting from peristaltic activity. A film taken 24 hours after administration of contrast should be used to demonstrate that all the contrast has reached the large intestine.

If a barium study is to be performed to demonstrate displacement of the GI tract during the investigation of an abdominal mass or diaphragmatic rupture then it is more economical to omit the initial films and take radiographs 30-45 mins following administration by which time the stomach and most of the small intestine should be visualised.

Evaluation: The contrast study should be evaluated for the following features:

i) The onset time and rate of gastric emptying. This usually starts within 15 minutes but may be delayed in normal nervous animals up to 30-45 minutes. Anything beyond this should be regarded as abnormal. The stomach is usually more or less empty within 1-2 hours and completely empty of barium within 4 hours.

ii) The rate of passage through the small intestine. Barium should reach the large intestine within 4 hours.

iii) The presence of localised or generalised dilation of the intestinal lumen or stomach.

iv) Dilution and/or flocculation of the barium suspension indicative of the retention and pooling of gastro-intestinal secretions.

v) The presence of mucosal roughening or irregularities particularly in the antral and pyloric region of the stomach.

vi) The presence of filling defects either within the lumen and suggestive of radiolucent foreign bodies or attached to the wall and indicative of proliferative mural or mucosal lesions.

vii) An assessment of the thickness of the stomach wall.

viii) Displacement of the GI tract in relation to other abdominal viscera or abdominal wall including the diaphragm.

The Large Intestine

Indications:
- Tenesmus
- Melaena
- Chronic diarrhoea
- Identification of the large intestine in relation to caudal abdominal/intra-pelvic masses etc.

Technique

A thorough, non-irritant, cleansing enema should be given at least 2-3 hours prior to examination. A dilute suspension of barium sulphate - usually 20% w/v made up by diluting 100% suspension with lukewarm water or saline - should be administered slowly either by an enema pump, or by a gravity feed tube and funnel. Alternatively, a Foley catheter can be inserted into the terminal rectum and the barium slowly injected by a large volume syringe. Administration should be continued until the colon is fully distended. The volume of contrast required is usually about 10 ml per kg body weight.

If the animal is sedated or anaesthetised, and this is preferable for this technique as it does not interfere with the results, leakage of contrast may occur and this can be prevented by securing the cuffed catheter with a purse-string suture round the anus.

Radiographs should be taken in lateral and ventrodorsal projection. The contrast may then be removed from the colon which is then distended with air and the radiograph repeated to produce a double contrast study which will allow much better evaluation of mucosal detail.

Evaluation: The contrast study should be evaluated for the following features:

i) Mucosal irregularities. The normal mucosa of the dog and cat is smooth and featureless.
ii) Luminal narrowing. Beware of localised narrowing immediately cranial to the pelvic brim due to colonic spasm.
iii) Displacement of the colon/rectum by an associated mass lesion in the adjacent organs/ tissues.

NB. It is important to realise that contrast studies of the large intestine are frequently disappointing in the investigation of chronic diarrhoea and have to some extent been superseded by endoscopy.

III: CONTRAST RADIOGRAPHY OF THE URINARY TRACT

In contrast to the investigation of the alimentary tract deep sedation or anaesthesia is not contra- indicated for urinary tract investigations providing the clinical condition of the subject permits. Indeed, anaesthesia is of value in ensuring accurate positioning for serial radiographs and lessens the likelihood of adverse reactions to intravenous contrast media such as nausea and retching.

Kidneys and Ureters - Intravenous Urography (IVU)

The kidneys and ureters can be studied following the intravenous injection of water-soluble iodine containing media which are readily excreted by the kidneys. This technique is termed intravenous or excretory urography - IVU.

Indications:
- The identification of the kidneys for the evaluation of renal size, shape and position
- Urinary incontinence
- The investigation of haematuria or pyuria NOT arising from the lower urinary tract.

Technique
There are two basic techniques for obtaining diagnostic IVU's.
i) The low volume, rapid injection technique used with or without abdominal compression
ii) The high volume, drip infusion technique

The former is preferred for the investigation of the kidneys, the latter is preferred by some people for the demonstration of the ureters.

Whichever technique is used the subject should, whenever possible, be prepared by starving for 24 hours and a cleansing enema administered 2-3 hours prior to examination to empty the colon and so prevent extraneous shadows from obliterating radiographic detail.

i) Low volume, rapid injection IVU
The patient is placed in dorsal recumbency ideally using some form of cassette tunnel if no Bucky tray is available. This will permit the taking of serial radiographs without having to disturb positioning until adequate opacification of the urinary tract has been achieved when lateral views may be required.

If compression is to be used, two pads should be placed over the ventral abdominal wall immediately in front of the pubis and a broad band tightened across the caudal abdomen to compress the bladder and ureters and so delay the passage of contrast from the renal pelvis and proximal ureter.

This may produce artefactual distension and distortion of the renal pelvices and ureters. Further films should be taken following the release of the compression and this should be done as soon as the renal pelvis and proximal ureters have been examined in order to evaluate the distal ureter. Adequate examinations can often be carried out without the use of compression.

A total dose of 600-800mg iodine per kg body weight is injected intravenously as rapidly as possible. Using 60-70% contrast medium (300-400mg I/ml) this will be a dose of 2ml per kg.

The initial film should be taken immediately on completion of the injection to demonstrate arterial opacification of the renal parenchyma.

Subsequent films should then be taken at 1, 5, 10, 15 and 20 minutes. Although both ventrodorsal and lateral views are ideal it is more convenient to take the initial views in VD projection and then take lateral views when adequate opacification has been achieved.

ii) High volume, drip infusion IVU
The contrast agent used is identical to the previous technique but is made up into a more dilute solution - 150mg I/ml - this may be purchased at a concentration ready for infusion or may be diluted with dextrose or saline from more concentrated formulations. A total dose of 1200 mg iodine per kg body weight (8ml per kg) should be infused over 10 to 15 minutes through an intravenous catheter.

The positioning is the same as above but without the use of compression.

Radiographs should be taken at 5, 10 and 15 minutes after the start of infusion. Again both views should be used.

This technique is particularly valuable for the investigation of ureteric conditions. For ureteric ectopia it is important to demonstrate the point of entry of the ureters into the bladder. This is best achieved by first performing a pneumocystogram to help highlight the bladder neck and to provide a radiolucent background against which to visualise the ureters.

Evaluation: The contrast study should be evaluated for the following features:-
  i)   Renal size, shape and position
  ii) Renal architecture - particularly the renal pelvis. This varies quite widely and the various normal appearances should be recognised
  iii) The size and position of the ureters particularly their entry into the bladder

Bladder - Cystography

Indications:
• Persistent haematuria
• Dysuria
• Urinary retention
• Urinary incontinence
• The identification, localisation and integrity of the bladder shadow.

Technique
The animal should be prepared wherever possible so that the terminal portion of the colon is empty. Either deep sedation or anaesthesia is necessary to facilitate positioning and restraint and to ensure satisfactory radiation safety. Plain films should be taken before the contrast examination.

The bladder is catheterised and thoroughly drained of urine. In bitches a rigid catheter should not be used as this produces distortion of the bladder neck and may cause damage to the bladder during positioning for radiography.

There are three main types of direct cystography that may be employed - negative contrast or pneumocystography, positive contrast cystography and double contrast cystography.

i) Pneumocystography
The bladder is inflated with air until moderately distended and firm as judged by gentle abdominal palpation. The air may be introduced either with a syringe and three way tap or by the careful use of a rubber bulb insufflator.

In some cases it may be difficult to maintain adequate filling of the bladder due to leakage of air round the catheter in which case the radiograph must be taken immediately on completion of inflation or during continuous inflation taking care to ensure protection of personnel.

Frequently the lateral view of the caudal abdomen will provide sufficient information on which to base a diagnosis but this should be supplemented by a ventrodorsal view where indicated.

NB. Inadequate filling of the bladder may lead to artefactual bladder wall thickening which may mimic pathological changes. However, in an anaesthetised animal care must be taken not to damage the bladder by over-inflation.

ii) Positive contrast cystography
This technique is similar to that above but the bladder is filled with dilute water-soluble contrast medium. Usually 5-10% w/v provides adequate opacification and the volume injected will range from 50-300ml depending on the size of the animal.

This technique provides better mucosal detail than does pneumocystography but small intra-luminal lesions or calculi may be masked by the contrast.

iii) Double contrast cystography
This technique provides optimum mucosal detail with least risk of masking intra-luminal lesions. 5-15ml of 20% contrast medium is injected into the empty bladder immediately followed by inflation with air as for a pneumocystogram and then the required films taken. The contrast medium coats the mucosal surface and the residual puddle of contrast on the dependent wall of the bladder will highlight any small radiolucent masses or calculi which may be missed by other techniques.

iv) Intravenous cystography
This technique can be employed in those situations where catheterisation is either not possible or is contra-indicated for any reason. It is possible to use the same procedure as for low volume, rapid-infusion IVU with radiographs of the bladder being taken after at least 30 mins. It is advisable to roll the animal gently from side to side to ensure thorough mixing of the contrast-laden urine with any urine which may have been in the bladder initially.

The results are often not as informative as the previously described techniques since the radiographer has less control over the degree of opacification or degree of bladder filling.

Evaluation: The contrast study should be evaluated for the following features:-
  i)   The size, shape and position of the bladder
  ii) Bladder wall thickness - localised or generalised

iii) Irregularities of the mucosal surface - localised or generalised

iv) Presence of intra-luminal opacities either free within the lumen or attached to the wall

v) Leakage of contrast into the peritoneal cavity

Urethra - Retrograde Urethrography and Vagino-Urethrography

Indications:
- Persistent haematuria
- Dysuria
- Urinary incontinence
- Urinary tract obstruction
- Evaluation of prostatic disease
- Lesions of the os penis
- Urethritis and urethral neoplasia.

Technique
Retrograde urethrography should be performed in those cases where a urethral lesion is the initial clinical diagnosis, following cystography where no abnormalities have been found, or to evaluate more fully a lesion already demonstrated by cystography.

i) Retrograde urethrography in the male dog
A urinary catheter is placed in the penile urethra and an injection of 5-10ml contrast medium made while occluding the urethral opening around the catheter. Contrast media containing 150-200mg iodine per ml are usually adequate and the contrast medium may be mixed thoroughly with KY lubricant jelly prior to injection. This enables the contrast to remain within the urethra for a longer period of time to facilitate radiography.

A lateral radiograph is generally the most informative and should be made immediately at the end of the injection of contrast. The hind legs should be pulled cranially to demonstrate the ischial urethra and caudally to demonstrate the penile and pelvic urethra.

If the prostatic urethra is to be examined then the catheter should be advanced so that the tip lies just distal to the prostate gland.

Ventrodorsal views may be of value in the identification of compression or displacement of the intra-pelvic urethra and in the evaluation of some prostatic lesions.

Evaluation: The films should be evaluated for the following features:
i) Mucosal irregularities or strictures
ii) Intraluminal defects caused by calculi - care must be taken to ensure that air bubbles do not become trapped in the contrast as these will mimic calculi

iii) The presence of abnormal extravasation of contrast material into the periurethral tissues or prostate gland

iv) Irregularity or stricture of the prostatic urethra

ii) Retrograde vagino-urethrography in the bitch
A Foley catheter with the lumen pre-filled with contrast medium to prevent the introduction of air bubbles and the tip cut off is inserted into the vestibule and the bulb inflated. In larger bitches a pair of tissue forceps may be required to hold the vulval lips closed to prevent the bulb slipping out. Alternatively, a dog catheter, similarly pre-filled with contrast, can be positioned in the vestibule and the vulval lips held closed with a pair of gentle bowel clamps. This latter method has the advantage that the whole of the vagina is filled with contrast and there is no risk of the inflated bulb of the Foley catheter obscuring a lesion or obstructing the urethral orifice.

Contrast medium (150-200mg I per ml) is introduced at a dose rate of approximately 1ml per kg. This fills both the vagina as far cranially as the cervix as well as the urethra, and in some cases partially outlines the bladder. Care must be taken not to use excessive pressure so that the vagina is not injured.

A lateral radiograph is usually the only view of value in this technique and is taken on completion of the injection. It should be processed and evaluated before the contrast is withdrawn and the catheter removed in case there has been inadequate filling.

Evaluation: The contrast study should be evaluated for the following features:
i) Mucosal irregularities or strictures. Note there is always marked narrowing of the lumen between the vestibule and cranial vagina
ii) Luminal defects caused by calculi or vaginal tumours
iii) The presence of abnormal communications of the ureters with either the urethra or vagina indicative of ureteral ectopia
iv) The location of the bladder neck and shape of the vesico-urethral junction in the assessment of sphincter mechanism incompetence

IV: CONTRAST RADIOGRAPHY OF THE SPINE - MYELOGRAPHY

Indications:
- Ataxia
- Paresis or paralysis in which a spinal cord lesion is suspected
- Spinal pain
- Neurogenic incontinence.

Technique

A low osmolar, non-ionic, water-soluble contrast agent is ESSENTIAL to prevent adverse toxic effects on the CNS. This is injected into the subarachnoid space and mixes with the cerebrospinal fluid (CSF) surrounding the cord. Iohexol (Omnipaque) or iopamidol (Niopam) are the contrast media of choice as they have virtually eliminated the side effects - convulsions and arachnoiditis - occasionally encountered with metrizamide (Amipaque).

The contrast may be introduced into the subarachnoid space following either cisternal or lumbar puncture. The cisternal route is most commonly used and most easily performed. Details of the technique for lumbar puncture are available (Douglas, Herrtage & Williamson, 1987).

The dose of contrast medium depends on both the size of the subject and the suspected site of the lesion. Cervical lesions generally require less contrast when administered by the cisternal route than do lumbar lesions. A dose rate of 0.3ml per kg body weight is usually quoted but often a minimum dose of 1.5-2.0 ml is required in small subjects up to a maximum dose of 8-9ml in larger animals. Both iohexol and iopamidol are usually used at a concentration of 300mg I per ml which is mildly hypertonic.

General anaesthesia is essential and if intravenous anaesthetic agents are being used the patient should be intubated to ensure a patent airway. The animal is placed in lateral recumbency - left or right depending on the preference of the operator - and the skin caudal to the occipital crest clipped and surgically prepared.

The head is held by an assistant with the nose positioned at right angles to the neck and the sagittal plane parallel to the table top. A 21-23 gauge needle - spinal or hypodermic - is inserted in the midline at the level of the cranial edge of the wings of the atlas. The needle should be directed towards the lower jaw with the bevel facing caudally.

The choice between a spinal or hypodermic needle is one of personal preference. A spinal needle is less likely to be blocked by tissue but can be too flexible to permit accurate redirection once the stylet has been removed. Hypodermic needles are easier to direct and are quite satisfactory although the bevel is longer and therefore there is the potential risk of injury to the cord in small subjects.

If a tilting table is available some workers prefer to have this tilted 10-15 degrees head up to ensure flow of contrast caudally. However, other people find this unnecessary and encounter no problems.

The needle should be advanced slowly. Resistance will be felt as the tip penetrates the ligamentum flavum followed by a slight 'popping' sensation as it enters the cisterna magna. Cerebrospinal fluid should then flow freely from the needle hub and may be collected for laboratory examination. If blood appears the needle should be withdrawn and the procedure reattempted with a clean needle.

It is advisable for those inexperienced in this technique to practise on recently euthanased animals before attempting the procedure in clinical cases.

The contrast medium is injected slowly over 1-2 mins ensuring that the needle tip remains steady in the subarachnoid space (GENTLE suction on the syringe plunger will result in a flow of CSF swirling back into the syringe). The injection should be terminated if any back pressure is experienced. At the completion of the injection the needle and syringe are removed. Radiographs may be taken immediately or following a few minutes with the subject tilted head up at 30-45 degrees.

Lateral radiographs should be taken at each level of the spine until either a normal study is confirmed or a lesion is detected. If a lesion is identified then further collimated lateral and ventrodorsal views centred at this level should be taken.

Evaluation: The contrast study should be evaluated for the following features:-

i)   Demonstration of even dorsal, ventral and lateral contrast columns outlining the subarachnoid space.

ii) Evidence of complete or partial obstruction to the flow of contrast.

iii) Displacement or deviation of the contrast columns.

iv) Divergence of the contrast columns indicative of intra-medullary lesions, cord swelling, or cord compression in the other plane.

v)   Variation in width of the contrast columns or filling defects.

vi) Outlining by the contrast columns of extra-dural masses.

These features are illustrated in Chapter 6.

V: OTHER CONTRAST TECHNIQUES

The following procedures are used less frequently and may require more specialised equipment or contrast media. They can, however, provide valuable additional diagnostic information in selected cases.

The procedures are outlined below but more precise information may be obtained from the references and texts indicated.

Angiography

This is the radiographic demonstration of portions of the vascular system by the injection of a water-soluble contrast agent either intravenously or intra-arterially. The examination is most satisfactory if a catheter can be placed in a blood vessel close to the region to be examined. For some examinations a single radiograph taken immediately at the termination of the injection provides adequate diagnostic information (e.g. portal venography) but films taken serially at intervals of 0.5-2 seconds are necessary for other studies (e.g. angiocardiography). These require the use of some form of rapid film changer.

Angiocardiography

This can be used to demonstrate congenital or acquired lesions of the heart. It is essential to obtain a bolus of contrast within the heart. This is best achieved by injecting the contrast as rapidly as possible through a catheter positioned close to the heart via the jugular vein - non-selective angiocardiography - or directly into a specific cardiac chamber or great vessel - selective angiocardiography.

Non-selective angiocardiography can be performed relatively easily provided some method of obtaining serial films is available. Selective angiocardiography requires that the positioning of the tip of the catheter is monitored by either image-intensified fluoroscopy or by periodic spot films.

Careful planning prior to the investigation and continuous monitoring of the patient during the examination are essential to ensure the safety and quality of the procedure.

The dose of contrast used depends on the purpose of the study but as a general rule it is better to use a smaller volume of high concentration contrast than larger volumes of lower density. Five to ten ml of medium containing 420 mg I per ml is often adequate although a dose rate of 1 ml/kg is often recommended. It is also essential to use as large a catheter as possible to ensure very rapid delivery of the bolus contrast.

Cerebral Arteriography and Cavernous Sinus Venography

These two techniques can both be used to demonstrate space-occupying lesions within the cranial cavity but require considerable experience in radiological interpretation. For both techniques it is preferable to use the low osmolar contrast agents because of the reduced likelihood of side effects.

Cerebral arteriography requires the catheterisation of the internal carotid or vertebral artery, a technique facilitated by the use of image intensified fluoroscopy.

Cavernous sinus venography is much simpler and requires the cannulation of the angular vein - a branch of the facial vein - just in front of the medial canthus of the eye - and injection of contrast to outline the orbital sinus, cavernous and petrosal sinuses on the floor of the cranial cavity. This technique can be used to demonstrate tumour masses associated with the floor of the cranial cavity e.g pituitary tumours.

Portal Venography

This technique will assist in the confirmation of the diagnosis in cases of congenital and acquired portosystemic shunts and assist in the management of these cases. A variety of methods have been described but the simplest, and that which gives the most consistent results, is direct cannulation of a jejunal vein.

A loop of jejunum is identified at laparotomy and an intravenous cannula tied in place in one of the jejunal veins. The animal is placed in lateral recumbency and 5 - 10 ml of water-soluble contrast medium injected as rapidly as possible. A radiograph of the abdomen and caudal thorax centred over the last rib is obtained immediately on completion of the injection.

In a normal animal the contrast will be seen outlining the portal vein and its branches within the liver. In cases of porto-systemic shunts the contrast will outline the shunt communicating directly with either the caudal vena cava, azygos vein, velar omental veins or occasionally the renal capsular veins.

Arthography

This can be performed by the injection of a small volume, 1-1.5ml of water-soluble contrast medium and/or by the use of air to produce positive, negative or double contrast studies.

The contrast medium is injected into the joint cavity and will demonstrate the articular surfaces and outline the joint capsule. This technique is of limited value and seldom reveals more than the information that can be obtained from a well positioned and exposed plain radiograph.

In practice its use is limited almost exclusively to the shoulder where it is occasionally of value in evaluating fully cases of osteochondritis dissecans.

Bronchography

This technique is used for outlining the bronchial tree in order to demonstrate bronchial obstruction, bronchiectasis and displacement of bronchi by extraneous masses. It can also be used to outline the granulomatous nodules in cases of infection by Filaroides osleri.

The contrast agent used is an aqueous suspension of propyliodine (Dionosil aqueous - Glaxo Ltd). The technique is to anaesthetise the subject lightly and then introduce the contrast medium by a fine catheter at the base of the trachea via the endotracheal tube. The animal is in lateral recumbency with the side to be investigated down. Following introduction of the contrast the subject is then positioned so as to distribute the contrast into the mainstem bronchi of the dependent lungfield and films in lateral and dorsoventral planes taken after 3 - 5 minutes.

The technique is simple but the indications are very limited especially as fibreoptic bronchoscopy has become more widely available.

Cholecystography

There are several organic iodine preparations which can be administered either orally or by intravenous injection which are preferentially excreted by the liver and thus used to outline the bile ducts and gall bladder (Herrtage and Dennis, 1987). There are, however, few indications for the use of these techniques in veterinary practice.

Dachrocystorinography

This procedure has been used to delineate the nasolacrimal apparatus in the dog and cat. Its use is indicated where the cause of abnormal lacrimal drainage needs to be established or in the investigation of facial masses possibly involving the lacrimal drainage structures.

The technique involves cannulation of one of the puncta in the eye, occlusion of the other punctum and injection of a small volume of contrast medium. Although standard 280 mg I per ml water-soluble media may not remain in the duct system long, they should be adequate and it is unwise to use more viscous material in case they result in iatrogenic blockage of the duct.

Hysterosalpingography

The outlining of the uterus (hysterography) and in a few cases the Fallopian tubes (salpingography) has been described but has few clinical applications.

Lymphangiography

Either oily iodine containing contrast agents (Lipiodol - May and Baker) or the routine water-soluble media can be used for outlining the lymphatic system.

The water soluble media outline the lymphatic vessels in much the same way as in venography or arteriography. However, the lymphatic vessels have to be identified by the injection of methylene blue into the interstitial tissues distal to the region of interest, and the vessels then surgically cannulated and the films taken during the injection of contrast medium.

Lipiodol can be injected subcutaneously distal to the region of interest and it will then be drained over a period of hours or days into the regional lymph nodes thus giving an indication of their size, position and function.

Pneumoperitoneography

This technique has been used, along with a variety of special radiographic positions, in an attempt to obtain better visualisation of the abdominal viscera. Air, carbon dioxide or nitrous oxide are the contrast media used to distend the peritoneal cavity.

The anaesthetised patient is placed in dorsal recumbency and a needle placed into the peritoneal cavity through or slightly to the right side of the umbilicus. A check should be made by pulling back on the syringe plunger that neither the intestine nor spleen has been penetrated. If the needle is correctly positioned there

should be no resistance to the injection of air. The chosen gas is then introduced slowly until the abdominal cavity is moderately but not excessively distended.

The radiographs taken will depend on the location of the organs it is wished to outline, but the general principle is to use a horizontal beam and position the subject so that the gas rises to surround the organ of interest while the other viscera fall away under the influence of gravity. Thus, to outline the bladder and uterus the pelvis and caudal abdomen is elevated.

This procedure is again of limited value and should only be used when there is inadequate inherent radiographic contrast on the plain film and other contrast techniques are inappropriate. Especial attention should be paid to radiation safety whenever horizontal beam projections are utilised.

Sialography

This involves the cannulation of the relevant salivary ducts and the injection of contrast medium to outline the glands and ducts and any lesions or defects associated with them. Investigation of sialocoeles by this method was instrumental in the identification of the sublingual salivary gland as the gland most likely to be involved but its use in clinical cases is seldom indicated. This procedure may also be used in the investigation of masses thought to be due to salivary neoplasia in either the sublingual, submandibular or parotid glands.

Very fine 23 - 25 gauge cannulae are required and 0.5 - 1 ml of water-soluble media containing 300 - 400 mg I per ml should be used.

The Demonstration of Sinus Tracts

Either water-soluble or oily contrast media can be injected into discharging sinuses to demonstrate their full extent and in some cases may help to outline otherwise radiolucent foreign bodies. The oily media produce a dense clear shadow but may mask small filling defects whereas the water-soluble media may diffuse into the tissues and fail to give a sharp outlining of the sinus tract. The radiographic views used will depend on the region under investigation.

REFERENCES

Douglas SW, Herrtage ME and Williamson HD (1987) Contrast media techniques. In: *Principles of Veterinary Radiography* pp241-286 4th Edition Balliere Tindall, London.

Herrtage ME and Dennis R (1987) Contrast media and their use in small animal radiology. *J. Small Animal Practice*. **28**, 1105-1114.

Dennis R and Herrtage ME (1989) Low osmolar contrast media - a review. *Vet. Rec.* **30**, 2-12.

CHAPTER EIGHT

Diagnostic Ultrasound

Frances Barr

CONTENTS

I: THE PHYSICS OF ULTRASOUND

A) Production of the Image

Diagnostic ultrasound makes use of high frequency sound waves. The frequency range used is usually between 2 and 10 MHz, which is considerably higher than the frequency range audible to the normal human ear (20 - 20,000 Hz).

The ultrasound transducer contains one or more crystals with piezo-electric properties. When a voltage is applied across such a crystal, it undergoes mechanical deformation and thus produces sound of a characteristic high frequency. The transducer is designed to produce short, regular pulses of sound.

When the transducer is placed in contact with the body surface, the sound travels through the tissues. Different tissues have a different resistance to the passage of sound, or **acoustic impedance**. Whenever the sound reaches an interface between tissues of differing acoustic resistance, part of the sound is reflected, and part continues on into deeper tissues. When the difference in acoustic resistance is great (eg. air/soft tissue or bone/soft tissue) then much of the sound is reflected and little continues into deeper tissues. When the difference in acoustic resistance is small (eg. soft tissue/soft tissue) then a smaller proportion is reflected and more passes on into deeper tissues.

The returning echoes are detected by the same transducer. Since sound is emitted in pulses, this leaves ample time between pulses for the crystal to act as a receiver. When the returning echoes impinge on the crystal, they cause mechanical deformation. Due to the piezo-electric properties of the crystal, this deformation results in the production of a small electrical signal.

The electrical signals produced by the returning echoes are analysed according to their strength and the site of origin within the tissues (calculated by the time delay between emission of the sound signal and detection of the returning echo). After analysis, an image is displayed on the screen.

B) Image Display Modes

A Mode (Figure 1)
This was the earliest display mode, and is now rarely used. A graphical display is used, with the horizontal axis representing the depth from which the echo originates, and the vertical axis representing the strength of the echo.

This display mode gives only limited information about major tissue boundaries.

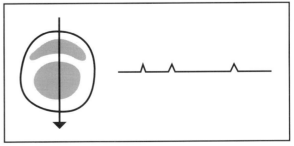

Figure 1.

B Mode (Figure 2)

This is the display mode most commonly used now. Multiple scan lines are used instead of the single scan line in A mode scanning. The returning echoes are represented as a dot on the screen, with the position on the screen representing the point of origin within the tissues, and the brightness of the dot representing the strength of the echo. This allows a two dimensional cross sectional image to be built up, representing a slice through the tissues in the plane of the beam. The image is continuously updated, thus allowing the movement of structures to be seen - so called real time scanning.

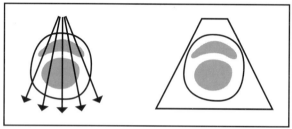

Figure 2.

M Mode (Figure 3)

This display mode is used to show movement of structures on the frozen image, and so finds most use in cardiology. A single scan line is selected from the B mode image, usually by means of a cursor. Echoes from this scan line are represented on a vertical line on the left of the screen as dots, with the brightness of the dot representing the strength of the echo and the distance along the line the depth of origin. As this vertical line scrolls across the screen, the image is continuously updated, showing the movement of all structures along the line.

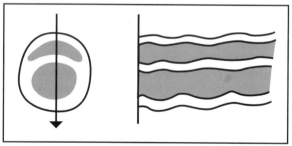

Figure 3.

C) Transducer Characteristics

1) Design

There are two main types of ultrasound transducer;

a) Linear array transducer: Crystals are arranged in a line along the surface of the transducer, and are activated sequentially to produce a rectangular sound beam. These types of transducer have the advantage of allowing a wide field of view, facilitating recognition of the relationships between structures. Very superficial tissues are particularly well

seen. They have the disadvantage of requiring a relatively large contact area between the skin and the transducer, and may be awkward to manipulate. Thus the linear array transducers are far from ideal for examination of thoracic or cranial abdominal structures.

b) Sector transducer: Mechanical sector transducers contain a single oscillating crystal or a small number of crystals mounted on a rotating wheel. Phased array transducers contain a number of crystals which are fixed in position, and activated sequentially. In each case, a fan shaped sound beam is produced. Phased array transducers have the advantage of higher image quality, and the lack of moving parts means a reduction in wear and tear. However, they tend to be considerably more expensive. The fan shaped beam of the sector transducer does not allow good visualisation of very superficial structures. However, they require only a small contact between the transducer and the skin, and are very manoeuvrable. In general therefore, the sector transducer is the preferred transducer type for use in small animals.

There are variations of these two main transducer types. Perhaps the most common is the curved linear transducer - basically a linear array transducer arranged with a convex rather than a flat scanning surface.

2) Frequency

The frequency of sound produced by the transducer is characteristic of the crystal or crystals within it. Low frequencies (2-3.5 MHz) of sound will penetrate well into soft tissues but will not produce image resolution of the highest quality. Such transducers are therefore selected when tissue penetration is vital, eg. the deeper abdominal and thoracic structures in large/giant breed dogs. High frequencies (7.5-10 MHz) produce optimal image resolution but are limited in tissue penetration. These transducers are selected for superficial structures where image detail is of paramount importance, eg. the eye.

For general small animal work, a 7.5 MHz transducer should allow satisfactory examination of thoracic and abdominal organs in cats and small dogs, superficial soft tissues and the eye. A 5 MHz transducer should provide adequate sound penetration to allow examination of the deeper abdominal and thoracic structures in medium sized and large dogs. Giant breed dogs may be a problem unless you are able to drop down to a 3.5 MHz transducer.

3) Focussing

Irrespective of the design of the transducer, focussing of the sound beam is essential, as the unfocussed sound beam diverges rapidly with consequent loss of image resolution. The focal zone of the transducer is that part of the sound beam where focussing, and therefore image quality, is optimal (Figure 4). Complex diffraction patterns can occur in the near field, or Fresnel zone. Beyond the focal zone, the Fraunhofer zone, the beam diverges rapidly and resolution decreases.

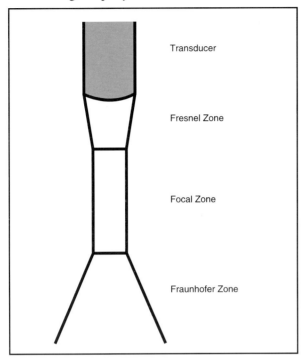

Figure 4.

This is of practical relevance as you should always aim to place the tissues of interest within the focal zone. If the tissues are deep to the focal zone, try gentle pressure on the abdominal wall to decrease the distance between the transducer and the structure of interest. If the tissues are too superficial, use an echolucent stand-off to increase the distance between the transducer and the structure of interest.

Annular array transducers are now available. In these transducers, the crystal is divided into concentric rings of varying thickness. Different frequencies of sound are produced, allowing focussing of the sound beam over a greater depth than is otherwise possible.

D) Equipment Controls

The image acquired on the screen can be altered in a number of ways to optimise its quality.

1) The power control on the machine alters the total sound output by the transducer, and thus the overall quantity of sound returning as echoes. Increasing the power therefore gives an overall brighter image, while decreasing it darkens the image. In general it is best to keep the power as low as possible without losing details of the structures being imaged.

2) The gain controls do not affect sound output, but alter the electronic amplification of the returning echoes. Increasing overall gain thus has a similar effect on

the image as increasing the power, and results in increased image brightness. However, the gain can be altered selectively in different parts of the image. It is usually necessary to have a lower gain for near field echoes and a higher gain for far field echoes, as the greater the distance of tissue crossed, the greater the loss of sound through absorption and scatter. In practical terms, the gain controls are used to achieve a uniform brightness across the depth of field.

3) Some machines have pre- and post-processing controls. These allow alteration of the grey scale on the moving and frozen images respectively, allowing accentuation of selected features of the image. These controls should be used with great care, however, as it is possible to produce image artefacts.

The number and complexity of the controls on an ultrasound machine vary greatly. Some or all of the following controls, in addition to those described above, may be found:

1) On-off switch.
2) Transducer selection (linear array/sector; frequency)
3) Display mode selection (B mode/M mode).
4) Depth selection. This allows you to choose the depth of tissues you wish to view. If only superficial tissues are viewed, the image is effectively magnified. Some machines also have zoom controls, allowing magnification of any part of the image.
5) Freeze frame.
6) Electronic callipers.
7) Beam angle. With wider beam angles, the field of view is clearly improved, but this results in either a reduced frame rate or inferior resolution. Use a wide angle for initial orientation, then reduce the angle for optimal image quality.
8) Frame rate. Select a slower frame rate for improved image resolution, or a faster frame rate for more accurate evaluation of movement.
9) Split frame. It may be possible to display two images side by side - either two cross-sectional images, or one cross-sectional and one M Mode image.
10) ECG.
11) Doppler (see below).

E) Doppler Techniques

Doppler ultrasonography allows the measurement of the velocity of blood flow in vessels or chambers of the heart. In addition, the character of the blood flow (laminar or turbulent) can be defined, and pressure gradients estimated.

The principle behind Doppler ultrasonography is straightforward. High frequency sound is emitted by the transducer and passes into the tissues of the body. When the reflecting interface is moving with respect to the transducer, there is a change in the wavelength and a corresponding change in the frequency of the reflected sound. This frequency change, termed the Doppler shift, depends on the frequency of emitted sound, the velocity of the reflecting surface and the velocity of sound in the tissues. When the reflecting surface is not moving parallel to the transducer, then only the vector component in that direction is considered, giving rise to an estimated velocity which is less than the actual velocity. Therefore the angle of incidence of the sound beam must also be considered. There are a number of different forms of Doppler imaging.

1) Continuous wave Doppler

A continuous beam of ultrasound is emitted by the transducer. The returning echoes are received by a separate crystal, and the frequency compared with that of the transmitted sound. The frequency shift may be displayed audibly and/or graphically. This system allows the measurement of a wide range of velocities, but provides no information as to the position of the reflector within the tissues.

2) Pulsed wave Doppler

As with conventional two-dimensional imaging, the sound is emitted in pulses, and the same crystal acts both as transmitter and receiver. Since the delay between transmission and detection is related to the depth of the reflecting structure, positional information is available with this technique. However, the pulsatile transmission limits the maximum velocity which may be measured.

3) Duplex Doppler

In this system, pulsed wave Doppler is combined with two-dimensional imaging, with simultaneous display of the images on the screen. Most duplex systems use two transducers within a single probe.

4) Colour flow Doppler

Velocity information is added to the two-dimensional image as colour, with the colour and intensity depicting the direction and magnitude of the velocity. Such a technique provides a huge amount of information about function as well as anatomy, but is currently very expensive.

F) The Biological Safety of Diagnostic Ultrasound

The effects of diagnostic ultrasound on living tissues have been investigated intensively. There have been no substantiated reports of adverse clinical effects in man despite widespread use of the technique for more than 15 years. Early reports of chromosomal damage to human leucocytes after diagnostic exposure were not confirmed. It is known that high intensity ultrasound can damage DNA in vitro and impair cell growth, but the doses required are far in excess of those used clinically. In the light of present knowledge therefore, it seems that diagnostic ultrasound is safe for both operator and patient.

II: THE ULTRASOUND EXAMINATION

A) Basic Examination Technique

It is important to select an appropriate part of the body surface for the ultrasonographic examination. Clearly it is sensible to choose an area of skin overlying the structures of interest, so that the depth of tissues which are to be traversed may be minimised. However, it is essential to avoid interposition of bone or gas filled structures - both bone and gas will block the sound beam and at worse will prevent visualisation of deeper tissues at all, and at best will impair image quality.

Once the scanning site has been selected, careful skin preparation is essential. The skin should be clipped and then cleaned with surgical spirit to remove excess grease and dirt. Liberal quantities of acoustic gel should then be applied, both to the skin surface and the transducer. The transducer may then be placed on the skin surface and the examination may begin. If concentric white lines are noted on the resulting image, this is an indication of poor contact, and the preparation of the site should be repeated.

B) Basic Interpretation of the Ultrasound Image

The following terms may be used when describing an image:

Echogenic; echodense; hyperechoic Appears white

Moderately echoic

Hypoechoic

Echolucent; anechoic Appears black

Bone or mineral and gas tend to produce intensely bright echoes with a shadow beneath the surface (see artifacts below). Some soft tissues such as fibrous tissue and, in some instances, fat tend to be hyperechoic. Other soft tissues, such as muscle, are less echoic. Fluid, irrespective of its nature, tends to be anechoic. Occasionally, fluid containing particles or air bubbles will appear moderately echoic, but may be differentiated from solid tissue by the swirling movement of the echoes.

Assess the shape and contour of any structures you can see. Evaluate the overall echogenicity, or brightness, of tissues, together with the texture or pattern of the echoes. In some complex structures, such as the kidney, it is important to assess the overall architecture. Finally, if relevant, examine the movement of structures. Make sure that you evaluate the area in more than one plane of section.

It is vital to appreciate that ultrasonographic changes are rarely specific. In addition, the absence of detectable changes does not preclude disease. The ultrasonographic examination should always be interpreted in the light of the history, physical examination and the results of other diagnostic procedures. Even so, histological examination of the relevant tissues will often be required for a definitive diagnosis.

The following image artifacts can be confusing unless they are recognised as such;

1) Acoustic enhancement: an area of increased brightness immediately below a fluid filled structure (Figure 5)

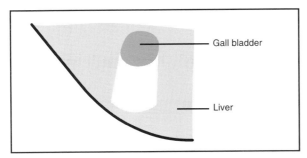

Figure 5.

2) Acoustic shadowing: an area of darkness with no image details immediately below a hyperechoic surface (Figure 6). Seen at the surfaces of bone, mineral or gas due to the highly relective nature of these surfaces.

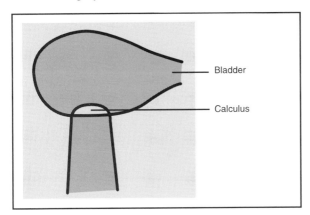

Figure 6.

3) Mirror image: an apparent mirror image of all or part of an organ. Seen at highly reflective interfaces due to internal reverberation of echoes, eg. a mirror image of the liver on the other side of the diaphragm due to reverberation at the interface between diaphragm and air filled lung; eg; a mirror image of the heart due to reverberation between the far side of the heart and the air filled lung.

4) Reverberations: streams of bright parallel lines (Figure 7). Seen once again at highly reflective interfaces, such as the lung/diaphragm interface, due to reverberation of echoes between the tissues and the transducer.

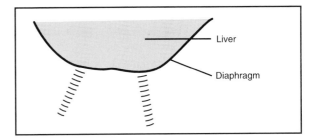

Figure 7.

C) The Liver

Technique
The liver may be scanned with the animal in dorsal or lateral recumbency. Nervous or distressed animals may be scanned standing. Clip an area of hair from the xiphisternum to about halfway between the xiphisternum and the umbilicus. Extend this area several inches on each side of the midline. Place the transducer just behind the xiphisternum and angle the beam craniodorsally. Sweeps can be made from side to side and up and down to image the whole liver.

In deep-chested dogs or animals with very small livers it may be necessary to image the liver from a right intercostal approach - clip the hair over the ventral third of the last 4-5 ribs on the right. Place the transducer in an intercostal space, altering the position until the liver can be clearly seen.

Normal Appearance
The reference point is the diaphragm - a thin echogenic line which moves with respiration. The liver lies between the skin surface and the diaphragm. It should be finely granular and even in texture, and is usually only moderately echoic (mid to dark grey). Solitary white patches in an otherwise orderly liver are normal, and probably represent hepatic ligaments and fissures. To the right the gall bladder may be seen - a rounded anechoic structure with a thin well defined wall. Also to the right may be seen the caudal vena cava. This is also anechoic. It will look round in cross section but becomes tubular in longitudinal section, and can be followed through the diaphragm. Small intrahepatic vessels may be seen as anechoic channels. Portal veins generally have echogenic walls whereas hepatic veins usually do not. Hepatic arteries and bile ducts are not usually visible in the normal animal. To the left the stomach may be identified as an ill defined heterogeneous mass if it contains food and/or gas, or an anechoic mass if it contains a lot of fluid.

Abnormal Findings

1) Focal parenchymal lesions may be hypoechoic or hyperechoic. Less commonly, "bulls-eye" lesions with a hyperechoic centre and a hypoechoic periphery may be seen. In small animals, such foci are usually neoplastic, but other possibilities include abscesses, infarcts, haematomata and nodular hyperplasia.

2) Diffuse parenchymal disease can be more difficult to detect. A diffuse heterogeneity of the parenchyma may be associated with diffuse neoplasia or advanced cirrhosis. More difficult are the conditions which may give rise to an overall change in echogenicity without any disruption of the normal even echotexture, eg. fatty infiltration may cause an increase in overall echogenicity with increased attenuation of the sound beam; some cases of hepatic lymphosarcoma are reported to cause an overall decrease in hepatic echogenicity.

3) Gall stones may be seen as echogenic foci which cast acoustic shadows, lying in the dependent part of the gall bladder. Abnormal thickening of the gall bladder wall can be due to inflammatory change or oedema. Polypoid changes of the mucosa are occasionally seen as an incidental finding in normal dogs. Extra-hepatic biliary obstruction will cause dilation of the gall bladder and common bile duct, followed by dilation of the intrahepatic bile ducts. Dilated bile ducts tend to be more tortuous, and to branch rather more irregularly, than blood vessels.

4) Hepatic veins tend to become fatter and more prominent in cases of right sided heart failure. Abnormal tortuous vessels may be seen within the liver parenchyma in cases of patent ductus venosus or hepatic arterio-venous fistulae. Primary porto-systemic shunts which are extra-hepatic may be more difficult to recognise, depending on the precise position and size of the shunting vessel.

D) The Spleen

Technique
The spleen is variable in position and may be difficult to find in the normal animal, especially in cats. The animal should be placed in dorsal or right lateral recumbency. A large area of the ventral abdomen between xiphisternum and umbilicus should be clipped. The head of the spleen can usually be found next to the stomach by placing the transducer parallel to the last rib on the left, several inches from the midline. Once the head is found, the rest of the spleen can be followed obliquely across the ventral abdomen or running down the left flank.

Normal Appearance
The spleen is more densely textured than the liver and so generally appears more echogenic (whiter). Vessels (anechoic channels) may be seen entering the parenchyma at the hilus, but otherwise vessels are rarely seen. The outline of the spleen should be smooth and well defined.

Abnormal Findings

1) Focal abnormalities within the parenchyma may be hypoechoic or, more commonly, of mixed echogenicity. They often protrude from the surface of the spleen, and may be highlighted by the presence of free abdominal fluid (anechoic). Such masses are usually neoplasms or haematomata.

2) A diffuse decrease in echogenicity has been described in association with splenic torsion.

E) The Kidneys

Technique
In most dogs, renal imaging is best performed with the animal in lateral recumbency, with the kidney to be imaged uppermost. Clip an area of hair a few inches square just behind the last rib on the left, and over the last two intercostal spaces on the right, just below the sublumbar muscles. The kidney lies superficially in each case.

In small dogs and cats, renal imaging can also be performed satisfactorily with the animal in dorsal recumbency and the transducer placed on the appropriate part of the ventral abdominal wall.

Normal Appearance
The normal kidney is smooth and well defined, although each pole may be slightly indistinct. The capsule may be seen as a thin echogenic line. The cortex is finely granular and is moderately hypoechoic (dark grey). Normally the renal cortex is less echoic than the liver, which in turn is less echoic than the spleen. The renal medulla is virtually anechoic and is divided into sections by the diverticula. The renal pelvis is intensely echogenic due to its high fat and fibrous tissue content - fluid is not visible within the normal renal pelvis. It may be difficult to see the whole of the right kidney at once because of rib shadowing.

Abnormal Findings

1) Dilation of the renal pelvis causes the normal echogenic knot to become a ring or 'C' shape, with a central anechoic area. As the dilation progresses, the central anechoic area expands, and the surrounding parenchyma becomes compressed until, in extreme cases, a thin walled bag of fluid is seen. Dilation of the ureter is often not appreciated. Renal calculi, irrespective of their mineral composition, appear as echogenic foci which cast acoustic shadows.

2) Focal parenchymal lesions may be seen as either rounded or wedge shaped lesions of an abnormal echogenicity and texture. Cysts typically are anechoic, with well defined walls and distal acoustic enhancement. Other lesions, such as neoplasms, abscesses, and infarcts may be of increased, decreased or mixed echogenicity.

3) Diffuse parenchymal disease most commonly gives rise to an overall increase in the echogenicity of the renal cortex, when compared with the liver. There may also be blurring of the normal cortico-medullary architecture, and irregularity of the renal outline. Neoplasms are often not detected until relatively advanced, and have commonly replaced all normal renal tissue by the time of examination, resulting in an irregularly shaped mass of mixed echogenicity.

F) The Bladder and Prostate

Technique
The animal can be examined in dorsal or lateral recumbency. An area of hair is clipped from the caudal ventral abdomen - in the midline in the cat or bitch, and to one side of the prepuce in the dog. The transducer is placed near the pubis and moved cranially until the bladder is identified. The bladder should be examined carefully in several planes of section. To examine the prostate in the dog, move caudally to the neck of the bladder and thence to the prostate. If the prostate is difficult to see or situated within the pelvis, you may be able to push it gently forward with a finger per rectum. Examinations of both bladder and prostate are most easily performed when the bladder is full.

Normal Appearance
The normal full bladder is smooth and well defined with anechoic contents. The normal smooth outline can be indented by a full colon or rectum dorsally.

The normal prostate is usually smooth and symmetrically rounded, but may not be very well defined from the periprostatic tissues. It is moderately hypoechoic and evenly granular in texture, except for a central echogenic linear structure termed the hilar echo. Small rounded anechoic foci less than one cm in diameter are seen quite frequently, and are usually small intraprostatic cysts of no clinical significance.

Abnormal Findings

1) Cystic calculi are easily seen as echogenic masses which cast an acoustic shadow and lie in the dependent portion of the bladder. Other intraluminal masses are hypoechoic, usually irregular in shape, and are highlighted by the surrounding anechoic urine. Neoplasms and polyps are adherent to the wall and so remain fixed in position even if the position of the animal is changed. Free blood clots will alter position as the animal moves, but those adherent to the wall can only be differentiated from soft tissue masses by sequential examinations. Diffuse thickening of the bladder wall may occur due to cystitis or neoplasia - but remember

that the bladder wall may appear artifactually thickened if the bladder is not distended.

2) Focal fluid filled lesions in the prostate are commonly seen. If these are less than one centimetre in diameter, they are rarely of clinical significance. Larger lesions, which can be rounded or irregular in shape, may represent intra-prostatic cysts, haematomata or abscesses.

3) Diffuse heterogeneity of the prostatic parenchyma can be associated with acute prostatitis (usually with an overall decrease in echogenicity) or with neoplasia or chronic prostatitis (usually with an overall increase in echogenicity). Prostatic hyperplasia causes little detectable change in the ultrasonographic appearance of the prostate other than for an increase in size.

4) Para-prostatic cysts are fluid filled masses with a varying soft tissue component, which may be adjacent to the bladder and prostate, but are distinct from these organs.

G) The Uterus

Technique
First of all locate the bladder, as described above. The cervix will lie dorsal to the bladder. The transducer may then be moved slowly cranially, making sweeps from side to side until the umbilicus is reached. The procedure can then be repeated if necessary, moving back towards the bladder.

Normal Appearance
The normal non-gravid uterus is not usually visible although the cervix may be seen dorsal to the bladder as a smooth, oval, hypoechoic mass. Pregnancy can be diagnosed with certainty from 28 days gestation onwards. Gestational sacs containing fluid (black) and foetal tissue (grey/white) will be seen, and foetal heart beats and generalised foetal movements detected. As pregnancy progresses, the differentiation of foetal organs may be recognised. It is not possible to assess foetal numbers with accuracy.

Abnormal Findings
Foetal death is first detected by an absence of foetal heart beats, followed by a gradual loss of foetal structure until only amorphous collections of debris, surrounded by fluid, are visible. Fluid distension of the uterine body and horns in the absence of foetal structures is indicative of pyometra, haematometra or hydrometra. Uterine neoplasms may be identified as a mass in the caudal abdomen, but unless they are surrounded by intra-uterine fluid they may be difficult to localise with certainty. Abscessation or granuloma formation of the uterine stump may be detected as a

mass between the bladder and the colon, depending on the size of the lesion.

H) The ovaries

Technique

The normal ovary is located caudal to the ipsilateral kidney, and tends to drop ventrally, suspended by the mesovarium, when the animal is standing. This is the region to search identifying the kidney first, then moving caudally and ventrally.

Normal Appearance

The normal ovary is difficult to detect in the dog and cat, particularly if the animal is not in oestrus. Around the time of oestrus, follicles may be detected in the ovary as anechoic areas bordered by relatively hyperechoic walls - but the ultrasonographic appearance of the ovary cannot be used to determine the time of ovulation.

Abnormal Findings

Large polycystic ovaries often fall into the mid or ventral part of the caudal abdomen. A well circumscribed mass with fluid contents and internal septa is typically seen. Ovarian tumours may also appear cystic, but may have a varying soft tissue component.

I) The testes

Technique

Examination of the scrotal testicle is straightforward as the transducer may be placed directly over the organ. If the transducer is placed in a pre-scrotal position, then both testes may be imaged side by side. If it is necessary to search for a non-scrotal testicle, then begin by searching the inguinal area systematically, proceeding to examine the abdomen from the region of the inguinal ring, to the bladder, to the ipsilateral kidney.

Normal Appearance

The normal testicle is smooth, well defined and oval. The parenchyma is evenly granular and of moderate echogenicity, with an echogenic spot or line in the centre. The adjacent epididymis is somewhat coarser in texture and irregular in outline.

Abnormal Findings

1) Focal masses within the testicle may be hypoechoic, hyperechoic or of mixed echogenicity, and usually represent neoplasms. However, abscesses, granulomas, cysts and haematomata may also occur.

2) Enlargement of the epididymis rather than the testicle is seen in epididymitis. A collection of small fluid filled cysts adjacent to the testicle may represent distension of the spermatic cord or a varicocoele.

J) The Gastro-Intestinal Tract

Technique

The gastro-intestinal tract does not, in general, lend itself to ultrasonographic examination, as the presence of solid ingesta or faecal material and the accumulation of intra-luminal gas impair image quality. However, useful information can be gleaned from examination of those parts of the tract which are fluid filled.

In order to investigate the stomach and duodenum, the animal should be starved for 12 hours, but allowed to drink just prior to the examination. The transducer should be placed behind the costal arch, to the left of the midline, and angled cranio-dorsally. Once the gastric fundus has been identified, the transducer can be moved to the right to image the antrum and pylorus, and then caudally to follow the duodenum. The rest of the gastro-intestinal tract can be imaged from the ventral abdominal wall.

Ultrasonographic examination of the gastro-intestinal tract should be performed before the administration of barium, as this will interfere with image quality.

Normal Appearance

The fluid filled stomach is a well circumscribed structure. The contents are anechoic, but often contain echogenic particles representing air bubbles or food particles which can be seen swirling around. Peristaltic activity may be apparent. The pylorus is often seen as a distinct rounded mass of mixed echogenicity caudal to the liver, to the right of midline. Fluid filled small intestine can be seen in longitudinal and transverse section as anechoic tubes, with a central hyperechoic stripe. Peristaltic activity may be seen.

If a high frequency transducer (7.5-10 MHz) is available, then detail of the gastric and intestinal wall can be appreciated. Five distinct layers can be identified:

1) Hyperechoic inner layer - interface between the mucosa and lumen.
2) Hypoechoic layer - mucosa.
3) Hyperechoic middle layer - submucosa.
4) Hypoechoic layer - muscle.
5) Hyperechoic outer layer - boundary between serosa and the peritoneal cavity.

Abnormal Findings

1) Abnormal fluid distension of the stomach and/or intestinal loops may be seen in cases of paralytic or obstructive ileus. Foreign bodies may also be identified provided they are outlined by fluid. Gaseous distension of the gastro-intestinal tract usually prevents a useful examination.

2) Subtle abnormalities in wall thickness and structure will not generally be detected, but gross lesions may be seen. The thickness of the wall will be increased and the normal layered architecture disrupted. Eccentric thickening around the lumen is usually suggestive of neoplasia.

3) An intussusception has a very characteristic appearance, with one section of bowel seen enclosed within a second section.

K) The Pancreas

Technique
The normal pancreas is difficult to image as it has poorly defined margins, and is often obscured by gas or solid material in the adjacent stomach, duodenum and colon. A high frequency transducer (5-7.5 MHz, depending on the size of the patient) is essential.

The animal should be placed in left lateral recumbency, and the transducer placed under the right 13th rib and angled dorsally, with the sound beam approximately parallel to the spine. Once the right kidney has been identified, the transducer is moved slowly medially until the descending duodenum is found.

The right pancreatic lobe lies dorsal and medial to the descending duodenum. If bowel gas is a problem, turn the animal over onto its right side, and repeat the procedure, placing the transducer between the animal and the table top. The left pancreatic lobe is more difficult to find. Start with the transducer caudal to the left 13th rib, and search the region caudal to the stomach, medial to the spleen and cranial to the left kidney.

Normal Appearance
The normal pancreas is often not seen clearly. It has a homogeneous echogenic texture with poorly defined margins. The pancreatico-duodenal vein runs in the right lobe, parallel to the descending duodenum, and may therefore be a useful landmark.

Abnormal Findings

1) In severe haemorrhagic necrotizing pancreatitis, irregular hypo- and anechoic areas may be seen in the region of pancreas, representing collections of necrotic tissue and pus. The surrounding mesentery may be hyperechoic due to inflammation and oedema. The duodenum tends to be thick walled and atonic, and there may be an associated peritoneal effusion. Secondary biliary obstruction may be seen.

2) Pancreatic tumours may themselves be difficult to image, but metastatic nodules in local lymph nodes and liver may be seen. Once again, there may be a secondary biliary obstruction.

L) The Adrenal Glands

Technique
The normal adrenal glands will only be seen if high frequency transducers (5-7.5 MHz) are available to produce optimal image quality.

To image the left adrenal gland, place the animal in right lateral recumbency, and place the transducer behind the last rib on the left, below the sublumbar muscles. Image the aorta and caudal vena cava in longitudinal section, then follow the aorta cranially until the origin of the left renal artery is identified. The left adrenal gland lies ventral or ventro-lateral to the aorta, cranial to the left renal artery.

Repeat the procedure on the other side to image the right adrenal gland. The right adrenal gland is dorsal or dorso-lateral to the caudal vena cava, cranial to the origin of the right renal artery.

Normal Appearance
The normal adrenal glands are hypoechoic when compared with the surrounding perirenal fat. The right adrenal gland is wedge shaped, while the left is more often bilobed in shape.

Abnormal Findings
Adrenal tumours may be hyperechoic or isoechoic and result in a loss of the normal shape of the gland. Larger tumours may be of mixed echogenicity due to the presence of necrosis and haemorrhage. Remember to look for compression or invasion of the adjacent caudal vena cava.

M) The Heart

Technique
A small area of hair should be clipped from the lower thoracic wall over the apex beat on each side. At this site there is minimal interference from air filled lung. If a working surface with a cut-out is available, the animal should be placed on its side and the heart imaged from underneath. It is feasible to image the heart from above but there may be more interference from air filled lung, particularly in barrel chested dogs. It is also possible to examine the heart with the animal sitting or standing if it becomes distressed in lateral recumbency.

Place the transducer in an intercostal space over the apex beat on the right, and angle the transducer craniodorsally. With the plane of the beam approximately parallel with the sternum, a short axis view of the heart will be achieved. Rotation of the transducer through 90° should produce a long axis view. The precise position and angulation of the transducer will vary between individuals, depending on body confirmation and the size and shape of the heart. By altering the plane of section of the beam, all the cardiac chambers, the valves and outflow tracts can be identified. Repeat the examination from the left side of the thorax if necessary. If available, connect the ECG so that the ultrasonographic appearance can be correlated with the stage of the cardiac cycle. Use the M mode display in order to obtain a more objective assessment of myocardial and valvular motility.

Normal Appearance

You should try to identify the right and left ventricles, the right and left atria, the interatrial and the interventricular septum, the right and left atrio-ventricular valves, the aortic outflow and the pulmonary outflow. The structures normally visible on some of the standard planes of section from the right and left thoracic wall are shown below (Figures 8-12). Since movement of structures can be seen it is possible to make an assessment of cardiac motility.

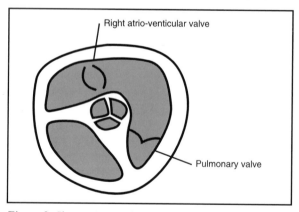

Figure 8: Short axis view from the right (near the apex).

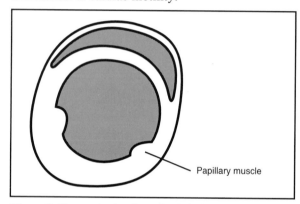

Figure 9: Short axis view from the right (near the base of the heart).

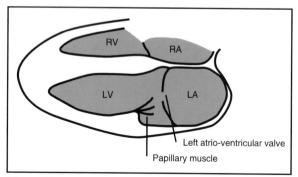

Figure 10: Long axis view from the right (optimised for the left atrium).

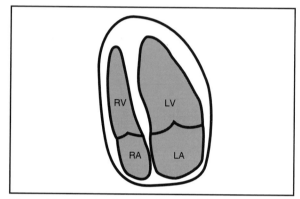

Figure 11: Long axis view from the right (optimised for the aortic outflow).

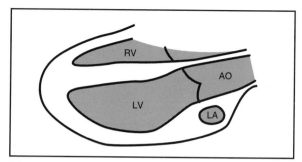

Figure 12: Four chamber view from the left.

N) The Eye

Technique

Examination of the eye is usually tolerated well by both dogs and cats. If the eye is painful, it is helpful to instil a few drops of topical local anaesthetic first. Place the transducer directly on the cornea or the 3rd eyelid - a satisfactory image is rarely achieved by imaging through the lids. Do not use spirit, but do use liberal quantities of acoustic gel. The commercial acoustic gels are not irritant to the cornea. Image the eye in both horizontal and vertical planes of section, swinging the beam up and down and from side to side to ensure that the whole area is examined. On completion of the examination, gently wipe away any excess gel.

Normal Appearance

The globe of the eye is anechoic, and smoothly rounded in shape. The lens is rarely seen clearly as its curved surfaces tend to scatter the reflected sound away from the transducer, but small bright echoes may be seen where the surface of the lens is perpendicular to the incident sound beam. The retina, choroid and sclera are not seen as separate layers, but as a single, smooth echogenic wall. A bright spot may be seen caudo-medially representing the optic disc. The retrobulbar tissues are composed of fat, which is quite echogenic, and extraocular muscles, which are relatively hypoechoic. The retrobulbar tissues form an orderly cone, within which the hypoechoic track of the optic nerve may sometimes be identified.

Abnormal Findings

1) The position of the lens can be determined, and both anterior and posterior luxations identified. If the lens is cataractous, it is much more clearly delineated than normal, with a thick and continuous echogenic border.

2) Retinal detachment is seen as a thin echogenic line ballooning into the vitreous from the posterior wall of the globe. If the detachment is complete, then a typical appearance of "seagull's wings" is seen, with points of attachment at the optic disc and the ciliary body.

3) Intraocular masses are readily seen as they are highlighted by the anechoic vitreous. It is, however, difficult to differentiate an intraocular neoplasm from an intraocular blood clot on a single ulrasonographic examination. Sequential examinations should show gradual resolution of a clot.

4) Retrobulbar lesions disturb the normal orderly cone of the retrobulbar tissues, and may cause deformation of the posterior aspect of the globe. It is not possible to differentiate a retrobulbar neoplasm from a retrobulbar abscess on ultrasonographic criteria alone, unless invasion of the globe can be demonstrated.

CHAPTER NINE

Radiography of Small Mammals, Birds and Exotic Species

R. Lee

INTRODUCTION

The following section is intended as an aid to the radiography of small animal species other than the dog and cat. It is not intended to cover the radiological signs of specific conditions and the reader is directed to more specialised texts for this purpose. However, it must be emphasised that the general principles of radiological interpretation contained in the previous chapters apply equally to these subjects.

It would be quite impossible to manually restrain any of the following species without contravening the basic priciples of radiation safety outlined in the next chapter, therefore it goes without saying that sedation or anaesthesia and the use of positioning aids is mandatory.

Although suggestions as to suitable sedatives and anaesthetics are made in some instances the reader is advised to consult either the Manual of Small Animal Anaesthesia or the Manual of Exotic Pets for details of the most appropriate agents and the appropriate doses.

For radiography of all of the species listed below it will not be necessary to use a grid and if available use should be made of high definition screens and films. This will permit maximum detail to be obtained of these subjects. For very small subjects use may be made of small dental non-screen film although the increased exposure factors required must be borne in mind.

Exposure factors will depend on the equipment being used and the particular film/screen combination but the relevant exposure values used for the cat, reduced according to the subject size, can be used as an initial guide.

Remember that many avian bones have relatively thin cortices and may contain air sacs so increasing their radiolucency.

I: SMALL MAMMALS

Due to the small size of these subjects it is generally satisfactory to take whole body radiographs rather than individually positioned films of particular regions. It will also normally be possible to select exposure factors that will permit evaluation of both the skeletal and soft tissue structures.

With the use of appropriate sedation mammals, smaller than rabbits are best positioned in ventral recumbency and the legs secured with adhesive tape either to the surface of the cassette or to a thin sheet of perspex. This latter procedure permits the animals to be easily repositioned should further films be required (Figure 9.1).

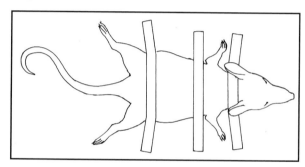

Figure 9.1: *Small mammal secured in ventral recumbency on a sheet of perspex for a DV view.*

For lateral views they can again be positioned either on the cassette or perspex, perferably using the same side in order to standardise technique, and held with adhesive tape. The dependent leg should be slightly more advanced that the non dependant leg and marked for identification on the plate (Figure 9.2).

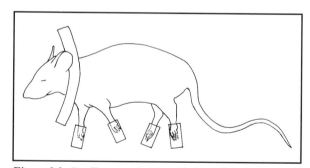

Figure 9.2: *Small mammal secured in lateral recumbency.*

The use of perspex tubes has been suggested for the positioning of small mammals but has the disadvantage that poor images for the evaluation of the thorax and abdomen result due to the superimposition of the flexed limbs. It is, however, a method that can be used for barium studies where it may be undesirable to use general anaesthesia (Figure 9.3).

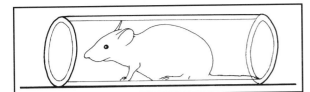

Figure 9.3: Perspex tube used for straining a conscious small mammal.

Rabbits can be radiographed in the equivalent positions used for the cat utilising foam sponges and ties as appropriate and radiolucent troughs for the DV and VD of the thorax and abdomen respectively. Care must be taken to ensure adequate anaesthesia in this species however, as serious self inflicted spinal injuries may result if they struggle or kick whilst restrained (Figure 9.4).

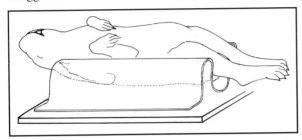

Figure 9.4: Rabbit positioned in a trough for a VD view of the body.

II: BIRDS

Depending on size either whole body radiographs or radiographs of specific regions such as the wing or leg may be taken.

For whole body radiography the bird should be positioned on a sheet of perspex in dorsal recumbency with the wings extended and the legs drawn caudally. The wings, neck and legs can be secured with adhesive tape. Masking tape is the most satisfactory as this does not damage the feathering as much as sellotape or zinc oxide tape. It is important to ensure that the bird is positioned absolutely symmetrically with the sternum overlying the spine and both wings equally extended (Figure 9.5).

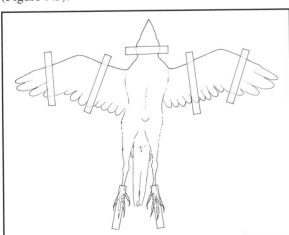

Figure 9.5a: Bird positioned on a perspex sheet in dorsal recumbency for a VD view of the body or wings

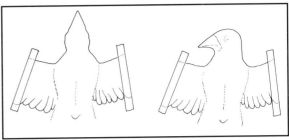

Figure 9.5b: Positioning of the head for a lateral or VD view.

Radiographs of the head can be taken in both the VD and lateral view whilst the bird is positioned as above. The flexibility of the avian neck permits repositioning of the head without any risk of damage.

In addition to the ventro-dorsal view, any radiographic evaluation of the body also requires the use of a lateral view. The bird should be positioned in lateral recumbency, perferably always on the same side for ease of interpretation. The wings should be extended above the body and secured with tape taking care not to compromise respiratory movement. The dependent leg is extended and secured whilst the non-dependent leg is retracted and secured (Figure 9.6).

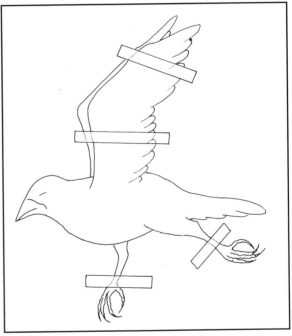

Figure 9.6: Bird positioned for a lateral view of the body or leg.

III: REPTILES

Snakes - it is most satisfactory to either sedate or anaesthetise using either Ketamine by i/m injection (20-100 mg/kg), Saffan either i/m (up to 15 mg/kg) or i/v (9 mg/kg) or Propofol i/v (10 mg/kg).

Small snakes may fit onto a single plate or may be coiled. Larger snakes will require more than one plate to be used in which case it is necessary to position numbered markers placed equidistantly from rostrum to cloaca to facilitate identification of the regions included on each plate (Figure 9.7).

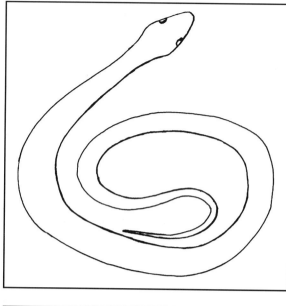

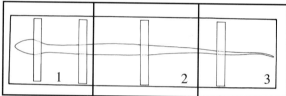

Figure 9.7: Alternative methods of positioning snakes for a DV view.

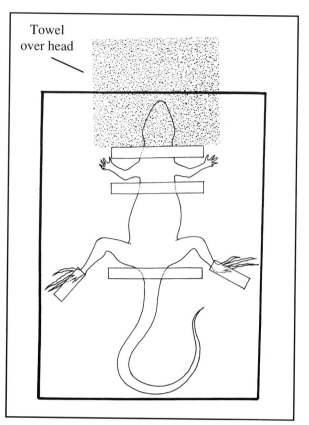

Figure 9.9: Lizard restrained in ventral recumbency for a DV view of the body or limbs.

An alternative method for small specimens is to position them in a perspex tube of appropriate diameter or if this is not available to use a sheet of clear X-ray film rolled into a tube. The advantage of this method of restraint is that it readily permits both DV and lateral views to be obtained with minimal repositioning of the subject (Figure 9.8).

Lizards and Iguanas and related species will often not require sedation if allowed to cool to room temperature - they should NOT, however, be put in a refrigerator! If the head is then covered with a thick towel and allowed to settle down they can then be positioned for either DV or VD views and restrained with adhesive tape to a sheet of perspex (Figure 9.9).

They will not, however, tolerate lateral recumbency. Lateral views if required have to be obtained by using a horizontal beam (Figure 9.10).

Tortoises and turtles can be restrained unanaesthetised with adhesive tape across the carapace; this will permit DV views of the whole body. Lateral and craniocaudal views will require the use of horizontal beam radiography (Figure 9.11).

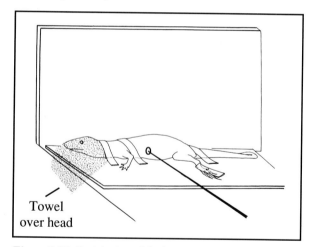

Figure 9.10: Positioning of the horizontal X-ray beam for a lateral view of a lizard.

For radiography of the limbs a short acting anaesthetic is advisable, e.g. i/v Propofol (14 mg/kg), to allow the limb to be drawn out of the shell and radiographed. Small non-screen dental films are useful for this purpose.

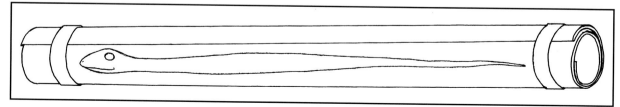

Figure 9.8: Restraint of a conscious snake in a tube made of rolled up X-ray film.

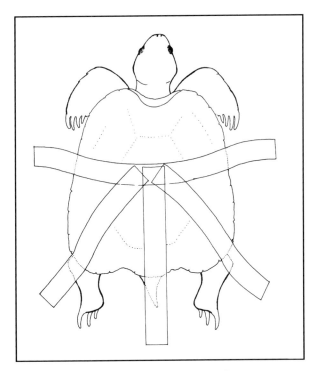

IV: NON-HUMAN PRIMATES

These will almost always require heavy sedation or anaesthesia and can then be positioned as for dogs. However, the DV/VD views of the thorax and abdomen may prove more valuable than the lateral views.

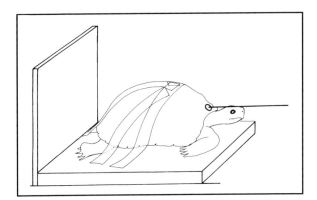

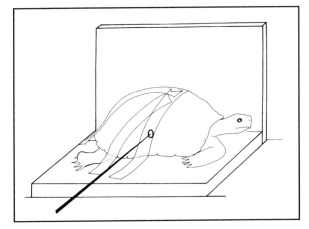

Figure 9.1: *Restraint of a tortoise for DV, lateral and Crcd views.*

CHAPTER TEN

Radiation Protection

P. M. Webbon

INTRODUCTION

X-rays are harmful. The short term effects, e.g. skin erythema, of prolonged exposure to X-rays have been known virtually since the production of X-rays, and some of their properties, were first recorded. The extent of the risk can be calculated or estimated and radiation protection procedures are intended to reduce the risk to a level where the potential hazard is both negligible relative to the benefits of the procedure and in keeping with other occupational hazards.

A Code of Practice 'Radiation Safety in Veterinary Practice' was first published in 1970 and amended in 1974. It was an advisory Code (rather like the Highway Code) and contained much good sense about veterinary radiography but some of its provisions were ignored in veterinary practices and institutions. This was particularly true of the requirement that 'animals should not be held for radiography unless other means of immobilisation are impracticable' and it was not uncommon for films referred for a second opinion to show images of fingers or hands, not always protected by lead gloves.

In 1985 the Ionising Radiation Regulations were passed. Together with an Approved Code of Practice (not to be confused with the 1974 Code of Practice which is now obsolete) the regulations lay down the general legal principles of radiation protection in all work activities. The body empowered to enforce the regulations is the Health and Safety Executive (HSE) through its inspectorate. An inspector for the HSE can, at any reasonable time, ask to inspect a practice's X-ray equipment and facilities as well as dosimetry records, local rules etc. It is worth bearing in mind that the Inspector may also use the opportunity to check on other aspects of safety such as autoclave service records.

A third, advisory, publication, 'Guidance Notes for the Protection of Persons against Ionising Radiation arising from Veterinary Use' replaces the 1974 Code of Practice and deals in a practical way, with radiography in veterinary practice. This booklet should be read by all persons involved in any form of veterinary radiography.

Whatever is the legal framework governing radiation protection, the basic rules remain the same.

The primary beam presents the most serious threat and no part of any person, protected or not, should be exposed to it. This can be achieved by reliably, and predictably, collimating the beam with a variable (light beam) diaphragm collimator and demonstrated by ensuring that the margins of the primary beam are visible on all films after processing. It is unacceptable to produce films on which no evidence of collimation is to be seen.

Protection from scatter is achieved by retiring as far as possible from the scatter producing patient, by shielding and by collimating the primary beam to reduce scatter production.

In general, exposure to personnel can be reduced by good radiographic technique : by reducing the need to repeat exposures, by good film processing and by using the fastest possible combination of films and intensifying screen.

Much of the rest of this chapter will deal with the implementation of the Ionising Radiation Regulations in small animal practice but this needs to be preceded by a short description of the hazardous effects of ionising radiation.

Biological Effects of Ionising Radiation

The principle which underlies diagnostic radiography is the differential absorption of the photons in an X-ray beam by different body tissues.

Those photons which pass unchanged through an animal have no effect on the animal's tissues but when X-ray energy is absorbed by a cell it results in ionisation and excitation of the atoms and molecules of the cell. This produces stable or unstable molecules and free radicals which may react with adjacent molecules and, directly or indirectly, exert a range of harmful effects on irradiated cells from impairment of function to genetic mutation or cell death.

The extent of the damage, which is cumulative, depends on the amount, rate and mechanism of energy absorption. The harmful cellular effects of ionising radiation may be manifested in varying ways in animals and man. These are recognised as either stochastic (probability of occurrence increases with the dose received) or non-stochastic effects (where the severity of the abnormality is dependent on the dose received but only occurs above a threshold dose). Examples of stochastic effects are carcinogenesis and induced genetic defects and of non-stochastic effects, cataract and cutaneous ulcers.

Radiation damage may affect either individuals who are the subjects of X-ray examinations or those responsible for conducting the examination. In veterinary practice, although no animal should be unnecessarily irradiated, the main concern of radiation protection is for the personnel involved.

Nevertheless, in certain circumstances protection of the animal patient may be indicated. For example, Wood *et al*, (1974) measured the scattered radiation dose to the scrotum (which was reflected out of the primary beam) of bulls undergoing hip radiography and concluded that it was sufficiently high to make shielding desirable. The standard dog hip dysplasia picture, under the BVA scheme, requires that the scrotum is irradiated in the primary beam and, in dogs intended for stud, a gonad guard may be a sensible precaution. The same could be true of bitches, but their numerical potential for contributing to the breed is less than for stud dogs.

The risk to the personnel involved in a radiographic procedure, although small, should not be underestimated. When radiaion protection procedures were less rigorously observed, O'Riordan (1970) recorded chronic, radiation-induced finger tip skin damage in 75 per cent of 41 staff in a group of veterinary practices. It is hoped that, if this survey were to be repeated, significantly less radiation damage would be revealed, but the potential risk still exists.

The Ionising Radiation Regulations

5(2)   'an employer shall not undertake... work with ionising radiation, unless... , he has notified the Executive of his intention to carry out such work...'

All practices with X-ray equipment should have notified the Health and Safety Executive that they own and use a diagnostic X-ray machine. Any who have not done so, or who buy an X-ray machine for the first time, should notify the Executive accordingly (see list of Area Offices at the end of the Chapter) with the following particulars (on headed notepaper or using HSE form 2522):

a)   Name and address of the employer
b)   Address of the practice premises
c)   That the business is a veterinary practice
d)   That the source of ionising radiation is a radiation generator
e)   That the X-ray machine will be used
   i)   at the address above only, or
   ii) it, or another machine, will be used at another address e.g. a branch surgery, or
   iii) it, or another machine, will be used for mobile radiography (usually of horses)
f)   The names of the people employed in the work
g)   The date of commencement of the work (which should be at least 28 days after the notification unless the Executive agree otherwise).

2(4)   'a trainee... (whether for profit or not) shall be treated as an employee... '

Students 'seeing practice' are therefore, for these purposes, considered as employees of the practice.

6(1)   'Every employer shall, in relation to any work with ionising radiation that he undertakes, take all necessary steps to restrict so far as reasonably practicable the extent to which his employees and other persons are exposed to ionising radiation'.

The practicability of exposure restriction will vary from case to case. Radiographs of a Miniature Dachshund with suspected thoracolumbar disc disease should be achieved with a dose to personnel so low that it is not measurable, and it would be very difficult to defend any technique other than general anaesthesia, the use of positioning aids, and withdrawal of personnel to a safe distance, perferably behind an adequate barrier (e.g. solid wall) but at least wearing a protective apron.

On the other hand, a Newfoundland with suspected cardiomyopathy and congestive heart failure may require, if all else fails, one, or even two, member(s) of staff to restrain and reassure the animal provided that they are as far as possible from the primary beam and suitably protected.

The aspect of veterinary radiography which has stimulated active debate for many years is the manual restraint of animals for radiography. Indeed, in the years between the publication of the 1974 Code and the passing of the 1985 Regulations some of the UK veterinary schools taught this as, if not the method of choice, at least the method of least inconvenience. The 1974 Code is, however, quite clear that animals should not be manually restrained unless any other alternative is impracticable and this same 'loophole' has to be written in the new legislation to take account of those cases where there is genuinely no practicable alternative.

The level of practicability is for the RPS (Radiation Protection Supervisor) to decide although the Principle is ultimately responsible and the RPA (Radiation Protection Adviser) must advise in general terms. If an animal is in pain such that it cannot be positioned easily for radiography without being held, e.g. for radiographs of a distal humeral epicondylar fracture, then general anaesthesia is indicated and should be followed by internal or external fixation. If the animal cannot be anaesthetised because of concurrent problems, e.g. pneumothorax, a specific radiographic diagnosis of its orthopaedic lesion is probably not required and can be postponed.

Most animals, that are not in acute pain, can be positioned for radiography with a combination of the skills of the radiographer, positioning aids such as foam pads and sandbags and judicious sedation when necessary (Webbon and France 1984). Those who deny that this is so have not taken the trouble to develop the necessary skills which are based on patience and compassion. A quiet environment is also necessary and makes doubly useful the restriction of entry to an X-ray room during radiography.

Animals which genuinely may need holding, more often to provide reassurance than restraint, are dogs in respiratory distress that panic if left on their side or sternum unattended, and some cats.

The 1985 Regulations effectively leave the decision regarding manual restraint to individual veterinary surgeons, but the law is flouted if 'practicable' is read as 'convenient'.

It is important to understand that the exposure to each staff member must be minimised, not just reduced. For example, if a practice manually positions animals, although they are anaesthetised, the dose to personnel is not minimised because positioning aids could be employed. It is not acceptable to rotate the staff involved, thereby reducing the dose to each staff member. The law clearly requires that the exposure to staff should be the minimum practicable.

This regulation also requires that the employer provides engineering controls and design features to reduce exposure, and provides safety features and warning devices. The way in which these requirements can be met are discussed in the following sections.

Equipment

Regulation 32 deals with the supply and specification of equipment.

X-ray machine: Regulation 32 makes it clear that any manufacturer or supplier of an X-ray machine must ensure that the equipment is safe and works correctly.

Tube head leakage must be minimal and with new machines this is usually so, but the leakage from variable diaphragm light beam collimators (LBD) fitted to machines less than 2 years old may be unacceptably high when it is investigated (Webbon and Ramsey, 1983). Significant leakage may be demonstrated from older machines, usually from the union of the tube head and beam limiting device, or from the beam limiting device itself.

Effective collimation of the primary beam is an integral part of radiation protection and in reality, the only satisfactory beam limiting device is an LBD collimator. Unfortunately, in some new machines the light beam does not predict accurately the path of the X-ray beam and may be inaccurate by several centimetres. This is important not least because the HSE Inspectorate has been advised to ensure that the margins of the primary beam are visible on the final, processed film. If the entire film is used, e.g. for a dog's abdomen, and the beam is collimated to leave a 1 cm margin, the X-ray beam must accurately follow the path of the light beam. Problems may also arise if the beam is collimated closely to radiograph e.g. a cat's tarsus. If the light beam is 2-3 cm inaccurate it would be possible to partially or completely miss the tarsus with the X-ray beam. It is the manufacturer's, or supplier's, duty to ensure that the safety features are functioning correctly.

There can be no excuse, or valid reason, for purchasing a new machine without a LBD collimator. Nevertheless, there are still in use some practices older machines which may be fitted with a cone, or selection of cones, or a rectangular aperture collimator. Practices using this type of equipment, which is not ideal but nevertheless safe, can continue to use it provided their System of Work ensures that it is used correctly. The size of the X-ray beam at the X-ray table top must be known for a given focus to film distance and animals must not be restrained manually. It is important that such practices aim to acquire more modern equipment as soon as possible within the financial constraints of the practice.

Additional safety features which should be checked are that the timer is accurate and reliably terminates the exposure, and a warning light, or meter, is fitted to indicate when the machine is connected to the main electrical supply and when X-rays are being generated. It is important to remember that if a machine is sold from one practice to another, the vendor is responsible for ensuring the safety of the machine and may need to employ a radiation protection adviser to do this.

One other important duty of the manufacturer/ supplier is to ensure that adequate operating instructions are supplied with the equipment. A survey of X-ray machines in veterinary practice (Webbon and Ramsey, 1983) found that that was not always achieved. It is certainly not satisfactory to provide an exposure chart copied from a textbook and little else.

A final point related to the X-ray machine is the siting of its connection to the electrical main. The last resort if a machine becomes dangerous e.g generates X-rays continuously, is to disconnect it from its main supply. It should be possible to do this quickly, easily and remotely from the machine. It should not be necessary to lean over the X-ray table, in the path of the primary beam, to reach the electricity socket or switch.

X-ray table: The 1970 Code of Practice for the Protection of Persons Exposed to Ionising Radiation from Veterinary Use (amended 1974) suggested that 'a 1 mm sheet of lead.., should be placed immediately under the cassette or film'.

To comply with Para 62 of the 1985 Code of Practice the X-ray table should be covered by 1mm of lead over an appropriate area. This does not take into account that veterinary practices may, indeed should, wish to use X-ray tables incorporating a moving grid and film tray, or even home made film trays to facilitate patient positioning. This requirement also implies that it is not unusual, in veterinary radiography, for personnel to stand close enough to the X-ray table for their legs to be in the primary beam during exposure. It is the author's opinion that the highest possible standards of veterinary radiography should have been enshrined in legislation while providing for the safe use of more basic facilities.

A large proportion of practices have, in reality, incorporated into the entire X-ray table, or one end of it, 1 mm of sheet lead. From the safety point of view this is satisfactory but it makes consistent positioning of a large dog difficult, during for example pelvic radiography or excretion urography, since the animal must be lifted to replace the cassette on the table top between exposures.

Warning Devices: The regulations require that, during radiography, accidental entry to the X-ray room should be very unlikely (see also Controlled Area). Additionally, the X-ray room should be permanently marked.

In practice every access door to the X-ray room should be marked with the standard trefoil radiation symbol, while restriction of entry during radiography may be satisfactorily achieved in a variety of ways. Some practices use simple signs reading 'X-RAYS. NO ENTRY' which are displayed during radiography. Others where, for example, access is via a corridor, have a hinged barrier bearing the same sign which blocks the corridor during radiography.

If the machine has a permanently wired electrical connection an ideal solution is to include in the circuit a red light which shows whenever the X-ray machine is turned on. A sign then is permanently displayed which reads,'X-RAYS. NO ENTRY WHEN LIGHT IS SHOWING'. (Not infrequently practices also have lights over the dark room door to show when it is occupied. This is confusing, especially as the lights are usually red, and should be discouraged).

Finally, some practices have a buzzer or bell warning which sounds when the X-ray machine is in use. In a busy practice, where the X-ray room is used for other purposes, this is a good system since it is difficult to ignore.

Shielding: The most useful aids to protection against scattered radiation are distance and shielding. The ideal arrangement is to have the control panel in the X-ray room behind a lead screen with a lead glass viewing window. This system is to be found in all teaching establishments but less frequently in veterinary practices, possibly due to shortage of space or, more likely, since lead screens are relatively expensive.

The 1970 Code of Practice defined a weekly work load of 30mA min above which a screen would be very desirable. In fact, it would be desirable whatever the work load, but increasingly essential as the work load increases.

A satisfactory, if less elegant, alternative is to leave the room and shelter behind a solid wall during the exposure. If personnel need (convenience is not sufficient justification) to remain in the X-ray room during the exposure they should wear a protective apron, ensuring that it is sufficiently long to cover the lower trunk and thighs.

It is also vital to consider the protection of other practice personnel and members of the public who may be in adjacent rooms and in general the following rules apply for the exposures and patients likely to be encountered in veterinary practice.

Adequate barriers to primary beam:

1) 4 $\frac{1}{2}$ inches of brickwork or concrete blocks
2) 1 mm of lead or its equivalent of lead rubber, glass or acrylic

NB: A 'typical' floor to a first floor room consisting of wooden joists with floorboards, or chipboard on their upper surface and plasterboard below is NOT an adequate barrier to primary radiation. Care must be taken, in a room which is not on the ground floor, to ensure that the beam is attenuated by a sufficiently large area of 1 mm of lead or its equivalent.

Adequate barriers to secondary (scattered) radiation:

1) 4 $\frac{1}{2}$ inches of brickwork, concrete blocks or thermally insulating blocks.
2) 0.5 mm of lead rubber, glass or acrylic.
3) A distance of 2 m from the edge of the primary beam plus a plasterboard, timber or glass partition or door.

Where the barrier separates the X-ray room from a public area, e.g. the waiting room or a public thoroughfare it is likely that a more substantial barrier would be advised by the RPA.

Controlled and Supervised Areas

The designation of a controlled or supervised area is, at least when reading the Regulations, a complicated matter. Basically, any area where the instantaneous dose rate is likely to exceed 7.5 uSv per hour, must be controlled. To put this in perspective (see also Dosimetry) 7.5 uSv is the level of exposure that might be measured during a conventional hip dysplasia radiograph at about 0.5 m from the edge of the primary beam. In theory, this could be repeated once a minute over an hour (producing a dose rate of 450 uSv/hour), in practice it might be repeated several times in an hour.

The controlled area can be calculated on this basis or, more usually, delineated by serial dose measurements. In reality, the simplest expedient is to designate the entire X-ray room a controlled area when the X-ray machine is connected to the main electricity supply. Paragraph 62 of the Approved Code of Practice defines conditions under which the controlled area may be defined without any measurement or the advice of an RPA.

These are:

a)   The only source of ionising radiation that may be operated at any one time in any room is a single piece of X-ray equipment specifically designed for X-ray diagnosis and that equipment is only used with the X-ray beam directed vertically downwards onto the table.

b)   The X-ray equipment is fitted with a light beam diaphragm or other device to ensure that the useful beam does not come within 10 cm of the edge of the table.

c)   The table is covered by 1 mm of lead over an area extending not less than 10 cm further in each direction than the largest area of useful beam.

d)   The equipment operates at less that 100 kV, and

e)   the work load of the X-ray equipment does not exceed 4mA minutes in any week.

The controlled area will then exist between the ceiling and floor in a vertical direction extending 1 metre out from each edge of the table.

It is easier to designate the entire room a controlled area than to try to indicate clearly the extent of a controlled area within the room. The only exception to this is where a fixed lead screen is available when the area behind the screen need not be controlled. This is very useful since unmonitored personnel, e.g. veterinary students, can retire behind the screen, out of the controlled area, while still observing the radiographic procedure.

Classified Workers

Part III of the Regulations stipulates that any person remaining in a controlled area during radiography must either be a Classified Person or obey a Written System of Work. This is attached to the Local Rules and the HSE must be satisfied that under the System of the Work no worker will receive an exposure in excess of three tenths of any dose limit.

Additionally, an employer must be able to demonstrate that this is the case, usually by all staff wearing personal dosemeters. In veterinary practice, no employees should be classified workers since no employee in any practice should ever approach three tenths of any dose limit.

Dosimetry

The Regulations only require that classified workers wear suitable personal dosimeters, but it is difficult for staff to work, legally, under a Written System of Work without also wearing personal dosemeters.

In veterinary practice personal dosimetry serves two purposes. It measures the exposure dose to personnel and monitors procedures. Dose limits should be irrelevant in veterinary practice. These dose limits are set making various assumptions that are not strictly applicable to veterinary practice. They are intended for a small number of radiation workers for whom the danger of radiation is their only real industrial hazard. The level of acceptable risk can then be equated with industrial injuries in other occupations. In veterinary practice radiation contributes only in part to the overall risk so that the only acceptable dose is that which is minimal, which when using thermoluminescent dosemeters (TLD) is recorded as 0.0 mSv. In the average practice it is satisfactory to wear a TLD for two months before changing it.

The radiation dose received by a worker wearing a thermoluminescent dosemeter is quoted as whole body and skin doses. This is calculated on the basis of the energy of the radiation absorbed by the dosemeter. A number of practices find that although their whole body dose records are consistently low, occasional skin dose readings in the region of 0.5 to 1.0 mSv are recorded. On investigation nothing can be found to explain the elevated reading which must then be concluded to be aberrant and due to 'thermal noise'.

Of more concern than single elevated skin dose readings are consistently higher skin and whole body readings for the same worker(s). These are again usually of the order of 0.5 to 1.0 mSv and as such, even if repeated monthly, would not exceed 3/10 of the appropriate dose limit. Nevertheless, they indicate a break down in procedure and should be thoroughly investigated.

To put dosimetry results in context it is valuable to consider the doses measured at various points during a 'typical' radiographic exposure as recorded by Webbon (1981) or Wrigley and Borak (1983). For a 17 kg dog and exposure factors of 60 kVp and 32 mAs to radiograph its pelvis and hips for hip dysplasia assessment, the doses would be in the order of:

Entry skin dose to the dog	1.5 mSv
Immediately outside the primary beam	0.04 mSv
25 cm away from the primary beam	0.008 mSv
35 cm away from the primary beam behind a 0.25 mm LE lead apron	0.00004 mSv

All staff involved in radiography should wear personal dosemeters the entire time that they are on duty in the practice, covered, when appropriate, by protective clothing. In busy practices, the RPA may advise that extremity (finger stall, finger strap or wrist strap) dosemeters are also worn.

Finally, the same dosemeters can be used for environmental monitoring. For example, if a room used for radiography joins the waiting room, even though dose measurements during a series of exposures indicate that the exposure rate is low in the waiting room, it is a wise precaution to fix a TLD to the wall in the waiting room to measure the accumulated dose over a period of time. Similar environmental monitoring would be appropriate in a room above the X-ray room.

Regulations 6(1) (quoted previously) makes it quite clear that it is the duty of an employer, i.e. the practice Principal(s), to ensure that radiation protection procedures are correctly followed. In deciding upon the procedures which are correct for each practice the Principal(s) will probably rely upon the advice of a Radiation Protection Adviser and the day-to-day implementation of the advice of the RPA is the responsibility of the practice Radiation Protection Supervisor. The responsibility of the Principal(s), RPA and RPS are summarised in Table 10.1.

Radiation Protection Adviser

Any practice with an X-ray machine that requires any member of staff to work in a controlled area must appoint a Radiation Protection Adviser. In effect this means all practices except those very few in which the controlled area is defined as in Paragraph 62 of the Approved code of practice (see earlier) and animals are never manually restrained.

Suitable people to act as Radiation Protection Advisers are

a)   Veterinary radiologists, holding the Diploma in Veterinary Radiology, with an active interest in radiation protection and the facilities and experience to apply the physics involved.
b)   A health physicist who has an active interest in veterinary radiology.

Once an RPA appointment has been made the Principal(s) must notify the HSE. The HSE will either approve and acknowledge the appointment or ask for more details of the qualifications and experience of the RPA in which case the RPA will ususally provide the

information directly to the HSE.

The duties of the RPA (which are summarised in Table 10.1) will differ with the nature of individual practices. In all cases, however, the RPA will need to draft local rules and a written system of work for each practice and provide a written report on the practice and its protection procedures. The report must be retained for inspection by the HSE and it is likely that the HSE Inspector will expect that recommendations in the report will have been acted upon.

Radiation Protection Supervisor

This will be a person appointed by the Principal(s) to take charge of routine protection procedures. In small practices the Principal will also be the RPS; in larger practices two Supervisors may need to be appointed, e.g. one to deal with small animals and the other horses or to supervise different sites. It is important to remember that it is the Principal(s) that retains the final responsibility for radiation protection and the RPS is appointed to assist the Principal(s) in discharging that responsibility.

Records

Good records of radiographic procedures are essential. Each radiographic exposure should be recorded with the following minimum details:

Date, Patient Identification, Owners name or case no., Breed, Projection, Exposure details, Personnel involved, Manual restraint.

This record can then be used to monitor various aspects of radiation protection, in addition to the monthly work load expressed in patient or exposure numbers or mA minutes. The RPA or RPS can, for example, easily see to what extent the radiographic work load is spread amongst staff and whether some members of a practice are more likely to restrain an animal manually than others. If an unexpectedly high reading on a dosemeter has to be investigated the period for which the dosemeter was worn can be searched to see if there is any logical reason, e.g. several barium studies on large dogs, to explain the higher reading.

This type of thorough record keeping requires a separate radiography day book and it is not satisfactory to record X-ray examinations only in the daily operating list.

Table 10.1:   Summary of Radiation Protection Responsibilities

---

PRINCIPAL OF PRACTICE:

Obtains	–	X-ray machine (NB supplier/manufacturer has a duty to ensure that it is working correctly and safely).
	–	'Guidance Notes for the Protection of Persons against Ionising Radiations arising from Veterinary Use'.
		(Approved Code of Practice for the Protection of Persons against Ionising Radiations arising from any Work Use).
Notifies	–	Health and Safety Executive.
Appoints	–	Radiation Protection Adviser.
		Radiation Protection Supervisor.

RADIATION PROTECTION ADVISER:

Check Room	–	Barriers to primary and secondary radiation		
	–	construction		
	–	size		
Check Procedures	–	Working routine		
	–	Monitoring	–	whole body
			–	extremity
			–	environmental
Check Equipment	–	Machine		
	–	Table		
	–	Protective clothing		
Advises/drafts	–	Local Rules		
	–	Written System of Work		
	–	Changes to	–	room
			–	procedures
			–	equipment
	–	Problems which may arise		
Check Training	–	Where necessary, staff in radiation protection procedures.		
Reports	–	On the practice to the Principle, advising changes where necessary.		

RADIATION PROTECTION SUPERVISOR:

Supervises	–	Procedures
		Monitoring
		Records
		Protective clothing.

Table 10.2:   Health and Safety Executive Area Officers

	Area	Address	Tel. No.	Local authority within each area
1)	SOUTH WEST	Inter City House Mitchell Lane, Victoria Street, Bristol, BS1 6AN	**01272 290681**	Avon, Cornwall, Devon, Somerset, Isles of Scilly Gloucestershire,
2)	SOUTH	Priestley House, Priestley Road, Basingstoke, RG24 9NW	**01256 473181**	Berkshire, Dorset, Hampshire, Isle of Wight, Wiltshire
3)	SOUTH EAST	3 East Grinstead House, London Road, East Grinstead, West Sussex RH19 1RR	**01342 26922**	Kent, Surrey, East Sussex, West Sussex
4)	LONDON N	Maritime House, 1 Linton Road, Barking, Essex IG11 8HF	**081-594 5522**	Barking & Dagenham, Barnet, Brent, Camden, Enfield, Ealing, Hackney, Haringey, Harrow, Havering, Islington, Newham, Redbridge, Tower Hamlets, Waltham Forest
5)	LONDON S	1 Long Lane, London SE1 4PG and Chancel House, Neasden Lane, London NW10 2UD	**071-407 8911** **071-459 8855**	Bexley, Bromley, City of London, Croydon, Greenwich, Hammersmith & Fulham, Hillingdon, Hounslow, Kensington & Chelsea, Kingston, Lambeth, Lewisham, Merton, Richmond, Southwark, Sutton, Wandsworth, Westminster.
6)	EAST ANGLIA	39 Baddow Road, Chelmsford, Essex CM2 0HL	**01245 284661**	Essex, Norfolk, Suffolk
7)	NORTHERN HOME COUNTIES	14 Cardiff Road, Luton, Beds, LU1 1PP	**01582 34121**	Bedfordshire, Buckinghamshire, Cambridgeshire, Hertfordshire
8)	EAST MIDLANDS	Belgrave House, 1 Greyfriars, Northampton NN1 2BS	**01604 21233**	Leicestershire, Northamptonshire, Oxfordshire, Warwickshire
9)	WEST MIDLANDS	McLaren Bldg, 2 Masshouse Circus, Queensway, Birmingham B4 7NP	**0121-200 2299**	West Midlands
10)	WALES	Brunel House, 2 Fitzalan Road, Cardiff CF2 1SH	**01222 473777**	Clwyd, Dyfed, Gwent, Gwynedd, Mid Glamorgan, Powys, South Glamorgan, West Glamorgan

Area	Address	Tel. No.	Local authority within each area
11) **MARCHES**	The Marches House, Midway, Newcastle-under-Lyme, Staffs, ST5 1DT	**01782 717181**	Hereford and Worcester, Salop, Staffordshire
12) **NORTH MIDLANDS**	Birkbeck House, Trinity Square, Nottingham NG1 4AU	**01602 470712**	Derbyshire, Lincolnshire, Nottingham
13) **SOUTH YORKSHIRE**	Sovereign House, 40 Silver Street, Sheffield S1 2ES	**01742 739081**	Humberside, South Yorkshire
14) **W & N YORKS**	8 St Pauls Street, Leeds, LS1 2LE	**01532 446191**	North Yorkshire, West Yorkshire
15) **GREATER MANCHESTER**	Quay House, Quay Street, Manchester M3 3JB	**0161-831 7111**	Greater Manchester
16) **MERSEYSIDE**	The Triad, Stanley Road, Bootle L20 3PG	**0151-922 7211**	Cheshire, Merseyside
17) **NORTH WEST**	Victoria House, Ormskirk Road, Preston PR1 1HH	**01772 59321**	Cumbria, Lancashire
18) **NORTH EAST**	Arden House, Regent Centre, Gosforth NE3 3JN	**0191-284 8448**	Cleveland, Durham, Northumberland, Tyne & Wea
19) **SCOTLAND EAST**	Belford House, 59 Belford Road, Edinburgh EH4 3UE	**0131-225 1313**	Borders, Central, Fife, Grampian, Highland, Lothian, Tayside and the island areas of Orkney & Shetland
20) **SCOTLAND WEST**	314 St Vincent Street, Glasgow G3 8XG	**0141-204 2646**	Dunfries and Galloway, Strathclyde and the Western Isles
NORTHERN IRELAND Health and Safety Inspectorate	Department of Economic Development, The Arches Centre, 13 Bloomfield Avenue, Belfast BT5 5HD	**01232 732411**	

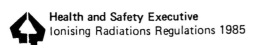

Health and Safety Executive
Ionising Radiations Regulations 1985

Notification of initial intention to work with ionising radiation or of significant changes in its use

Notes

1.   Under Regulations 5(2), 5(6) and Schedule 4 of the Ionising Radiations Regulations 1985 notification is required when an employer commences work with ionising radiation for the first time. Exemptions to this requirement are contained in Schedule 3 of the Regulations which is reproduced overleaf.

2.   Employers who undertake work with ionising radiation at premises other than their own will only need to notify that they are in that business and will not need to notify each subsequent address at which they do their work. However an exception to this would be where additional particulars are required by the Health and Safety Executive.

3.   Space is provided at 6 for the convenience of any employer who occupies several premises operating under the same name.

1.   Name and address of employer

Postcode

2.   Address of premises where, or from where, the work is to be carried on

Postcode

3.   Nature of business

4.   Do you intend to use

a)   sealed sources   Yes ☐   No ☐

b)   unsealed radioactive substances   Yes ☐   No ☐

c)   a radiation generator   Yes ☐   No ☐

or

d)   is the notification the result of exposure to the   Yes ☐   No ☐
     short lived daughters of radon 222?

5.   Mobile sources

a)   Is any work with ionising radiation involving
     any of the sources specified in 4 a),b)or c)   Yes ☐   No ☐
     carried on at any address other than the
     address shown in 2?

b)   If 'YES', state for what purpose.

6.   Multiple site employer

If the employer occupies premises other than those given above, completing this section will avoid the need to send a duplicate notification. Enter the details as shown at 4 & 5 against each address. Further details may be included on a separate sheet if necessary.

Address

i)   4 a) Yes ☐   No ☐
                                              b) Yes ☐   No ☐
                                              c) Yes ☐   No ☐
                                              d) Yes ☐   No ☐
                                           5 a) Yes ☐   No ☐
                                              b)

ii)   4 a) Yes ☐   No ☐
                                              b) Yes ☐   No ☐
                                              c) Yes ☐   No ☐
                                              d) Yes ☐   No ☐
                                           5 a) Yes ☐   No ☐
                                              b)

continued overleaf

Address

iii)

4 a) Yes ☐   No ☐

b) Yes ☐   No ☐

c) Yes ☐   No ☐

d) Yes ☐   No ☐

5 a) Yes ☐   No ☐

b)

iv)

4 a) Yes ☐   No ☐

b) Yes ☐   No ☐

c) Yes ☐   No ☐

d) Yes ☐   No ☐

5 a) Yes ☐   No ☐

b)

7. Anticipated commencement date of work with ionising radiations.

8. Is this a new notification or a significant change in use? (state which)

Signature   Date

Name   Telephone no.

The completed form should be returned to

The Health and Safety Executive

or, in the case of work offshore, to

Dept of Energy (PED)
Thames House South
Millbank
London SW1P 4QJ

Ionising Radiations Regulations 1985 – Schedule 3

Work not required to be notified under Regulation 5 (2)

Work with ionising radiation shall not be required to be notified in accordance with Regulation 5(2) when the only such work being carried out is in one or more of the following categories –

a)   no radioactive substance having an activity concentration of more than 100 Bqg^{-1} is involved;

b)   the quantity of radioactive substance does not exceed the quantity specified in column 2 of Schedule 2;

c)   timepieces and instruments containing or bearing radioluminescent paint are kept or used where effective means are taken to prevent contact with or leakage of any radioactive substance;

d)   articles containing or bearing radioluminescent paint are manufactured or repaired and where the only liquid radioluminescent paints, (if any) at the premises where the work is carried on are paints containing less than the following quantities of the following radionuclides:-

    (a) 2 GBq of tritium; or

    (b) 100 MBq of promethium 147;

e)   gas mantles containing compounds of thorium are stored or used;

f)   a radiation generator is operated or used which does not under normal operating conditions cause a dose rate of more than 1μSvh^{-1} at a distance of 100mm from any accessible surface and is of a type approved by the Health and Safety Executive for the purposes of this sub-paragraph;

g)   an apparatus containing a radioactive substance is involved which does not under normal operating conditions, cause a dose rate of more than 1μSvh^{-1} at a distance of 100mm from any accessible surface and is of a type approved by the Health and Safety Executive for the purposes of this sub-paragraph;

h)   the work involves the care of a person to whom a radioactive medicinal product, (within the meaning of the Medicines (Administration of Radioactive Substances) Regulations 1978 (SI 1978/1006)) has been administered; or

i)   the work is carried out on a ship, aircraft, hovercraft or hydrofoil by members of its crew.

APPENDIX I

The British Veterinary Association / Kennel Club HIP Dysplasia Scoring Scheme

All radiographs submitted under the B.V.A./K.C. Hip Dysplasia Scheme are assessed by means of a scoring system based on the radiographical features. The original B.V.A./K.C. Certification Scheme, which was set up in 1965 and recognised three categories of hip dysplasia: 'Pass', Breeders Letter' and 'Fail', is no longer available.

Procedure for the Submission of Radiographs to the Scheme

1) Each dog must be presented to the veterinary surgeon with its Kennel Club Registration Certificate and, if appropriate, its Transfer Certificate. Dogs must be at least ONE year of age, although there is no longer any upper age limit.

2) The radiograph must be taken with the dog in dorsal recumbency and with the hind limbs extended so that the femora are parrallel to each other and to the other top. The stifles should be rotated inwards so that the patellae are centred between the femoral condyles. General anaesthesia or heavy sedation must be used to facilitate positioning and to obviate the need for manual restraint.

3) The Kennel Club Registration number of the dog, the date the film was taken and a right or left marker MUST be radiographed onto the film using lead letters or X-rite tape, OR photographed on to the film with a light marker before the film is processed. This information may not be added after the radiograph has been processed. The K.C. registration number appears at the top right hand corner of the K.C. Registration Certificate.

4) The veterinary surgeon then sends to the British Veterinary Association, 7 Mansfield Street, LONDON, W1M 0AT:-

a) the radiograph
b) the combined declaration form and scoring sheet (Fig 1) completed and signed by the owner and veterinary surgeon. Supplies of these forms are available from B.V.A.
c) a cheque made payable to the B.V.A. for the submission fee.

5) The B.V.A. panel of scrutineers check that film quality and patient positioning are adequate for an accurate assessment and then score the hips. In the event of an X-ray being rejected by the scrutineers because because of poor film quality or incorrect positioning a further charge will be made for the examination of a repeat film. Each hip is assessed and scored on the nine radiological features listed on the combined declaration form and scoring sheet (Fig. 1). Each feature is given a score between 0 and 6 (except for one, the caudial acetabular edge, the maximum score for which is five). This gives a maximum possible score of 53 for each hip and a total score ranging from 0 to 106 for each dog, the higher the total score the greater the degree of abnormality.

6) The radiograph and two copies of the completed scoring sheet are returned to the owner. Where an appeal is made against the score given, the radiograph may be re-submitted on the payment of a further fee. The radiograph will then be re-scored by the chief scrutineer whose decision is final.

7) The B.V.A. will send the details and results of all Kennel Club registered dogs to the Kennel Club for publication in the Kennel Gazette. Dogs not registered with the Kennel Club may be scored, but their details and results will not be sent to the Kennel Club for publication.

BRITISH VETERINARY ASSOCIATION/KENNEL CLUB
HIP DYSPLASIA SCHEME

To: British Veterinary Association
        7 Mansfield Street
        LONDON W1M OAT

KC Reg No:

PLEASE TYPE OR USE BLOCK CAPITALS FOR ALL INFORMATION   (Please use Black Ink)

Date radiograph taken ....

Breed ....

Sex .... Date born ....

KC Registered Name ....

Name of owner .... Address ....

....

Sire:		PGS	
		PGD	
Dam:		MGS	
		MGD	

I hereby declare that:
(a)   The particulars above are correct and relate to the dog submitted for radiographic examination
(b)   The dog has not previously been submitted for scoring
(c)   I give permission for a copy of the certificate to be sent to the geneticist retained by the breed society or other representative body
(d)   I give permission for the results of the examination to be used at a future date for the purpose of statistical research
(e)   I give permission for the results to be published

DELETION OF ANY OF THESE ITEMS INVALIDATES THE FORM

Owner's signature .... Date ....

Veterinary surgeon submitting radiograph (BLOCKS) ....

Address ....

....

Date .... Signed .... MRCVS

Film quality: Satisfactory/too thin/too dark/extraneous marks

Position: Satisfactory/tilted laterally left/right/femora not sufficiently extended/femora not evenly extended

HIP JOINT	Right	Left
Norberg angle		
Subluxation		
Cranial acetabular edge		
Dorsal acetabular edge		
Cranial effective acetabular rim		
Acetabular fossa		
Caudal acetabular edge		
Femoral head/neck exostosis		
Femoral head recontouring		
TOTALS (max possible 53 per column)		

The current BVA fee is £19.30 inclusive of VAT per dog and a reduced fee of £15.40 inclusive of VAT per dog for five or more dogs for the same owner

Total Score (max possible 106)

I HEREBY CERTIFY that the above-named animal was examined under the rules of the BVA/KC Hip Dysplasia Scheme

on .... (date)   Signed .... (Scheme Secretary)

Signed .... (Scrutineer)

Fig 1: Submission form and scoring sheet.

Comment

The main advantage of the Scoring Scheme is that it allows a mean score to be calculated for each breed (Fig. 2). The mean score for any breed represents the overall hip status of the breed since it is calculated from all the recorded scores both high and low. The larger the number of dogs scored from that breed the more accurate the mean score will be. Thus, dogs wish to control hip dysplasia should only breed with animals below the breed mean. In addition, the hip status within a breed can be monitored over a period of time to show any change. The hip score results are updated periodically and are published in the veterinary and lay press. For information to be properly utilised the scoring sheets should be submitted to the breed geneticist for analysis.

BVA/KENNEL CLUB HD Scheme Breed Mean Scores

LIST 1:   HIPS SCORES BY BREED (BVA)   TO 22.4.1994
This covers scoring under BVA/KC and the (now defunct)BVA/GSDL schemes. Dogs resident outside Britain but scored by the BVA are included. This latter is a very small number of animals.

A: BREEDS WITH 1000 OR MORE SCORED (11)

Bearded Collie	1126	0 - 78	11.09
Bernese Mountain Dog	1805	0 - 102	16.14
Border Collie/working sheepdog	2251	0 - 89	12.96
English Setter (10)	1070	0 - 95	20.41
Flat-Coated Retriever	1818	0 - 78	9.18
German Shepherd Dog (15)	19980	0 - 106	18.55
Golden Retriever (11)	13291	0 - 106	19.91
Gordon Setter (6)	1020	0 - 104	25.68
Labrador Retriever	15530	0 - 103	16.41
Newfoundland (4)	1339	0 - 106	32.90
Rottweiler	5803	0 - 99	13.92
GROUP TOTAL	65033		

B: BREEDS WITH 500 TO 999 SCORED   (8)

Belgian Shepherd Dog*	636	0 - 104	11.57
Dobermann	560	0 - 70	10.10
Japanese Akita	817	0 - 73	11.12
Old English Sheepdog (8)	820	0 - 100	21.42
Samoyed	624	0 - 94	12.66
Siberian Husky	848	0 - 30	5.87
Weimaraner	672	0 - 89	13.37
Welsh Springer Spaniel (14)	574	0 - 104	18.62
GROUP TOTAL	5551		

C: BREEDS WITH 100 TO 499 SCORED   (32)

Airedale Terrier (19)	463	0 - 91	17.80
Boxer	201	0 - 64	16.31
Briard (7)	338	0 - 99	23.78
Brittany (16)	126	0 - 74	18.35
Bullmastiff (5)	378	0 - 104	30.34
Cavalier King Charles Spaniel	202	2 - 91	16.41
Chesapeake Bay Retriever	159	0 - 52	12.09
Chow Chow	483	0 - 102	14.39
Clumber Spaniel (1)	348	0 - 102	44.56
Cocker Spaniel	123	5 - 60	16.48
Elkhound	207	0 - 61	14.43
English Springer Spaniel	278	0 - 74	12.89
German Short-Haired Pointer	156	0 - 57	9.40
German Wire-Haired Pointer	120	0 - 53	10.38
Giant Schnauzer	109	0 - 66	13.73
Great Dane	145	0 - 59	12.08
Hungarian Puli (12)	193	1 - 102	18.79
Hungarian Vizsla	176	2 - 58	12.52
Irish Setter	402	0 - 100	15.49
Irish Water Spaniel (18)	312	0 - 102	17.81
Italian Spinone	241	0 - 89	17.12
Large Munsterlander	169	0 - 88	16.71
Leonberger	143	0 - 56	11.80
Mastiff	120	0 - 81	17.41
Polish Lowland Sheepdog	166	5 - 59	17.34
Pyrenean Mountain Dog	212	0 - 94	12.67
Rhodesian Ridgeback	418	0 - 72	12.09
Rough Collie	426	0 - 89	12.79
St Bernard (9)	131	0 - 70	20.62
Soft-Coated Wheaten Terrier	111	2 - 51	12.78
Standard Poodle	182	4 - 74	16.36
Tibetan Terrier (17)	369	0 - 90	18.23
GROUP TOTAL	7607		

D: BREEDS WITH 40 TO 99 SCORED   (17)

Alaskan Malamute	80	2 - 66	14.31
Anatolian Shepherd Dog	91	0 - 68	13.42
Australian Shepherd Dog	86	2 - 29	10.27
Bouvier des Flandres (20)	99	4 - 70	17.73
Curly-Coated Retriever	89	1 - 50	10.47
Dalmatian	48	0 - 39	9.70
Field Spaniel	48	0 - 51	16.17
Hovawart	78	0 - 79	10.93
Irish Red & White Setter	65	0 - 52	10.17
Irish Wolfhound	58	0 - 86	5.99
Keeshond	40	3 - 63	12.52
Maremma	85	2 - 83	13.34
Otterhound (2)	87	4 - 102	40.77
Shetland Sheepdog (13)	67	2 - 100	18.76
Sussex Spaniel (3)	58	10 - 101	38.74
Swedish Vallhund	68	2 - 28	12.71
Tibetan Mastiff	51	3 - 45	14.14
GROUP TOTAL	1197		

E: BREEDS WITH 10 TO 39 SCORED   (21)

Afghan Hound	30	0 - 54	9.04
Beagle	12	10 - 31	17.83
Bichon Frise	15	4 - 19	10.66
Bloodhound	17	8 - 62	23.47
Hungarian Komondor	16	4 - 72	18.12
Japanese Shiba Inu	20	0 - 35	10.55
Kerry Blue Terrier	37	4 - 53	16.80
Malinois	17	0 - 60	11.58
Miniature Poodle	13	6 - 58	17.46
Miniature Schnauzer	14	4 - 32	13.08
Norwegian Buhund	28	2 - 42	11.89
Nova Scotia Duck Tolling Retriever	28	0 - 43	12.83
Pointer	16	0 - 20	10.01
Pug	14	10 - 53	24.78
Saluki	36	0 - 14	4.68
Schnauzer	21	6 - 70	24.37
Shar-Pei	15	6 - 51	13.87
Smooth Collie	31	0 - 17	5.36
Staffordshire Bull Terrier	14	7 - 23	13.71
Tibetan Spaniel	28	2 - 31	11.51
Welsh Corgi(Pembroke)	11	12 - 50	25.00
GROUP TOTAL	433		

F: BREEDS WITH <10 BUT REACHING THIS TOTAL WITH LIST 2 (3)

Australian Cattle Dog	7	7 - 16	11.00
Bulldog	6	10 - 51	34.33
Bull Terrier	9	4 - 12	8.56
GROUP TOTAL	22		

GRAND TOTAL (92 BREEDS) 79821

* Groenendael/Tervueren only

Figures in brackets after breed name is rank order for worst 20 breeds (1 = worst). Breeds with 40+ only.

This tabulation is made on an Elonex PC433 kindly donated by Leander International (Arden Grange) to whom grateful acknowledgement is made. It was originally printed on a Hewlett Packard Deskjet 500.

Starting date of the scheme was June 1978 for GSD with all other breeds being included by December 1983.

Fig 2: B.V.A. / K.C. Hip Dysplasia Scheme mean scores.

APPENDIX II

Reading List and References

READING LIST
This reading list is included as a guide to the reader who wishes to obtain more specific information about the topics covered in this manual. It is not necessarily exhaustive but will hopefully be a useful introduction to the current literature.

BOOKS AND COLLECTED ARTICLES
Atlas of Radiographic Anatomy of the Dog, Cat and Horse. Ed. 1V. Vols. 1 and 2. H Schebitz and H Wilkens. Paul Parey, Berlin & Hamburg. 1986.
Christensen's Introduction to the Physics of Diagnostic Radiology. Curry TS, Dowdey JE and Murray RC. Lea and Febiger, Philadelphia. 1990.
Diagnostic Radiology of the Dog and Cat. Ed. II. JK Kealy. WB Saunders Co., London 1987.
Diseases of the Thorax - Radiographic Diagnosis. Suter PF and Gomez JA (1987) Iowa State University Press, Ames.
Principles of Veterinary Radiography. Ed. IV. SW Douglas, ME Herrtage and HD Williamson. Balliere Tindall, London 1987.
Radiology in Veterinary Orthopaedics. JP Morgan. Lea and Febiger, Philadelphia. 1973.
Radiographic Positioning of Small Animals. GD Ryan. Lea and Febiger, Philadelphia. 1981.
Radiographic Technique in Veterinary Practice. JW Ticer. WB Saunders Co., London 1984.
Radiological Refreshers: A series of articles by various authors published in the *Journal of Small Animal Practice* between 1973 and 1981.
Safe radiography. Chemical restraint to assist radiographic positioning. (1989). *J. Small Animan practice*. 30, 270-272.
Small Animal Radiology: a diagnostic atlas and text. RL Burk and N Ackerman. Churchill Livingstone, New York, 1987.
Techniques of Veterinary Radiography. Ed. IV. JP Morgan, S Silverman and WJ Zontine. Iowa State University Press 1993.
The Radiological Diagnosis in Canine and Feline Emergencies. SE Olsson. Lea and Febiger, Philadelphia. 1973.
Textbook of Veterinary Diagnostic Radiology. Edited by DE Thrall. Ed II. WB Saunders Co., Philadelphia 1993.
The Veterinary Clinics of North America. 4:4 Radiology. WB Saunders Co., London 1974.
The Veterinary Clinics of North America. 12:2 Radiology, 2. WB Saunders Co., London 1982.
Veterinary Radiological Interpretation. SW Douglas and HD Williamson. Heinemann, London 1970.

Additional Invaluable Aids to Radiological Interpretation
Anatomy of the Domestic Animals (any edition). S Sisson and JD Grossman. WB Saunders Co.
Miller's Anatomy of the Dog. Ed. III. HE Evans. WB Saunders Co., Philadelphia, 1993.

REFERENCES

RADIOGRAPHIC QUALITY
Lee R (1984) Radiography problems and reasons for poor quality. *In Practice*, 6 (5), 154-160.

PHARYNX LARYNX TRACHEA AND OESOPHAGUS

General
Gibbs C (1986) Radiographic examination of the pharynx, larynx and soft tissue structures of the neck in dogs and cats. *Veterinary Annual* 26, 227-241.

Pharynx and larynx
Gaskell CJ (1974) The radiographic anatomy of the pharynx and larynx of the dog. *Journal of Small Animal Practice*. 15, 89-100.
Glen JB (1972) Canine salivary mucocoeles: results of sialographic examination and surgical treatment of 50 cases. *Journal of Small Animal Practice*. 13, 515-526.
Lee R (1974) Radiographic examination of localised and diffuse soft tissue swellings in the mandibular and pharyngeal area. *Vet. Clin. N Amer.* 4 (4), 723-740.

Trachea
Beaumont PR (1982) Intra-tracheal neoplasia in two cats. *Journal of Small Animal Practice*. 23, 29-35.
Brouwer GJ et al (1984) Tracheal rupture in a cat *Journal of Small Animal Practice*. 25, 71-76.
Done SH et al (1976) Observations on the pathology of tracheal collapse in the dog. *Journal of Small Animal Prac.* 17, 783-791.
Gourley IMG et al (1970) Tracheal osteochondroma in a dog; a case report. *Journal of Small Animal Practice*. 11, 327.
Harvey CE (1989). Inherited and congenital airway conditions. *Journal of Small Animal Practice* 30, 184-187.

Oesophagus
Carb AV et al (1973) Oesophageal carcinoma in the dog. *Journal of Small Animal Practice*. 14, 91-99.
Houlton JEF et al (1985) Thoracic oesophageal foreign bodies in the dog: a review of 90 cases. *Journal of Small Animal Practice*. 26, 521-536.
Kleine LJ (1974) Radiologic examination of the oesophagus in dogs and cats. *Vet. Clin. N Amer.* 4 (4), 663-686.
Pearson H (1966) Foreign bodies in the oesophagus. *Journal of Small Animal Practice*. 7, 107-116.
Pearson H (1970) The differential diagnosis of persistent vomiting in the young dog. *Journal of Small Animal Practice*. 11, 403-415.
Pearson H et al (1978) Oesophageal diverticulum formation in the dog. *Journal of Small Animal Practice*. 19, 341-355.
Pearson H et al (1978) Reflux oesophagitis and stricture formation after anaesthesia: a review of seven cases in dogs and cats. *Journal of Small Animal Practice*. 19, 507-519.
Squires RA (189). Oesophageal obstruction by a hairball in a cat. *Journal of Small Animal Practice* 30.

SKULL

Bennett D *et al* (1976) Mechanical interference with lower jaw movement as a complication of skull fractures. *Journal of Small Animal Practice.* 17, 747-751.

Frew DJ and Dobson JM (1992). Radiological assessment of 50 cases of incisive or maxillary neoplasia in the dog. *Journal of Small Animal Practice* 33, 11-18.Gibbs C (1976) Traumatic lesions of the skull (Radiological Refresher - 7) *Journal of Small Animal Practice.* 17, 551-554.

Gibbs C (1977) Traumatic lesions of the mandible (Radiological Refresher - 9) *Journal of Small Animal Practice.* 18, 51-54.

Gibbs C (1978) Ear disease (Radiological Refresher - 11) *Journal of Small Animal Practice.* 19, 539-545.

Gibbs C (1978) Dental disease (Radiological Refresher - 13) *Journal of Small Animal Practice.* 19, 701-707.

Gibbs C, *et al* (1979) The radiographic features of intra-nasal disorders in dogs: a review of 100 cases. *Journal of Small Animal Practice.* 20, 515-535.

Harvey CE (1971) Traumatic frontal mucocele in the dog: a case report. *Journal of Small Animal Practice.* 12, 399-403.

Jaggy A *et al* (1991). Occipitoatlanto-axial malformation with atlantoaxial subluxation in a cat. *Journal of Small Animal Practice* 32, 366-372.

Johnson KA *et al* (1994). Maxillary central giant cell granuloma in a dog. *Journal of Small Animal Practice* 35, 427-430.

Lane JG (1982) Disorders of the canine temporo-mandibular joint. *Veterinary Annual* 22, 167-180.

Morgan JP and Miyabayashi T (1991). Dental radiology: Ageing changes in permanent teeth of Beagle dogs. *Journal of Small Animal Practice* 32, 11-18.

Mould JRB (1990). Cholesterol granumloma of the maxilla in a dog. *Journal of Small Animal Practice* 31, 208-211.

Sarkiala E *et al* 1993). Clinical, radiological and bacteriological findings in canine periodontitis. *Journal of Small Animal Practice* 34, 265-270.

Smith KC *et al* (1993). Odontoma in a juvenile Boxer: Clinical, radiographic and pathological findings. *Journal of Small Animal Practice* 34, 142-145.

Sullivan M *et al* (1986) The radiological features of aspergillosis of the nasal cavity and frontal sinuses of the dog. *Journal of Small Animal Practice.* 27, 167-180.

Sullivan M, Lee R and Skae CA (1987) The radiological features of sixty cases of intra-nasal neoplasia in the dog. *Journal of Small Animal Practice.* 28, 575-586.

Sullivan M (1989). Temperomandibular ankylosis in a cat. *Journal of Small Animal Practice* 30, 401-405.

Thomas RE (1979) Temporo-mandibular joint dysplasia and open-mouth jaw locking in a Basset Hound: a case report. *Journal of Small Animal Practice.* 20, 697-701.

Zontine WJ (1974) Dental radiographic technique and interpretation. *Vet. Clin. N Amer.* 4 (4), 741-762.

THORAX

General

Bright RM *et al* (1990). Hiatal hernia in the dog and cat: A retrospective study of 16 cases. *Journal of Small Animal Prac.* 31, 244-250.

Burnie AG *et al* (1989). Gastro-oesophageal reflux and hiatus hernia associated with laryngeal paralysis in a dog. *Journal of Small Animal Practice* 30, 414-416.

Darke PGG *et al* (1977) Acute respiratory distress in the dog associated with paraquat poisoning. *Vet Rec.* 100, 275-277.

Douglas SW (1970) Radiology of the normal canine thorax. *Journal of Small Animal Practice.* 11, 669-678.

Gaskell CJ *et al* (1980) Respiratory disease in cats. *In Practice* 2 (6), 5-14.

Johnston SA *et al* (1993). Pectus excavatum and left to right intracardiac shunt in a kitten. *Journal of Small Animal Practice* 34, 577-581.

O'Dair HA *et al* (1991). Aquired immune-mediated myasthenia gravis in a cat associated with a cystic thymus. *Journal of Small Animal Practice* 32, 198-202.

Stead AC (1972) Radiological features of post-road accident chest injuries. *The Veterinary Annual.* 13, 113-117.

Waldron DR *et al* (1990). Oesophageal hiatal hernia in 2 cats. *Journal of Small Animal Practice* 31, 259-263.

Williams JM (1990). Hiatal hernia in a Shar-pei. *Journal of Small Animal Practice* 31, 251-254.

The Lungs

Barr FJ *et al* (1986) The radiological features of primary lung tumours in the dog: a review of 36 cases. *Journal of Small Animal Practice.* 27, 493-505.

Barr FJ *et al* (1987) Primary lung tumours in the cat. *Journal of Small Animal Practice.* 28, 1115-1125.

Biery DN (1974) Differentiation of lung diseases of inflammatory or neoplastic origin from lung disease in heart failure. *Vet. Clin. N Amer.* 4 (4), 711-721.

Brownlie S *et al* (1986) Bronchial foreign bodies in four dogs. *Journal of Small Animal Practice.* 27, 239-245.

Corcoran BM *et al* (1991). Pulmonary infiltration with eosinophils in 14 dogs. *Journal of Small Animal Practice* 32, 494-502.

Critchley KL (1976) Torsion of a lung lobe in the dog. *Journal of Small Animal Practice.* 17, 391-394.

Dobbie GR *et al* (1986) Intrabronchial foreign bodies in dogs. *Journal of Small Animal Practice.* 27, 227-238.

Gurin SR *et al* (1993). Cavitating mycotic pulmonary infection in a German shepherd dog. *Journal of Small Animal Practice* 34, 36-39.

Herrtage ME *et al* (1985) Congenital lobar emphysema in two dogs. *Journal of Small Animal Practice.* 26, 453-464.

Lee R (1976) Patterns of pulmonary disease on thoracic radiographs in dogs and cats. *The Veterinary Annual* 16, 178-186.

Lord PF (1976) Alveolar lung disease in small animals. *Journal of Small Animal Practice.* 17, 283-303.

Moon M (1992). Pulmonary infiltrates with cosinophilia. *Journal of Small Animal Practice* 33, 19-23.

O'Sullivan SP (1989). Paraquat poisoning in the dog. *Journal of Small Animal Practice* 30, 361-364.

Sardinas JC *et al* (1994). Toxoplasma pneumonia in a cat with incongruous serological test results. *Journal of Small Animal Practice* 35, 104-107.

Scott-Moncrieff JC *et al* (1989). Pulmonary squamous cell carcinoma with multiple digital metastases in a cat. *Journal of Small Animal Practice* 30, 696-699.

Suter PF *et al* (1974) Radiographic differentiation of disseminated pulmonary parenchymal disease in dogs and cats. *Vet. Clin. N Amer.* 4 (4), 687-710.

Tennant BJ And Haywood S (1987) Congenital bullous emphysema in a dog: a case report. *Journal of Small Animal Practice.* 28, 109-116.

Thrall DE (1979) Radiographic diagnosis of metastic pulmonary neoplasia. *Comp. contd. Edn. Pract. Vet.* 1, 131-139.

Wheeldon EB *et al* (1977) Chronic respiratory disease in the dog. *Journal of Small Animal Practice.* 18, 229-246.

Pleural Cavity

Fagin B (1989). Using radiography to diagnose traumatic diaphragmatic hernia. *Vct. Med.* 84, 662-672.

Gibbs C (1973) Radiological features of intra-thoracic neoplasia in the dog and cat. *The Veterinary Annual* 14, 199-208.

Grandage J (1974) The radiology of the dog's diaphragm. *Journal of Small Animal Practice.* 15, 1-17.

Gruffydd-Jones TJ *et al* (1979) Clinical and radiological features of anterior mediastinal lymphosarcoma in the cat: a review of 30 cases. *Vet. Rec.* 104, 304-307.

Jones BR *et al* (1975) Spontaneous pneumomediastinum in the racing greyhound. *Journal of Small Animal Practice.* 16, 27-33.

Kealy JK *et al* (1981) Radiology of the mediastinum. (Radiological Refresher - 17) *Journal of Small Animal Practice.* 22, 717-729.

Malik R *et al* (1991). Pyothorax associated with a Mycoplasma species in a kitten. *Journal of Small Animal Practice* 32, 31-34.

Robertson S *et al* (1983) Thoracic empyema in the dog: a report of 22 cases. *Journal of Small Animal Practice.* 24, 103-119.

Sullivan M and Lee R (1989). Radiological features of 80 cases of diaphragmatic rupture. *Journal of Small Animal Practice* 30, 561-566.

Cardiovascular

Bright JM *et al* (1992). Feline hypertrophic cardiomyopathy: Variations on a theme. *Journal of Small Animal Practice* 33, 266-274.

Cobb MA and Brownlie SE (1992). Intrapericardial neoplasia in 14 dogs. *Journal of Small Animal Practice* 33, 309-316.

Cornelius L *et al* (1985) Kinking of the intrathoracic caudal vena cava in four dogs. *Journal of Small Animal Practice.* 26, 67-80.

Darke PGG (1980) Cardiac disease syndromes in dogs and cats. *In Practice* 2 (3), 5-12.

Darke PGG (1989) Congenital heart disease in dogs and cats. *Journal of Small Animal Practice* 30, 599-607.

Gibbs C *et al* (1982) Idiopathic pericardial haemorrhage in the dog: a review of 14 cases. *Journal of Small Animal Practice.* 23, 483-500.

Gruffydd-Jones TJ *et al* (1986) Cardiomyopathy and thromboembolism in cats. Veterinary Annual 26, 348-360.

Hill BL (1981) Canine idiopathic congestive cardiomyopathy. *Comp. cont. Edn. Pract. Vet.* 3, 615.

Lee R (1975) The radiographic diagnosis of heart disease in the dog. (Radiological Refresher - 3) *Journal of Small Animal Practice.* 16, 207-209.

Luis Fuentes V *et al* (1991). Purulent pericarditis in a puppy. *Journal of Small Animal Practice* 32, 585-588.

Luis Fuentes V (1992). Feline heart disease: An update. *Journal of Small Animal Practice* 33, 130-137.

Malik R *et al* (1993). Valvular pulmonic stenosis in Bull mastiffs. *Journal of Small Animal Practice* 34, 288-292.

Matic SE (1988) Congenital heart disease in the dog. *Journal of Small Animal Practice.* 29, 743-759.

Pion PD and Kittleson MD (1990). Taurine's role in clinical practice. *Journal of Small Animal Practice* 31, 510-518.

Selcer BA *et al* (1988). Hyperadrenocorticism: Radiographic diagnosis. *Vet. Radiol.* 29, 35-36.

Stepien RL and Bonagura JD (1991). Aortic stenosis: Clinical findings in 6 cats. *Journal of Small Animal Practice* 32, 341-350.

Suter PF (1981) The radiographic diagnosis of canine and feline heart disease. *Comp. cont. Edn. Pract. Vet.* 3, 411.

Van Den Broek AHM *et al* (1987) Cardiac measurements on thoracic radiographs of cats. *Journal of Small Animal Practice.* 28, 125-135.

ABDOMEN

General

Blaxter AC *et al* (1988) Congenital porto-systemic shunts in the cat: a report of nine cases. *Journal of Small Animal Practice.* 29, 631-645.

Gibbs C, *et al* (1972) Radiological features of inflammatory conditions of the canine pancreas. *Journal of Small Animal Practice.* 13, 531-544.

Gibbs C (1981) Radiological features of liver disorders in dogs and cats. *The Veterinary Annual* 21, 239-250.

Harris SJ *et al* (1984) Obstructive cholelithiasis and gallbladder rupture in a dog. *Journal of Small Animal Practice.* 25, 661-667.

Huntley K *et al* (1982) Radiological features of canine Cushings syndrome: a review of 48 cases. *Journal of Small Animal Practice.* 23, 369-380.

Lamb CR (1989). Dilation of the pancreatic duct: An ultrasonographic finding in acute pancreatitis. *Journal of Small Animal Practice* 30, 410-413.

Lee R (1978) Contrast media and techniques 1 and 11 (Radiological refreshers - 12 and 14) *Journal of Small Animal Practice.* 19, 589-592 and 774-777.

Lee R and Leowijuk C (1982) Normal parameters in abdominal radiology of the dog and cat. *Journal of Small Animal Practice.* 23, 251-269.

Rochlitz, I (1984) Feline Dysautonomia (the Key-Gaskell/dilated pupil syndrome): a preliminary review. *Journal of Small Animal Practice.* 25, 587-598.

Root CR (1974) Interpretation of abdominal survey radiographs. *Vet. Clin. N Amer.* 4 (4), 763-803.

Rothuizen J *et al* (1982) Congenital porto-systemic shunts in 16 dogs and 3 cats. *Journal of Small Animal Practice.* 23, 67-83.

Stead AC *et al* (1983) Splenic torsion in dogs. *Journal of Small Animal Practice.* 24, 549-554.

Suter PF *et al* (1970) The diagnosis of injuries to the intestines, gallbladder and bile ducts in the dog. *Journal of Small Animal Practice.* 11, 575-584.

Weaver AD (1976) Radiological diagnosis and prognosis of primary abdominal neoplasia in the dog. *Journal of Small Animal Practice.* 17, 357-363.

Gastro-Intestinal tract

Brovida C and Castagnaro M (1989). An unusual case of hydronephrosis in a bitch. *Journal of Small Animal Practice* 30, 367-370.

Davies JV and Read HM (1990). Urethral tumours in dogs. *Journal of Small Animal Practice* 31, 131-136.

Farrow CS (1982) Radiographic appearance of parvovirus enteritis. *J Am. vet. med. Ass.* 180, 43-47.

Fonda D *et al* (1989). Gastric carcinoma in the dog: A clinical pathological study of 11 cases. *Journal of Small Animal Practice* 30, 353-360.

Frendin J, Funquist B and Stavenborn B (1988) Gastric displacement in dogs without clinical signs of acute dilation. *Journal of Small Animal Practice.* 29, 775-779.

Funquist B (1979) Gastric torsion in the dog. 1. Radiological picture during non-surgical treatment related to the pathological anatomy and to the further clinical course. *Journal of Small Animal Practice.* 20, 73-91.

Gibbs C *et al* (1973) The radiological diagnosis of gastro-intestinal obstruction in the dog. *Journal of Small Animal Practice.* 14, 61-82.

Gibbs C, *et al* (1986) Localised tumours of the canine small intestine: a report of 20 cases. *Journal of Small Animal Practice.* 27, 507-519.

Gomez, JA (1974) The gastrointestinal contrast study. *Vet. Clin. N Amer.* 4 (4), 805-841.

Happe RP (1981) pyloric stensis caused by hypertrophic gastritis in three dogs. *Journal of Small Animal Practice.* 22, 7-17.

Miyabayashi T and Morgan JP (1991). Upper gastrointestinal examinations: A radiographic study of clinically normal Beagle puppies. *Journal of Small Animal Practice* 32, 83-88.

Murray M *et al* (1972) Primary gastric neoplasia in the dog: a clinicopathological study. *Vet. Rec.* 91, 474-479.

Pearson H (1970) The differential diagnosis of persistent vomiting in the young dog. *Journal of Small Animal Practice.* 11, 403-415.

Pearson H *et al* (1974) Pyloric and oesophageal dysfunction in the cat. *Journal of Small Animal Practice.* 15, 487-501.

Root CR *et al* (1969) Contrast radiography of the upper gastrointestinal tract in the dog. *Journal of Small Animal Practice.* 10, 279-286.

Thomas, RE (1982) Gastric dilation and torsion in small and miniature breeds of dog: 3 case reports. *Journal of Small Animal Practice.* 23, 271-279.

Thrall DE *et al* (1976) Irregular intestinal margination in the dog: normal or abnormal? *Journal of Small Animal Practice.* 17, 305-312.

Van Bree H And Sackx A (1987) Evaluation of radiographic liver size in twenty seven normal deep-chested dogs. *Journal of Small Animal Practice.* 28, 693-703.

Urogenital system

Ackerman N (1981) Radiographic evaluation of the uterus: a review, *Vet, Radiol.* 22, 252-257.

Allen WE *et al* (1980) Two cases of incontinence in cats associated with acquired vagino-ureteral fistula. *Journal of Small Animal Practice.* 21, 367-371.

Allen WE *et al* (1985) Contrast radiographic study of the vagina and uterus of the normal bitch. *Journal of Small Animal Practice.* 26, 153-166.

Biewenga WJ *et al* (1978) Ectopic ureters in the cat: a report of two cases. *Journal of Small Animal Practice.* 19, 531-537.

Burnie AG *et al* (1983) Urinary bladder neoplasia in the dog: a review of seventy cases. *Journal of Small Animal Practice.* 24, 129-143.

Farrow CS *et al* (1976) late term foetal death in the dog: early radiographic diagnosis. J Am. Vet. Radiol. Soc. 17, 11-17.

Holt PE *et al* (1982) Canine ectopic ureter: a report of 29 cases. *Journal of Small Animal Practice.* 23, 195-208.

Holt PE *et al* (1983) Disorders of urination associated with canine intersexuality. *Journal of Small Animal Practice.* 24, 475-487.

Holt PE *et al* (1984) An evaluation of positive contrast vagino-urethrography as a diagnostic aid in the bitch. *Journal of Small Animal Practice.* 25, 531-549.

Kneller SK (1974) Role of the excretory urogram in the diagnosis of renal and ureteral disease. *Vet. Clin. N Amer.* 4 (4), 843-861.

Park RD (1974) Radiographic contrast studies of the lower urinary tract. *Vet. Clin. N Amer.* 4 (4), 863-887.

Pearson H *et al* (1971) Urinary tract abnormalities in the dog. *Journal of Small Animal Practice.* 12, 67-84.

Pearson H *et al* (1980) Urinary incontinence in the dog due to accidental uretero-vaginal fistulation during hysterectomy. *Journal of Small Animal Practice.* 21, 287-291.

Stead AC *et al* (1976) The canine urinary bladder and prostate. (Radiological Refresher - 8) *Journal of Small Animal Practice.* 17, 629-634.

Stone EA *et al* (1978) Radiographic interpretation of prostatic disease in the dog. *J Am. Anim. Hosp. Ass.* 14, 115-118.

Thrall DE (1981) Radiographic aspects of prostatic disease in the dog. *Comp. cont. Edn. Pract. Vet.* 3, 730.

Weaver AD (1980) Prostatic disease in the dog. *The Veterinary Annual* 20, 82-93.

Webbon PM (1979) Radiology of the canine kidney. *The Veterinary Annual.* 19, 144-151.

White RAS *et al* (1987) The diagnosis and management of paraprostatic and prostatic retention cysts in the dog. *Journal of Small Animal Practice.* 28, 551-574.

ORTHOPAEDICS

General

Brearley MJ and Jeffery N (1992). Cryptococcal osteomyelitis in a dog. *Journal of Small Animal Practice* 33, 601-604.

Dunn JK *et al* (1992). Successful treatment of 2 cases of metaphyseal Osteomyelitis in the dog. *Journal of Small Animal Practice* 33, 85-89.

Lamb CR *et al* (1993). Radiographic diagnosis of an expansile bone lesion in a dog. *Journal of Small Animal Practice* 34, 239-241.

Morgan JP (1975) Systematic radiographic interpretation of skeletal disease in small animals. *Vet. Clin. N Amer.* 4 (4), 611-626.

Vaughan LC (1979) Muscle and tendon injuries in dogs. *Journal of Small Animal Practice.* 20, 711-736.

Wigney DI *et al* (1990). Osteomyelitis associated with Penicillium verruculosm in a German shepherd dog. *Journal of Small Animal Practice* 31, 449-452.

Skeletal Development

Havewinkel HAW (1989). Nutrition in relation to skeltal growth deformities. *Journal of Small Animal Practice* 30, 625-630.

Mooney CT and Anderson TJ (1993). Congenital hypothyroidism in a boxer dog. *Journal of Small Animal Practice* 34, 31-35.

Smith RN (1960) Radiological observations on the limbs of young greyhounds. *Journal of Small Animal Practice.* 1, 84-90.

Smith RN (1963) Fusion of ossification centres in the cat. *Journal of Small Animal Practice.* 10, 523-530.

Watson ADJ *et al* (1991). Osteochondral-dysplasia in Bull terrier litter mates. *Journal of Small Animal Practice* 32, 312-317.

Generalised Diseases

Bennett D (1976) Nutrition and bone disease in the dog and cat. *Vet. Rec.* 98, 313-321.

Bennett D (1987) Immune based non erosive inflammatory joint disease of the dog. 1. Canine sytemic lupus erythematosus. *Journal of Small Animal Practice.* 28, 871-890.

Bennett D and Kelly DF (1987) Immune-based non erosive inflammatory joint disease of the dog. 2. Polyarthritis/polymyositis syndrome. *Journal of Small Animal Practice.* 28, 891-908.

Bennett D (1987) Immune based non erosive inflammatory joint disease of the dog. 3. Canine idiopathic polyarthritis. *Journal of Small Animal Practice.* 28, 871-890.

Bennett D (1987) Immune-based erosive inflammatory joint disease of the dog: canine rheumatoid arthritis. 1. Clinical, radiological and laboratory investigations. *Journal of Small Animal Practice.* 28, 779-798.

Bennett D and Nash AS (1988) Feline immune based polyarthritis: a study of thirty-one cases. *Journal of Small Animal Practice.* 29, 501-523.

Bennett D and Taylor DJ (1988) Bacterial infective arthritis in the dog. *Journal of Small Animal Practice.* 29, 207-230.

Biery DN *et al* (1975) Radiographic appearance of rheumatoid arthritis in dogs. *J Amer. Anim. Hosp. Ass.* 11, 607-612.

Brodey RS (1979) Aspects of canine hypertrophic osteoarthropathy. *Veterinary Annual* 19, 178-187.

Canfield PJ *et al* (1994). Multifocal idiopathic pygranulomatous bone disease in a dog. *Journal of Small Animal Practice* 35, 370-373.

English PB (1969) A case of hyperostosis due to hypervitaminosis A in a cat. *Journal of Small Animal Practice.* 10, 207-212.

Grondalen J (1976) Metaphyseal osteopathy (hypertrophic osteodys-trophy) in growing dogs. A clinical study. *Journal of Small Animal Practice.* 17, 721-735.

Hunt JM *et al* (1980) The complications of diaphyseal fractures in dogs: a review of 100 cases. *Journal of Small Animal Practice.* 21, 103-119.

Johnston KA *et al* (1988) Vitamin D dependent rickets in a St. Bernard dog. *Journal of Small Animal Practice.* 29, 657-666.

Kramers P *et al* (1988) Osteopetrosis in cats. *Journal of Small Animal Practice.* 29, 153-164.

Lamb CR (1990). The double cortical line: A sign of osteopenia. *Journal of Small Animal Practice* 31, 189-192.

Reid RA *et al* (1983) Generalised osteomyelitis in a dog: a case report. *Journal of Small Animal Practice.* 24, 687-694.

Stead AC *et al* (1983) Panosteitis in dogs. *Journal of Small Animal Practice.* 24, 623-635.

Stead AC (1984) Osteomyelitis in the dog and cat. *Journal of Small Animal Practice.* 25, 1-13.

Vaughan LC (1975) Complications associated with internal fixation of fractures in dogs. *Journal of Small Animal Prac.* 16, 415-426.

Vaughan LC (1976) Growth plate defects in dogs. *Vet. Rec.* 98, 165-168.

Bone 'Tumours'

Biery DN *et al* (1976) Bone cysts in the dog. *J Am. vet. Radiol. Soc.* 917, 202-213.

Finnie JW *et al* (1981) Multiple cartilagenous exostoses in a dog. *Journal of Small Animal Practice.* 24, 597-602.

Gibbs C *et al* (1984) The radiological features of osteosarcoma of the appendicular skeleton in dogs: a review of 74 cases. *Journal of Small Animal Practice.* 25, 177-192.

Gibbs C *et al* (1985) The radiological features of non-osteogenic bone tumours in the appendicular skeleton of the dog: a review of 34 cases. *Journal of Small Animal Practice.* 26, 537-553.

Hay CW *et al* (1994). Multilobular tumour of bone at an unusual location in the axilla of a dog. *Journal of Small Animal Practice* 35, 633-636.

May C and Newsholme SJ (1989). Metastasis of feline pulmonary carcinoma presenting as multiple digital swelling. *Journal of Small Animal Practice* 30, 302-310.

Mcglennon NJ *et al* (1988) Synovial sarcoma in the dog - a review. *Journal of Small Animal Practice.* 29, 139-152.

Webbon PM *et al* (1978) Bone tumours (Radiological refresher - 10) *Journal of Small Animal Practice.* 19, 251-256.

FORELIMB

General

Houlton JEF (1984) Osteochondrosis of the shoulder and elbow joints in dogs. *Journal of Small Animal Practice.* 25, 339-413.

Koma LMPK and Stead AC (1987) Angiographic examination of the forelimb in dogs with abnormal growth of the distal radius and ulna. *Journal of Small Animal Practice.* 28, 1065-1072.

Shoulder

Bittegeko SBP *et al* (1993). Infectious epiphysitis and arthritis in a puppy. *Journal of Small Animal Practice* 34, 571-575.

Clayton-Jones DG *et al* (1975) The shoulder joint (Radiological Refresher - 4) *Journal of Small Animal Practice*. 16, 523-526.

Muir P and Johnson KA (1994). Supraspinatus and biceps brachii tendinopathy in dogs. *Journal of Small Animal Practice* 35, 239-243.

Van Bree H (1990). Evaluation of the prognostic value of positive contrast shoulder arthrography for bilateral osteochondritis lesions in dogs. *Am. J. Vet. Res.* 51, 1121-1125.

Vaughan LC *et al* (1968) Osteochondritis dissecans of the head of the humerus in dogs. *Journal of Small Animal Practice*. 9, 283-294.

Vaughan LC *et al* (1969) Congenital dislocation of the shoulder joint in the dog. *Journal of Small Animal Practice*. 10, 1-3.

Elbow

Campbell JR (1979) Congenital luxation of the elbow in dogs. *The Veterinary Annual*. 19, 229-236.

Cockett PA *et al* (1985) The repair of humeral condylar fractures in the dog: a review of 79 cases. *Journal of Small Animal Practice*. 26, 493-520.

Culvenor JA *et al* (1982) Avulsion of the medial epicondyle of the humerus in the dog. *Journal of Small Animal Practice*. 23, 82-89.

Denny HR *et al* (1980) The surgical treatment of osteochondritis dissecans and ununited coronoid process in the elbow joint. *Journal of Small Animal Practice*. 21, 323-331.

Denny HR (1983) Condylar fractures of the humerus in the dog: a review of 123 cases. *Journal of Small Animal Practice*. 24, 185-197.

Guthrie S (1989). Use of a radiographic scoring technique for the assessment of dogs with elbow osteochondrosis. *Journal of Small Animal Practice* 30, 639-644.

Guthrie S *et al* (1991). Microfocal radiography as an aid to the diagnosis of canine elbow osteochondrosis. *Journal of Small Animal Practice* 32, 503-508.

Kene ROC *et al* (1982) Radiological features of congental elbow luxation/subluxation in the dog. *Journal of Small Animal Practice*. 23, 621-630.

Puglisi TA *et al* (1987). Stress radiography of the canine humeral joint. *J. Am. Anim. Hosp. Ass.* 24, 235-240.

Read RA *et al* (1990). Fragmentation of the medial coronoid process of the ulna in dogs: A study pf 109 cases. *Journal of Small Animal Practice* 31, 330-334.

Robins GM (1980) Some aspects of the radiological examination of the canine elbow. *Journal of Small Animal Practice*. 21, 417-428.

Webbon PM *et al* (1976) The elbow. (Radiological Refresher - 6) *Journal of Small Animal Practice*. 17, 395-401.

Forearm

Clayton-Jones DG (1970) Disturbance in the growth of the radius in dogs. *Journal of Small Animal Practice*. 11, 453-468.

O'Brien TR *et al* (1971) Epiphyseal plate injury in the dog: a radiographic study of growth disturbance in the forelimb. *Journal of Small Animal Practice*. 12, 19-36.

Ramadan RO *et al* (1978) Premature closure of the distal ulnar growth plate in dogs: a review of 58 cases. *Journal of Small Animal Practice*. 19, 647-667.

Carpus and Foot

Campbell JR (1976) Carpal injuries. (Radiological Refresher - 5) *Journal of Small Animal Practice*. 17, 179-182.

Bennett D *et al* (1985) Sesamoid disease as a cause of lameness in young dogs. *Journal of Small Animal Practice*. 26, 567-579.

Miller A *et al* (1990). Luxation of the radial carpal bone in four dogs. *Journal of Small Animal Practice* 31, 148-154.

HINDLIMB

General

Carmichael S *et al* (1989). Single condylar fractures of the distal femur in the dog. *Journal of Small Animal Practice* 30, 500-504.

Ramadan RO *et al* (1979) Disturbance in the growth of the tibia and femur in dogs. *Vet. Rec.* 104, 433-443

Pelvis and Hips

Anon: (1974) Radiological features of hip dysplasia (Radiological Refresher) *Journal of Small Animal Practice*. 15, 475-478.

Barr ARS *et al* (1987) Clinical hip dysplasia in growing dogs: the long-term results of conservative management. *Journal of Small Animal Practice*. 28, 243-252.

Brass W (1989). Hip dysplasia in dogs. *Journal of Small Animal Practice* 30, 166-170.

Denny HR (1971) Simultaneous epiphyseal separations and fractures of the neck and greater trochanter of the femur in the dog. *Journal of Small Animal Practice*. 12, 613-621.

Denny HR (1978) Pelvic fractures in the dog: a review of 123 cases. *Journal of Small Animal Practice*. 19, 151-166.

Henricson B *et al* (1966) On the aetiology and pathogenesis of hip dysplasia: a comparative review. *Journal of Small Animal Practice*. 7, 673-688.

Lawson DD (1963) The radiographic diagnosis of hip dysplasia in the dog. *Vet. Rec.* 75, 445-456.

Lee R (1970) A study of the radiographic and histological changes occurring in Legge-Calve-Perthes disease (LCP) in the dog. *Journal of Small Animal Practice*. 11, 621-638.

Lee R (1976) Proximal femoral epiphyseal separation in the dog. *Journal of Small Animal Practice*. 17, 669-679.

Madsen JS and Svalastroga E (1991). Effect of anaesthesia and stress on the radiographic evaluation of the coxofemoral joint. *Journal of Small Animal Practice* 32, 64068.

Madsen JS *et al* (1991). Delayed ossification of the femoral head in dogs with hip dysplasia. *Journal of Small Animal Practice* 32, 351-354.

Pérez-Aparicio FJ and Fjeld TO (1993). Coxofemoral luxations in cats. *Journal of Small Animal Practice* 34, 345-349.

Pérez-Aparicio FJ and Fjeld TO (1993). Femoral neck fractures and capial epiphyseal separations in cats. *Journal of Small Animal Practice* 34, 445-449.

Smith GK *et al* (1990). New concepts of coxofemoral joint stability and development of a clinical stress-radiographic method for quantitating joint laxity in the dog. *J.A.V.M.A.* 196, 59-70.

Stifle

Arnbjerg J and Heje NI (1993). Fabellae and popliteal sesamoid bones in cats. *Journal of Small Animal Practice* 34, 95-98.

Bennett D *et al* (1988) A reappraisal of anterior cruciate ligament disease in the dog. *Journal of Small Animal Practice*. 29, 275-297.

Denny HR *et al* (1980) Osteochondritis dissecans of the canine stifle joint. *Journal of Small Animal Practice*. 21, 317-322.

Gregory SP and Pearson GR (1990). Synovial osteochondromatosis in a Labrador retriever bitch. *Journal of Small Animal Practice* 31, 580-583.

Houlton JEF and Meynink SE (1989). Medial patella luxation in the cat. *Journal of Small Animal Practice* 30, 349-352.

MacPherson GC and Allan GS (1993). Osteochondral lesion and cranial cruciate ligament rupture in an immature dog stifle. *Journal of Small Animal Practice* 34, 350-353.

Morgan JP (1969) Radiological pathology and diagnosis of degenerative joint disease of the stifle joint of the dog. *Journal of Small Animal Practice*. 10, 541-544.

Pond MJ (1973) Avulsion of the extensor digitorum longus muscle in the dog: a report of 4 cases. *Journal of Small Animal Practice*. 14, 785-796.

Read RA *et al* (1982) Deformity of the proximal tibia in dogs. *Vet. Rec.* 111, 295-298.

Strom H *et al* (1989). Osteochondritis dissecans on the lateral femoral trochlear ridge in a dog. *Journal of Small Animal Practice* 30, 43-44.

Hock

Carlisle CH and Reynolds KM (1990). Radiographic anatomy of the tarsocrural joint of the dog. *Journal of Small Animal Practice* 31, 273-279.

Carlisle CH *et al* (1990). Radiographic signs of osteochondritis dissecans of the lateral ridge of the trochlea tali in the dog. *Journal of Small Animal Practice* 31, 280-286.

Denny HR (1981) Osteochondritis dissecans of the hock joint in the dog. *Veterinary Annual* 21, 224-228.

Holt PE (1974) Ligamentous injuries to the canine hock. *Journal of Small Animal Practice.* 15, 457-474.

Ness MG (1993). Metatarsal III fractures in the racing Greyhound. *Journal of Small Animal Practice* 34, 85-89.

Rosenblum GP *et al* (1978) Osteochondritis dissecans of the tibio-tarsal joint in the dog. *Journal of Small Animal Prac.* 19, 759-767.

Robins GM *et al* (1983) Osteochondritis dissecans of the lateral ridge of the trochlea of the tibial tarsal bone in the dog. *Journal of Small Animal Practice.* 24, 675-685.

Schmökel HG *et al* (1994). Tarsal injuries in the cat: A retrospective study of 21 cases. *Journal of Small Animal Practice* 35, 156-162.

Sumner-Smith G and Kuzma A (1989). A technique for arthrodesis of the canine tarsocrural joint. *Journal of Small Animal Practice* 30, 65-67.

SPINE

General

Bennett D *et al* (1981) Discospondylitis in the dog. *Journal of Small Animal Practice.* 22, 539-547.

Denny HR *et al* (1982) Diagnosis and treatment of cauda equina lesions in the dog. *Journal of Small Animal Practice.* 23, 425-443.

Denny HR *et al* (1977) Cervical spondylopathy in the dog: a review of 35 cases. *Journal of Small Animal Practice.* 18, 1,17-132.

Denny HR *et al* (1988) Atlanto-axial subluxation in the dog: a review of thirty cases and an evaluation of treatment by lag screw fixation. *Journal of Small Animal Practice.* 29, 37-47.

Dyce J *et al* (1991). Canine "arachnoid cysts". *Journal of Small Animal Practice* 32, 433-437.

Gibbs C (1972) Radiological features of spinal lesions in dogs and cats. *The Veterinary Annual* 13, 107-112.

Griffiths IR (1972) Some aspects of the pathogenesis and diagnosis of lumbar disc protrusion in the dog. *Journal of Small Animal Practice.* 13, 439-447.

Houlton JEF and Jeffries AR (1989). Infective polyarthritis and multiple discospondylitis in a dog due to Erysipelothrix rhusiopathiae. *Journal of Small Animal Practice* 30, 35-38.

Ladds P *et al* (1970) Congenital odontoid process separation in two dogs. *Journal of Small Animal Practice.* 12, 463-471.

Larsen JS (1977) Lumbo-sacral transitional vertebrae in the dog. *J Am. Vet. Radiol. Soc.* 18, 76-79.

Lee R (1973) Intervertebral disc lesions in the dog. (Radiological Refresher - 1) *Journal of Small Animal Practice.* 14, 111-112.

Lee R (1984) Discospondylitis in the dog. *Veterinary Annual* 24, 281-285.

Lewis DG (1989). Cervical spondylo-myelopathy ("wobbler" syndrome) in the dog: A study based on 224 cases. *Journal of Small Animal Practice* 30, 657-665.

Lewis DG (1991). Radiological assessment of the cervical spine of the Dobermann with reference to cervical spondylo-myelopathy. *Journal of Small Animal Practice* 32, 75-82.

Lewis DG and Kelly DF (1990). Calcinosis circumscriptia in dogs as a cause of spinal ataxia. *Journal of Small Animal Practice* 31, 36-38.

Lewis RE (1974) Roentgen signs of the spine. *Vet. Clin. N Amer.* 4 (4), 647-662.

McKee WM *et al* (1989). Vertebral stabilisation for cervical spondylopathy using a screw and washer technique. *Journal of Small Animal Practice* 30, 337-342.

McKee WM *et al* (1990). Surgical treatment of lumbosacral discospondylitis by a distraction-fusion technique. *Journal of Small Animal Practice* 31, 15-20.

Mitten RW (1974) Vertebral osteomyelitis in the dog due to Nocardia-like organisms. *Journal of Small Animal Practice.* 15, 563-570.

Morgan JP *et al* (1989). Spondylosis deformans in the female Beagle dog: A radiographic study. *Journal of Small Animal Practice* 30, 457-460.

Morgan JP and Bailey CS (1990). Cauda equina syndrome in the dog: Radiographic evaluation. *Journal of Small Animal Practice* 31, 69-77.

Morgan JP (1968) Congenital abnormalities of the vertebral column of the dog: a study of the incidence and significance based on a radiographic and morphologic study. *J Am. Vet. Radiol. Soc.* 9, 21-28.

Ness MG (1994). Degenerative lumbosacral stenosis in the dog: A review of 30 cases. *Journal of Small Animal Practice* 35, 185-190.

Read RA *et al* (1983) Caudal cervical spondylomyelopathy (Wobbler syndrome) in the dog; a review of 30 cases. *Journal of Small Animal Practice.* 24, 605-621.

Schmid V and Lang J (1993). Mesuremeants on the lumbosacral junction in normal dogs and those with cauda equina compression. *Journal of Small Animal Practice* 34, 437-442.

Sharp NJH *et al* (1992). Radiological evaluation of "wobbler" syndrome – caudal cervical spondylomyelopathy. *Journal of Small Animal Practice* 33, 491-499.

Watt PR (1991). Degenerative lumbosacral stenosis in 18 dogs. *Journal of Small Animal Practice* 32, 125-134.

Wheeler SJ (1989). Diagnosis of spinal disease in dogs. *Journal of Small Animal Practice* 30, 81-91.

Wheeler SJ (1992). Atlantoaxial subluxation with abscence of the dens in a Rotweiler. *Journal of Small Animal Practice* 33, 90-93.

Wright JA (1979) Congenital and developmental abnormalities of the vertebrae. (Radiological Refresher - 15) *Journal of Small Animal Practice.* 20, 625-634.

Wright. JA *et al* (1979) The clinical and radiological features associated with spinal tumours in 30 dogs. *Journal of Small Animal Practice.* 20, 461-472.

Wright JA (1980) Neoplasia fractures and dislocations of the spine in the dog. (Radiological Refresher - 16) *Journal of Small Animal Practice.* 21, 129-138.

Wright JA (1980) Spondylosis deformans of the lumbo-sacral joint in dogs. *Journal of Small Animal Practice.* 21, 45-58.

Wright JA (1982) A study of osteophyte formation in the canine spine 1: spinal survey and 11; radiographic survey. *Journal of Small Animal Practice.* 23, 697-711 and 747-761.

Myelography

Cox FM *et al* (1986) The use of Iopamidol for myelography in dogs: a study of 27 cases. *Journal of Small Animal Practice.* 27, 159-165.

Hathcock JT *et al* (1988). Comparison of 3 radiographic contrast procedures in the evaluation of the canine lumbosacral spinal canal. *Vet. Radiol.* 29, 4-15.

Lamb CR (1994). Common difficulties with myelographic diagnosis of acute intervertebral disc prolapse in the dog. *Journal of Small Animal Practice* 35, 549-558.

McKee WM and Renwick PW (1994). Marsupialisation of an arachnoid cyst in a dog. *Journal of Small Animal Practice* 35, 108-111.

Olby NJ *et al* (1994). Correlation of plain radiographic and lumbar myelographic findings with surgical findings in thoracolumbar disc disease. *Journal of Small Animal Practice* 35, 345-350.

Webbon PM *et al* (1983) Contrast radiology of the spine of the dog. *Veterinary Annual.* 23, 247-253.

Wheeler SJ *et al* (1985) Iohexol myelography in the dog and cat: a series of 100 cases and a comparison with metrizamide and iopamidol. *Journal of Small Animal Practice.* 26, 247-256.

Wheeler SJ *et al* (1985) Myelography in the cat. *Journal of Small Animal Practice.* 26, 143-152.

Wright JA *et al* (1981) Metrizamide myelography in 68 dogs. *Journal of Small Animal Practice.* 22, 415-435.

CONTRAST MEDIA

Herrtage M and Dennis R (1988) Contrast media and their use in small animal radiology. *Journal of Small Animal Practice.* 28, 1105-1114.

EXOTIC SPECIES

Cooper JE *et al* (1976) Radiological examination of birds: a report of a small series. *Journal of Small Animal Practice.* 17, 799-808.

Gibbs C *et al* (1981) Radiological examination of the rabbit. I: head, thorax and vertebral column. *Journal of Small Animal Practice.* 22, 687-703.

Hinton MH *et al* (1982) Radiological examination of the rabbit. *II*: The abdomen. *Journal of Small Animal Practice.* 23, 687-696.

Holt PE (1978) Radiological studies on the alimentary tract in two Greek tortoises. *Vet. Rec.* 103, 198-200.

Jackson OF *et al* (1981) Radiology of tortoises, terrapins and turtles. *Journal of Small Animal Practice.* 22, 705-716.

Mcmillan MC (1986) Radiology of avian respiratory disease. *Comp. cont. Edn. Pract. Vet.* 8, 551-567.

Mcmillan MC (1986) Radiographic diagnosis of avian abdominal disorders. *Comp. cont. Edn. Pract. Vet.* 8, 616-637.

DIAGNOSTIC ULTRASOUND

Allen WE *et al* (1989). Hydrops fetalis diagnosed by real-time ultrasonography in a Bichon-frise bitch. *Journal of Small Animal Practice* 30, 465-4647.

Barr FJ (1992). Normal hepatic measurements in mature dogs. *Journal of Small Animal Practice* 33, 367-370.

Barr FJ (1992). Ultrasonagraphic assessment of liver size in the dog. *Journal of Small Animal Practice* 33, 359-364.

Barr FJ (1990). Evaluation of ultrasound as a method of assessing renal size in the dog. *Journal of Small Animal Practice* 31, 174-179.

Barr FJ *et al* (1990). Ultrasonographic measurement of normal renal parameters. *Journal of Small Animal Practice* 31, 180-184.

Darke PGG (1992). Doppler echocardiography. *Journal of Small Animal Practice* 33, 104-112.

Darke PGG *et al* (1993). Transducer orientation for Doppler echocardiography in dogs. *Journal of Small Animal Practice* 34, 2-8.

Elwood CM *et al* (1993). Clinical and echocardiographic findings in 10 dogs with vegtative bacterial endocarditis. *Journal of Small Animal Practice* 34, 420-427.

England GCW (1991). Relationship between ultrasonographic appearance, testicular size, spermatozoal output and testicular lesions in the dog. *Journal of Small Animal Practice* 32, 306-311.

England GCW (1992). Ultrasound evaluation of pregnancy and spontaneous embryonic resorption in the bitch. *Journal of Small Animal Practice* 33, 430-436.

England GCW and Allen WE (1990). Studies on canine pregnancy using B-mode ultrasound: Diagnosis of early pregnancy and the number of conceptuses. *Journal of Small Animal Practice* 31, 321-323.

England GCW *et al* (1990). Studies on canine pregnancy using B-mode ultrasound: Development of the conceptus and determination of gestational age. *Journal of Small Animal Practice* 31, 324-329.

Jensen AL *et al* (1994). Unusual ultrasonographic presentation of cholecystolithiasis in a dog. *Journal of Small Animal Practice* 35, 420-422.

Lamb CR (1990). Abdominal ultrasonography in small animals: Intestinal tract and mesentery, kidneys, adrenal glands, uterus and prostate. *Journal of Small Animal Practice* 31, 295-304.

Lamb CR (1990). Abdominal ultrasonography in small animals: Examination of the liver, spleen and pancreas. *Journal of Small Animal Practice* 31, 6-15.

Miyabayashi T *et al* (1990). Ultrasonographic appearance of torsion of a testicular seminoma in a cyptorchid dog. *Journal of Small Animal Practice* 31, 401-403.

Munro E and Stead C (1993). Ultrasonographic diagnosis of uterine entrapment in an inguinal hernia. *Journal of Small Animal Practice* 34, 139-141.

Stamoulis ME and Fox PR (1993). Mitral valve stenosis in 3 cats. *Journal of Small Animal Practice* 34, 452-456.

Vörös K *et al* (1991) Correlation of ultrasonographic and pathomorphological findings in canine hepatic diseases. *Journal of Small Animal Practice* 32, 627-634.

RADIATION PROTECTION

Ionising radiation safety (1992). *Journal of Small Animal Practice* 33, 47-49.

O'riordan MC (1970) X-ray hazards *In Practice. Vet. Rec.* 87, 640-642.

Webbon PM (1981) Radiology in veterinary science. *Br. vet. J.* 137, 349-357.

Webbon PM and France C (1984) *Atlas of Canine Surgical Techniques.* Ed. Bedford PGC, Blackwell Scientific Publications.

Webbon PM and Ramsay LJ (1983) Survey of X-ray machines in veterinary practice. *Vet. Rec.* 112, 224.

Wood AKW *et al* (1974) Gonadal dosage in radiography of the coxofemoral joint of the bull. *Australian Vet. J* 50, 130-131.

Wood AKW *et al* (1974) Radiation protection in equine radiography. *Australian Vet. J.* 50, 373-379.

The Ionising Radiations Regulations 1985. Statutory Instrument (1985) No. 1333. HMSO.

Approved code of Practice, The protection of persons against ionising radiation arising from any work activity. Health and Safety Commission, 1985. HMSO.

Guidance Notes for the Protection of Persons Against Ionising Radiations Arising from Veterinary Use. National Radiological Protection Board and Health and Safety Executive. (1988) HMSO.

Ionising Radiations Regulations (Northern Ireland 1985) Statutory Rules of Northern Ireland (1985) No.273. HMSO - Government Bookshop, Belfast.

Approved Code of Practice, The protection of persons against ionising radiation arising from any work activity. Health and Safety Agency for Northern Ireland, HMSO - Government Bookshop, Belfast.

APPENDIX III

Manufacturers of X-Ray Equipment, Films and Accessories

Agfa-Gevaert Ltd, 27 Great West Road, Brentford, Middlesex, TW8 9AX. Tel 0181 560 2131, Fax 0181 231 4947,

CGR Medical Ltd, Astronaut House, Hounslow Road, Feltham, Middlesex, TW14 9AD,

Centaur Services, Centaur House, Torbary Road, Castle Cary, Somerset,

Charles Hammer, 29-31 Danburg Street, Islington, London, N1 8LE,

CIBA Animal Health, Whittlesford, Cambridge, CB2 4QT. Tel 01223 833621, Fax 01223 836526,

Cuthbert Andrews, 5 High Street, Bushey Village, Watford, Herts.

Du Pont Ltd Wedgewood Way, Stevenage, Herts, SG1 4QN. Tel 01438 734 543,

Fuji Photo Film Ltd, Fuji Film House, 125 Finchley Road, London, NW3 6JH. Tel 0171 586 9351,

GEC Medical Equipment Ltd, PO9 Box 2, East Lane, Wembley, Middlesex,

HA West (X-ray) Ltd, 4 Watson Cres, Edinburgh, EH11 1ES. Tel 0131 337 7337

IGE Medical Systems Ltd X-ray Product Division, Coolidge House, 352 Buckingham Avenue, Slough, Berks SL1 4ER

Kodak Ltd, Health Science Division, PO Box 66, Station Road, Hemel Hempstead, Herts, HP1 1JU.

PLH Medical Ltd, Rembrandt House, Whippendell Road, Watford, Herts, WD1 7PR. Tel 01923 37521, Fax 01923 32216,

Philips Medical Systems, Kelvin House, 63-67 Glenthorne House, Hammersmith, London, W6 0LJ.

Progressive X-ray Ltd, Clarke Street, Guide Bridge, Ashton Under Lyne, Lancs, OL7 0LJ. Tel 0161 330 6721/2/3,

ROC Trading Ltd, Unit 2, MSH Industrial Estate, 100 Slade Green Lane, Slade Green, Erith, Kent. Tel 01322 351125, Fax 01322 351165,

Redmark Surgical Cradles, 6 Madley Close, Ashley Heath, Hale, Altrincham, Cheshire, WA14 3NJ. Tel 0161 928 0193, Fax 0161 926 9480,

SMR Ltd, Sumera House, 17 Station Road, Poulton-le Fylde, Lancs, FY6 7HU. Tel 01253 883282, Fax 01253 899026,

Siemens Ltd, Siemens House, Windmill Road, Sunbury on Thames, Middlesex, TW16 7HS.

Technical Medical Services, 13 Sandringham Drive, Bramcot Hill, Nottingham, NG9 3EA. Tel/Fax 0115 925 7724,

Todd Research, Robjohns Road, Chelmsford, Essex, CM1 3DP. Tel 01245 262233, Fax 01245 269409,

Vertec Scientific Ltd, 5 Comet House, Calleva Park Estate, Aldermaston, Reading, Berks, RG7 4QW.

Veterinary Drug Company, Common Road, Dunnington, York, Y01 5RU,

Veterinary Drug Company, Common Road, Dunnington, York, Y01 5RU.

Veterinary Radiological Ltd, 151 East Beech Road, Selsy, Chichester, West Sussex. Tel 01243 604696.

Veterinary X-Rays, Seer Green, Beaconsfield, Bucks, HP9 2QZ. Tel 012407 73713/71385, Fax 012407 71958.

WS Rothband Co Ltd, Albion Mill, Helmshore, Rossendale, Lancs, BB4 4JR. Tel 01706 830086. Fax 01706 830324.

Wardray Ltd, 15-19 Bakers Row, London, EC1R 3DT. Tel 0171 387 2666/8.

Wolverson X-ray & Electro-Medical Ltd, Walsall Street, Willenhall, West Midlands, WV13 2DY.

X-Ograph Ltd, Cotswold House, Malmesbury, Wilts, SN16 9JS. Tel 016662 4641.

X-ray Sales & Service, Vale Farm, Lydlynch, Sturminster Newton, Dorset, DT10 2SD. Tel 01258 73382.

3M UK plc, Information and Imaging Division, PO Box 1, Bracknell, Berks. Tel 01344 858676, Fax 01344 858248.

Index